Endorsements for *The Practical Handbook of Hearing Voices*

In a society where voice hearing  is a breath of fresh air to read *The Practica*... ges offer a smorgasbord of possibilities and a... ed without nuance or humility. This multi-v... ...pters exploring a range of topics, from language, ..., and spirituality to different therapeutic approaches. In reading it, with my own experiences as a voice hearer front and centre, I welcome this diversity and am hungry for more.
Rai Waddingham, Chair, English National Hearing Voices Network

Hearing voices is a normal human experience – and often a sane response to an overwhelming situation. Thanks to the survivor movement challenging harmful treatments for psychosis, we now have practical guides to coping and thriving with voices. This new volume is a potent antidote to a century of medical folly.
Will Hall, author of **The Harm Reduction Guide to Coming off Psychiatric Drugs** *and co-founder, Hearing Voices Network USA*

A superb book that provides readers with many lifetimes' worth of hard-won insights into voice hearing. Anyone who wants to better understand the experience of hearing voices should read it.
Simon McCarthy-Jones, Associate Professor in Clinical Psychology and Neuropsychology, Department of Psychiatry, Trinity College Dublin, and author of **Can't You Hear Them? The science and significance of voice hearing**

This ground-breaking book is the most important resource I have come across on the topic of voice hearing. It will be hugely useful to both trainee and qualified mental health professionals, as well as to people who hear voices, their friends and families. The book outlines in simple language the recent seismic shift in the field, away from the traditional approach that saw voices only as hallucinations, symptoms to be eliminated, and towards an appreciation that voice hearing is a common human experience that different people understand and approach in different ways. The book is a rich and exciting mine of conceptual and practical resources, documenting personal experiences, research and approaches to helping. It is the one volume that every voice hearer, and everyone who helps people who hear voices – or trains others to help them – should have on their shelf.
Anne Cooke, Clinical Director, Doctoral Programme in Clinical Psychology, Canterbury Christ Church University

The authors of *The Practical Handbook of Hearing Voices* are a who's who of the world of voice-hearing experience, scholarship and passionate engagement over more than three decades and together chart the first crucial steps of one of humankind's greatest journeys. Together they have turned a pathologised 'symptom' into a living, life-affirming, supportive set of communities, a range of practices, fresh understandings, relationships, justice and emancipation. They have found real direction within deep distress. You hold in your hand the opportunity to meet key members of that brave international community, which has transcended convention and brought hope where there was often none at all, to experience for yourself what they learned. This is the life's work of some simply astonishing ordinary people. Who 'lacks insight' now?! They changed my life and they will change yours too. Read this book!

Dr Jonathan Gadsby, Critical Mental Health Nurses' Network, Research Fellow, Birmingham City University

The Practical Handbook of Hearing Voices

THERAPEUTIC AND CREATIVE APPROACHES

Edited by
Isla Parker, Joachim Schnackenberg
and Mark Hopfenbeck

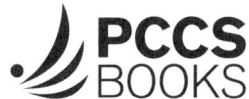

First published 2021

PCCS Books Ltd
Wyastone Business Park
Wyastone Leys
Monmouth
NP25 3SR
contact@pccs-books.co.uk
www.pccs-books.co.uk

This collection © Isla Parker, Joachim Schnackenberg
and Mark Hopfenbeck, 2021
The individual chapters © the contributors, 2021

All rights reserved.
No part of this publication may be reproduced, stored in a retrieval system, transmitted or utilised in any form by any means, electronic, mechanical, photocopying or recording or otherwise, without permission in writing from the publishers.

The authors have asserted their right to be identified as the authors of this work in accordance with the Copyright, Designs and Patents Act 1988.

The Practical Handbook of Hearing Voices:
Therapeutic and creative approaches

British Library Cataloguing in Publication data: a catalogue record for this book is available from the British Library.

ISBN Paperback 978 1 910919 91 0
ePub 978 1 910919 93 4

Cover design by Jason Anscomb

Typeset in-house by PCCS Books using Minion Pro and Myriad Pro
Printed in the UK by Short Run Press, Exeter

Contents

Foreword — ix
Marius Romme and Sandra Escher

Introduction — 1
Isla Parker, Joachim Schnackenberg and Mark Hopfenbeck

PART ONE – HEARING OUR VOICES

1. The Maastricht Approach: social and personal perspectives on hearing voices — 13
   Dirk Corstens

2. Hearing voices: why the words we use matter — 24
   Akiko Hart

3. Hearing voices groups — 30
   Peter Bullimore

4. Facilitating hearing voices groups — 39
   Sasha Priddy and Charlotte Howard

5. Painting has helped me to cope with my voices — 48
   Reshma Valliappan

6. Voices: victim to victor — 55
   Ron Coleman

7. The things they say — 64
   Aimee Wilson

8. Journey to recovery — 68
   Clifford O'Connor

9. Hearing voices in grief — 75
   Jacqueline Hayes

10. Spirituality, religion and voices — 85
    Christopher C.H. Cook

11. Voice hearing and cannabis: a harm-reduction approach — 94
    Rufus May and Kate Quinn

12. Black voices and the deafness of whiteness — 103
    Colin King

PART TWO – EMERGING SOCIAL AND THERAPEUTIC APPROACHES TO WORKING WITH VOICES

13. Voices, values and values-based practice: engaging with what matters in voice hearing — 113
    David Crepaz-Keay and Bill (K.W.M.) Fulford

14. An invitation to dialogue: what we can all learn from Open Dialogue and Hearing Voices Networks — 123
    Olga Runciman and Iseult Twamley

15. Medication and voices: reflections from a relational perspective — 136
    Dirk Corstens and Joachim Schnackenberg

16	Voice hearers at work *Caroline Moughton*	*152*
17	Navigating university as a voice hearer *Deborah Altman*	*169*
18	Experience focused counselling (Making Sense of Voices) *Joachim K. Schnackenberg, Oana-Mihaela Iusco and Senait Debesay*	*180*
19	Voice Dialogue *Ruth Lafferty and Rob Allison*	*194*
20	Experience focused counselling with children and young people who hear voices *Senait Debesay*	*203*
21	Understanding voices while living with dementia *David Storm and Ron Coleman*	*211*
22	How cognitive behaviour therapy can help people who are distressed by hearing voices *Mark Hayward*	*222*
23	Recovery-oriented cognitive therapy and distressing voices *Aaron Brinen*	*229*
24	AVATAR therapy: a digital therapy to help people with distressing voices *Mar Rus-Calafell and Tom Craig*	*237*
25	Relating therapy for voices: learning how to respond assertively in difficult relationships *Mark Hayward, Sheila Evenden and Angie Culham*	*246*
26	Meaning-making in voice hearing *Nicola Barclay, Guy Dodgson, and Anna Luce*	*256*
27	Responding to trauma dialogically: an introduction to peer-supported Open Dialogue *Mark Hopfenbeck*	*273*
28	A psychodynamic understanding of voice hearing *Christine Cox*	*283*
29	Compassion-focused therapy and the courage of compassionate relating to voices *Charles Heriot-Maitland*	*295*
30	Working with voices using the narrative genogram *Lykourgos Karatzaferis*	*305*
31	Mindfulness and hearing voices *Rufus May and Elisabeth Svanholmer*	*315*

PART THREE – CREATIVE APPROACHES TO WORKING WITH VOICES

32	Creative ways to engage with voices *Rufus May and Elisabeth Svanholmer*	*329*
33	Dramatherapy for people who hear voices *Louise Combes*	*341*

34	Dance movement psychotherapy and voice hearing: looking outward and inward *Mary Coaten*	*351*
35	Awesome metalcore therapy: using heavy metal music in therapeutic work with voices *Kate Quinn and Daniel Baines*	*359*
36	A safe space: sound therapy and hearing voices *Jane Ford*	*367*
37	How writing memoirs and poetry may help voice hearers *Isla Parker*	*376*
38	Finding an authentic voice: music therapy in multidisciplinary psychiatric support services *Stella Compton Dickinson*	*384*
	Conclusion *Isla Parker, Joachim Schnackenberg and Mark Hopfenbeck*	*395*
	Afterword *Gail A. Hornstein*	*399*
	Contributors	*403*
	Name index	*415*
	Subject index	*422*

Dedication

To the memory of Sandra Escher

Acknowledgements

I would like to thank first and foremost the many voice hearers and voices who have been kind enough to teach me about my ongoing need to continually discover how to love, respect and appreciate the true greatness and potential of every person, even if their life experience has suggested otherwise. I would particularly like to thank Ron Coleman and Karen Taylor, who were my first trainers, mentors and inspiration in the Hearing Voices Movement approach, when I first met them in 2000. I am also particularly grateful to Marius Romme and Sandra Escher, who supported and trained us in setting up a training schedule for the 'Making Sense of Voices' approach between 2006–2010. Dirk Corstens has also been particularly helpful in my development. Senait Debesay has been a true friend, colleague and personal and professional inspiration, both in how to live life well and in our instigation and development of our training and consultancy provision in the Making Sense of Voices approach, which we called experience focused counselling, since the year 2007. There have also been truly inspirational co-collaborators with lived experience in the provision of training, such as Suzanne Engelen, Oana-Mihaela Iusco and Christian Feldmann, to name but a few. My wise, insightful and patient trainers and mentors in Voice Dialogue, John Kent and Michael Zimmermann, must also not go unmentioned. Finally, my wife, Nicole – thank you for supporting me in learning about love. And my son, Laurence – thank you for meeting me in my vulnerability.

Joachim Schnackenberg

Foreword

Marius Romme and Sandra Escher

In 1987, when we were challenged by a person who was hearing voices to take her experience seriously rather than dismiss it as an expression of illness, we started listening in a very different way to what she and other voice hearers had to say. For a (then) professor of psychiatry in Maastricht (Marius Romme) and a science journalist and counsellor (Sandra Escher), this required a willingness to completely change our attitude and our approach. We formalised this change in our novel research and in our various social and political initiatives over the years that followed. This was the birth of what came to be known as the Hearing Voices Movement (HVM), and we could never have imagined what it was to become.

Now, 34 years later, it is with great joy and a zeal for an ongoing need for change that we feel ourselves part of a worldwide movement for fundamental, paradigmatic and ongoing change in our societies and mental health services. This book is one very important testimony to the many positive changes that have already taken place. It also points to the many things that still need to be transformed. Finding a new way of doing things has been so important for so many people along the way already, so that they could find a way out of what had previously been thought to be an inevitable future and life of chronic mental illness. It has been about saying that life does not have to be dominated by mental and emotional suffering, as well as by mental health services. That is what this new way of doing things is all about.

Our research, active engagement with and learning from voice hearers with often long-term mental health problems but also experiences of recovery and professional mental health service provision experiences, such as Ron Coleman, Jacqui Dillon, Eleanor Longden, Peter Bullimore, Antje Wilfer, Olga Runciman, Rachel Waddingham and many more, as well as our mutual learning with active mental health professionals such as Dirk Corstens, Rufus May, Karen Taylor, Paul Baker, Trevor Eyles, Marlene Weiterschan, Senait Debesay and Joachim Schnackenberg, to name but a very few, turned into the HVM. The HVM self-defines as a civil rights movement and has come to represent a central voice in the Recovery Movement. Recovery at its heart expresses the idea that it is possible for every person with a diagnosed mental health problem to define and live their lives as fully as is possible for people without such diagnoses.

Through our research and engagement with the HVM, we found that voices are clearly connected to the life history of a person; often related to trauma; possible to live with and live well; not pathological in nature, and that understanding the voices is a key to understanding the person's past and current distress. Voices could even turn out to be important messengers about an important part of the person's life experiences, or sources of knowledge and inspiration to help the person on their road to recovery. We speak here not of voices that had never been experienced as difficult by their hearers. We speak of voices that, on the surface, appeared to make life a real misery for those experiencing them; of voices heard by people who had been diagnosed with chronic schizophrenia, other mental health diagnoses and none. In summary, we found that it is not the voices (or similar experiences like visions, tastes, unwanted thoughts, non-shared realities (traditionally referred to as delusions in psychiatry)) that are the problem. Instead, they point to areas in the person's life that they may be experiencing as often overwhelmingly difficult and for which, to date, they have not felt able to find a solution.

The voices and other such experiences can become overwhelming and thus lead to difficulty in managing one's everyday life, simply because the person has not yet found a way to relate to them as constructively as they could. There are normally very good reasons why this has not been possible for some people, the main one being a lack of helpful accompaniment along the way. Such an understanding does, however, remain contrary to a prevailing biologically based view or belief of the meaninglessness of these experiences, which has been and remains prevalent today, even if it is starting to change in research and practice settings.

Many of the authors in this book are very well known to us through their experience and expertise in working towards fundamental change.

So, in summary we would say that, through our research and engagement with the HVM, we have found that voices are clearly connected to the life history of a person, and understanding the voices represents a key to understanding the person. If we take seriously what voice hearers and voices have to say and remember that every single person remains the author of their lives, then we can find good ways forward in the recovery process. Training may well be helpful in conveying many of the new insights, but the main focus has to remain one of openness to the voice hearer, the voices and also to our own fears and prejudices, which can so often get in the way. We trust that this book will further help to move on the urgently needed changes in our societies and mental health services.

Professor Marius Romme, Dr Sandra Escher
Amsterdam, 25 May, 2021

Introduction

Isla Parker, Joachim Schnackenberg and Mark Hopfenbeck

Our aim in *The Practical Handbook of Hearing Voices* is to explore what it means to hear a voice or voices and be distressed by the experience. We felt it was important to devote a whole book to this topic as – based on our practice experience – far from regarding hearing voices as just one of many problems or 'symptoms' produced by an assumed 'illness',[1] we have found that understanding voices in the here-and-now can actually be a key to understanding past and current distress in the person's life, and thus to finding ways forward in a process of recovery (Schnackenberg et al., 2018).

Although hearing voices (and having similar experiences, such as visions) has long fascinated and intrigued humankind, much of the dominant scientific and societal discourse of the past 180 years or so has seen these experiences firmly placed into pathologising and/or problematising frameworks of understanding. It has thus become, in the view of many, an entirely negative experience that should best be eradicated – one with no personal significance or value for the person or society. Within Western cultures, a more positive view of these experiences has largely been confined to societal niches, such as esoteric and certain religious understandings (Smith, 2007). That some people can live well with their voices and visions continues to be of little interest and consequence to most mainstream mental health services and practice, even if the scientific discourse is slowly waking up to this fact.

This dominant negative view of voices, visions and similar experiences within the scientific and psychiatric community has been largely the product of the influence of leading philosophers, academics, psychiatrists and psychologists. The

---

1. We use inverted commas here, and later around 'schizophrenia', to indicate that, based on the latest research and practice-based understanding, voices should no longer be considered to be signs of pathology, and that it also remains unclear and is becoming increasingly contested whether discrete mental illnesses, disorders or syndromes such as 'schizophrenia' exist or have even been discovered in the first place (Johnstone & Boyle, 2018).

views of people who themselves experience voices and visions have tended not to be actively consulted and nor have these negative hypotheses been tested in any meaningful research (McCarthy-Jones, 2013). This has started to change over the past three and a half decades, with the advent of large-scale population studies finding that most voice hearers do not need psychiatric input (Tien, 1991; Beavan et al., 2011), and with psychiatric researchers and practitioners like Romme and Escher (1989) asking voice hearers directly about their experiences. This led to the realisation that, in fact, voices should not be seen as signs of illness or a solely negative experience with no positive value for the individual or society. This book, with its editors' and contributors' diverse backgrounds in personal, lived, professional and research experience, is testimony to this change.

As a result of many of the latest insights and developments emerging in this fast-moving area of practice and research, it is now clear that some people who hear voices can be distressed by them, but this is not the case for every person who hears voices. Many people who hear voices, or have visions or other difficult-to-explain sensory experiences or hold distressing beliefs that are not shared by people around them, never come to the attention of the mental health services (Beavan et al., 2011; Linscott & van Os, 2013). Our focus in this book is on hearing voices when the voices are associated with distress. We now know from experience and from the research that it can be difficult to form a balanced relationship with voices. If this is the case, the voices can be experienced as overwhelming, and it can be quite difficult to cope with life at these times. This is when people who hear voices or have other unusual experiences can end up coming to the attention of mental health services (Corstens et al., 2008).

The understanding that it is not the voices or the other unusual experiences in themselves that are the problem but the way the experiencer and other people relate to them is still comparatively new and is often not well understood in traditional mental health services. In fact, it stands in contrast to the traditional understanding of voices as an indication of particular diagnoses of mental illnesses that are hypothesised to be primarily biologically based, such as 'schizophrenia'. Within this more traditional understanding, voices are often seen as bereft of personal meaning and are generally referred to as a 'hallucination':

> ... a sensory experience which occurs in the absence of external stimulation of the relevant sensory organ, but has the compelling sense of reality of a true perception, is not amenable to direct and voluntary control by the experiencer, and occurs in an awake state. (Laroi & Aleman, 2010, p.100)

The approach that has been and remains largely dominant in many mental health services is therefore to try to medicate the voices away, ignore them and advise people not to listen to what they say.

The insights and the various approaches presented in this book take a different view on the ability of the voice hearer to exert control over their experience and find personal meaning in the relationship with the voices. This is, in many cases, based on many years of experience in this field of practice, personal testimony and lately also on research. The contributors challenge the mainstream passive and pathologising or problematising depiction of hearing voices and demonstrate that positive change is indeed possible when the voice hearer finds ways of redressing the relationship with their voices. It is now also clear that it is common for voice hearers to have had very traumatic experiences that, for the most part, have at best not been noticed as relevant, and at worst, been ignored or dismissed by mental health services where trauma-sensitive paradigms and practices have not been adopted, particularly in relation to psychosis, hearing voices and similar experiences. It is also clear that biological causes and markers of voice hearing still elude researchers (McCarthy-Jones, 2013; Johnstone & Boyle, 2018).

One of the reasons why there have been these new insights into voice hearing in the last three to four decades, both in practice and in research, is the growing challenge to the traditional understanding of the effectiveness of the main medications used in this field – antipsychotics. The latest research now confirms what many voice hearers and some professionals have been asserting for some time: antipsychotics appear to be at best mildly helpful and only for a minority of voice hearers (Leucht et al., 2009; 2013; 2017). This needs to be weighed against the increasing awareness about possible negative long-term effects on body, brain, mortality rates and quality of life (Moncrieff, 2020). One example of recognising the consequent urgent need to change is a state-sponsored mainstream research project in Germany into 'antipsychotic induced brain changes'.[2] As a result of clear indications in the research of the potential long-term negative effects of antipsychotics, this project is investigating, for example, whether antipsychotics are on balance neurotoxic or neuroprotective and what approaches to treatment might mitigate their most harmful effects. They are thus investigating whether there are safer alternatives to the current guidelines on long-term maintenance therapy.

Many professionals and researchers still believe that diagnoses such as schizophrenia are chronic, life-long and need to be treated with long-term medication. However, many voice hearers and a growing number of other researchers and professionals disagree, and are presenting evidence that real recovery, as rated by the person concerned, is possible.

Key voices influencing the political, practice-based and research discourse of the last three and a half decades within and outside of psychiatry are the Recovery Movement and, most notably, the Hearing Voices Movement (HVM). These are civil rights movements that promote a de-pathologisation and emancipatory approach, fuelled by the insights, testimonies and activism of voice hearers, professionals and other allies. Most of these insights and the findings that emerged from the research of the co-founders of the HVM, Marius Romme and Sandra Escher, have now been confirmed in larger-scale studies (Corstens et al., 2014). These insights include the connection of voices with trauma; that hearing voices cannot be specifically linked

---

2. See www.apic.rwth-aachen.de/ and https://clinicaltrials.gov/ct2/show/NCT02435095

to specific diagnoses or any diagnosis; that the person's relationship with and what the voices say are key to understanding and living with them; that voices are not in themselves pathological but can even be helpful; that there is a strong connection to unwanted emotions, and, most importantly perhaps, that voice hearers can find a way to recover (even if it can be hard work) with their voices and even without long-term medication. Some notable testimonies of this are those of Jacqui Dillon, Ron Coleman, Peter Bullimore, Olga Runciman, Eleanor Longden and Antje Wilfer, among many more (Romme et al., 2009).[3]

The HVM has also contributed strongly to a much more varied understanding of voice hearing and how to live well and recover with the experience, in many cases with the help of voices rather than despite them (Romme et al., 2009). Thus, one of the many insights of the HVM is that voices can actually be a force for good (or be used as a force for good) if their positive intention has been identified or the relationship with them has positively changed (Schnackenberg & Burr, 2017). We also have a clearer understanding of just how varied and widely spread, both in clinical and non-clinical contexts, the experience of voice hearing can be (Woods, 2017). Research also confirms another long-known HVM insight: that the same or similar kinds of voices can occur across different diagnoses, and that there do not appear to be any diagnosis-specific differences in voice characteristics, as had previously long been assumed (Waters & Fernyhough, 2017).

Some people hear only one voice, while others hear two or more, or even hundreds. They may turn up in groups or crowds or be simply a felt presence and say nothing verbally at all. Voices can vary in loudness and location (Hayward et al., 2012), in the feelings they arouse, in their physicality and in what they actually say. From the perspective of the HVM, this varied expression makes sense, as voices have specific meaning in a person's life context. Voice hearers can therefore find, or be accompanied to find, additional meaning, and from this an improvement in their relationship with the voices through some of the processes and approaches described in this book. Other approaches focus primarily on the ability of the voice hearer to distance themselves assertively from the impact of their voices.

Our aim in this book is to contribute to the advancement of facilitating, accompanying and supporting voice hearers in finding their own way forward, outside (or alongside) current mainstream provision. Too many voice hearers say they are not helped by mainstream services (Romme et al., 2009). Too often they share 'not just a common experience of hearing voices but also a (frequently negative) experience of mental health services' (Woods, 2013, p.265). For these and a variety of other personal and scientific reasons, voice hearers often reject psychiatric labels such as schizophrenia (Woods, 2013, p.265) as stigmatising, based on unconvincing science and unhelpful (see Coleman, 2004, p.55–56; Johnstone & Boyle, 2018; Longden, 2009, p.143).

This is not to say that the mainstream primary focus on medication is never experienced as helpful. In Chapter 15, Dirk Corstens, a psychiatrist based in

---

3. See the Intervoice website for many more testimonies, at www.intervoiceonline.org

the Netherlands, outlines some approaches available in the mainstream that use medication to lessen the distress and anxiety that some voice hearers experience.

Unfortunately, however, the patient role may also cause problems for some people. For example, if individuals start to feel helpless and become passive and engage less with former activities so that their social network reduces, they may become isolated and lonely. As we write this introduction, living through lockdown during the Covid-19 pandemic has presented additional challenges, as voice hearers have had limited opportunities to mix socially with others. However, phone calls, online gatherings and social media, as well as permitted outdoor walks, may have helped some to have some social contact. The value of hearing voices or similar groups – as, for example, outlined in the chapters by Ron Coleman, Peter Bullimore, and Olga Runciman and Iseult Twamley – describe how voice hearers have been helped by hearing-voices groups to rebuild a life beyond the mental health system. Other voice hearers can be supportive to each other, as well as at times to their families and friends, and engage with a range of activities, including paid work.

Another important aspect considered in this book is the fact that people's beliefs and/or explanations about their voices may impact on how some voice hearers relate to the voice/s that they hear. For example, the person may have a spiritual explanation for the voices and feel that they are hearing the voice of God or the devil; they may link the voice with an abusive figure that they recognise from their past; for some people, the voice may be friendly and offer comfort at a difficult time, such as a bereavement. Some of the chapters will explore how relational frameworks such as the Maastricht Approach (also known as the HVM approach, or 'Making Sense of Voices' or 'experience focused counselling') are used to support voice hearers to develop more positive relationships with their voices in a variety of settings, whether personal, social or psychotherapeutic. For example, some may find it helpful to approach their voices as if they were family members or close acquaintances. This pattern of relating to the voice/s may enable the voice hearer to change the relationship to a different power dynamic where they feel more in control and less distressed and less anxious.

Considerable stigma and discrimination currently exist in society towards people who hear voices, and this may in part be associated with the perception of voices as meaningless and dangerous (Angermeyer & Matschinger, 2005). As Woods (2017) notes, the stigma associated with mental disorders in general, and particularly with receiving a diagnosis of 'schizophrenia' or 'psychosis', is, for some people, part of the distress of hearing voices (Corrigan & Rao, 2012; Goffman, 1990; McCarthy-Jones, 2013). Stigma and prejudice add to the difficulties experienced by voice hearers and their families, particularly if it leads to limited opportunities to find work or social acceptance. Chapter 16 outlines examples of 'reasonable adjustments' that might be helpful for voice hearers to find work and sustain a job.

In this book, we offer a range of perspectives from voice hearers, mental health professionals and researchers as to what approaches and strategies voice hearers may find helpful to live well with their voices. Some of the approaches have thus far only been applied primarily with people with a formal diagnosis of psychosis, such as schizophrenia. This includes, for example, cognitive behaviour therapy for psychosis. Others, such as the HVM approach and those that share its principles, can be used, irrespective of which diagnosis or whether any has in fact been given. It is also clear in its de-pathologising stance, the value of peer support, the possibility of seeing the contents and intentions of voices (once decoded) as sources of knowledge and even wisdom in some cases, and the need for trauma-sensitive work. In this way, it goes further and states that voices do not simply need to be managed or related to in a better way, but can actually become a force for good.

For the most part, such approaches do not yet form part of routine mental health service provision. However, some mainstream services in some Western countries are starting to open up to the idea of changing their practice and amending local and national guidelines to incorporate some of the approaches introduced in this book. Such paradigmatic shifts take time, but it is evident that, increasingly, mental health professionals do recognise that there is no quick, simple 'fix' for distressing voices and pills often do not stop the voices altogether – for some people, they may reduce distress and anxiety; for others, they are not helpful. Some voice hearers will find a particular therapy or approach useful; others may find that their voices, once better understood and related to, can be a source of real enrichment and recovery, and they would not want to lose them; others may prefer to play football or another sport, or even play a musical instrument. Voice hearers are individuals too, so they will have different experiences of hearing voices and will find different things helpful.

Moreover, hearing voices does not mean that you cannot live a fulfilling life or even become and remain famous. Famous past and current voice hearers include, for example, Brian Wilson of the Beach Boys. Another singer, Lady Gaga, has talked openly in the media about her experiences of hearing voices in childhood. She said:

> It's how I deal with my insanity. From when I was young I had voices in my head, and for the longest time I was drinking and doing a lot of drugs, and it was the clothing and the artistry that saved me. I get sheer joy out of creativity. (British Comedy Guide, 2013)

You can find a list of historical famous people who have heard voices on the Intervoice website.[4] Examples include Socrates, Joan of Arc, Mahatma Gandhi and the writer Charles Dickens. You will note that most of these were not known to have suffered with unusual mental distress.

This book does not favour one approach to working with voices over any other, although contributions from people in the HVM do feature more often. This is because the HVM approach has been so inspirational for so many experts-by-experience who have been vital in driving advances in our understanding of voices and visions. We wish to honour that, especially as we feel they continue

---

4. See www.intervoiceonline.org/about-voices/famous-people

not to be acknowledged or given a strong enough role in practice or in the scientific discourse. Importantly, many of the other approaches, such as cognitive behavioural approaches, also relate to or draw inspiration from the HVM approach, as can be seen in the respective chapters. Each approach described here is only one among many and what is needed is an openness towards what works for the individual. We do not want to replace one dominant paradigm (for example, the current pathologising and problematising approach) with another. It is also our aim that this book will contribute to a continuing dialogue between the different approaches presented here, as well as provide a greater sense of choice for those seeking help with their voices.

We are also aware that this book cannot hope to be definitive: we have not included some approaches, such as metacognitive training, acceptance and commitment therapy or the use of real-time MRI scans, as we are limited by space and these approaches are either very similar to others or still in the very early stages of development in relation to their application to hearing voices.

Some of the approaches described here were primarily tested in research settings and were driven more by professionals; others were developed and initially evaluated in practice settings. It should be pointed out that many services would first need to adapt their practices and how they are organised before they could properly offer some of the approaches that are on offer here. However, what is true, regardless of the respective setting, is that a mutually trusting relationship is necessary between the voice hearer, the voices and those working with them. This does not have to take years to develop, but many voice hearers say they have been in mental health services for many decades without any professional or other person ever taking an interest in their personal life history or traumatic experiences, let alone in any meaning that the voices could be conveying. It may, alas, not be easy for these people to start looking at areas of their lives that for so many years have been ignored or regarded with fear both by them and the people (including professionals) who were supposed to accompany them in their recovery processes. Voluntary engagement with any support on offer and a sense of safety are, of course, also key, but many services routinely use a degree of informal or formal force against people using their services, making it difficult to establish helpful, trusting and voluntary relationships.

In calling for the relationship to be acknowledged between voice hearing and trauma, we are not proposing that only highly trained professionals, like trauma therapists, should work with voice hearers. In fact, most trauma therapists have traditionally not been trained to work with people with voice hearing experiences as these experiences were thought to be biological in origin and therefore not amenable to the trauma-informed approach (with some notable exceptions, of course). We also feel that there should not be an automatic assumption that medication must be given first during phases of feeling acutely overwhelmed, as is common practice. This is not backed up by research findings, even if it is common practice and regularly found in guidelines (see Chapter 15 on medication). There are, for example, many accounts of people benefitting from the HVM approach in acutely overwhelming situations and in acute settings when medication had not made any positive difference.

We would like to offer a final thought on the significance of voices, based on our own HVM-inspired practice and insights. With the stubborn refusal of voices, visions and similar experiences to just go away with medication or to engage with voice hearers or those who accompany them in a way that they experience as constructive unless they are treated with a certain degree of respect and interest in what they have to say, such experiences have often pointed a finger at areas that the person would benefit from resolving in their own life. Exploration of the connection between voices and often untold traumatic experiences also helps to reveal untold suffering and holds up a truth-telling mirror to those experiencing the voices, to those accompanying the voice hearers and to a society that, although it has started to change in recent decades, still struggles to know how to deal well with its own frailties and transgressions and violence towards others. One could argue that, therefore, voices have both a personal and a societal function towards healing and thriving.

The contents

Each chapter in this book offers reflective learning points to help the reader consider and put into practice the approach it describes. The aim is to encourage voice hearers to expect person-centred support or accompaniment from mental health professionals, and for these professionals to be adequately trained to provide this.

Part one of the book, titled 'Hearing our voices', offers voice hearers' perspectives as to the experience and personal meaning of their voices and what has helped them to recover and live full lives, while hearing voices some of the time.

Part two, 'Emerging social and therapeutic approaches to working with voices', explores the non-medical models and techniques voice hearers, those close to them and mental health practitioners use to support voice hearers. They include approaches based on the HVM approach, those using cognitive therapy techniques, some that draw on other therapy models, such as psychodynamic theory, mindfulness and narrative therapy, and more practical support offered in, for example, workplaces and by legislation.

Part three, 'Creative approaches to workinmg with voices', describes innovative and experimental creative ways of working with voices using, for example, dance, drama and poetry, and how these can benefit voice hearers and help them to relate to their voices in more positive ways.

We hope readers will dip into the book to find a particular chapter or chapters when they would like advice or help on a particular aspect of voice hearing or a therapy or self-help strategy. In this respect, the book is a 'practical handbook' that offers practical suggestions, as well as sharing voice hearers' own experiences. We hope that you will find it interesting and helpful.

Isla Parker, Joachim Schnackenberg and Mark Hopfenbeck
February 2021

References

Angermeyer, M.C. & Matschinger, H. (2005). Causal beliefs and attitudes to people with schizophrenia: Trend analysis based on data from two population surveys in Germany. *British Journal of Psychiatry, 186*(4), 331–334.

Beavan, V., Read, J. & Cartwright, C. (2011). The prevalence of voice-hearers in the general population: A literature review. *Journal of Mental Health, 20*(3), 281–292.

British Comedy Guide (2013). *The Graham Norton Show: Series 14, Episode 5 – Lady Gaga, Jude Law, Greg Davies, June Brown.* [Online.] British Comedy Guide.

Coleman, R. (2004). *Recovery: An alien concept?* P&P Press.

Corrigan, P.W. & Rao, D. (2012). On the self-stigma of mental illness: Stages, disclosure, and strategies for change. *The Canadian Journal of Psychiatry, 57*(8), 464–469.

Corstens, D., Escher, S. & Romme, M. (2008). Accepting and working with voices: The Maastricht approach. In: A. Moskowitz, I. Schäfer, M.J. Dorahy (Eds.), *Psychosis, trauma and dissociation: Emerging perspectives on severe psychopathology* (pp.319–332). John Wiley & Sons.

Corstens, D., Longden, E., McCarthy-Jones, S., Waddingham, R. & Thomas, N. (2014). Emerging perspectives from the Hearing Voices Movement: Implications for research and practice. *Schizophrenia Bulletin 40*(Suppl.4), S285–S294.

Goffman, E. (1990). *Stigma: Notes on the management of spoiled identity.* Penguin Books.

Hayward, M., Strauss, C. & Kingdon, D. (2012). *Overcoming distressing voices: A self-help guide using cognitive behavioural techniques.* Robinson.

Johnstone, L., Boyle, M., with Cromby, J., Dillon, J., Harper, D., Kinderman, P., Longden, E., Pilgrim, D. & Read, J. (2018). *The Power Threat Meaning Framework: Towards the identification of patterns in emotional distress, unusual experiences and troubled or troubling behaviour, as an alternative to functional psychiatric diagnosis.* British Psychological Society.

Laroi, F. & Aleman, A. (2010). *Hallucinations: A guide to treatment and management.* Oxford University Press.

Leucht, S., Arbter, D., Engel, R.R., Kissling, W. & Davis, J.M. (2009). How effective are second-generation antipsychotic drugs? A meta-analysis of placebo-controlled trials. *Molecular Psychiatry, 14*(4), 429–447.

Leucht, S., Cipriani, A., Spineli, L., Mavridis, D., Orey, D., Richter, F., Samara, M., Barbui, C., Engel, R.R., Geddes, J.R., Kissling, W., Stapf, M.P., Lässig, B., Salanti, G. & Davis, J.M. (2013). Comparative efficacy and tolerability of 15 antipsychotic drugs in schizophrenia: A multiple-treatments meta-analysis. *The Lancet 382*, 951–962.

Leucht, S., Leucht, C., Huhn, M., Chaimani, A., Mavridis, D., Helfer, B., Samara, M., Rabaioli, M., Bächer, S., Cipriani, A., Geddes, J.R., Salanti, G. & Davis, J.M. (2017). Sixty years of placebo-controlled antipsychotic drug trials in acute schizophrenia: Systematic review, Bayesian meta-analysis, and meta-regression of efficacy predictors. *American Journal of Psychiatry, 174*(10), 927–942.

Linscott, R.J. & van Os, J. (2013). An updated and conservative systematic review and meta-analysis of epidemiological evidence on psychotic experiences in children and adults: On the pathway from proneness to persistence to dimensional expression across mental disorders. *Psychological Medicine, 43*, 1133–1149.

Longden, E. (2009). Eleanor Longden. In M. Romme, S. Escher, J. Dillon, D. Corstens & M. Morris (Eds.), *Living with voices: 50 stories of recovery* (pp.142–146). PCCS Books.

McCarthy-Jones, S. (2013). *Hearing voices: The histories, causes and meanings of auditory verbal hallucinations.* Cambridge University Press.

Moncrieff, J. (2020). *A straight talking introduction to psychiatric drugs* (2nd ed.). PCCS Books.

Romme, M.A.J. & Escher, A.D.M.A.C. (1989). Hearing voices. *Schizophrenia Bulletin, 15*(2), 209–216.

Romme, M., Escher, S., Dillon, J., Corstens, D & Morris, M. (2009). *Living with voices: 50 stories of recovery*. PCCS Books.

Schnackenberg, J., Burr, C., with Furrer, M., Iusco, O.M., & Debesay, S. (2017). *Stimmenhören und Recovery:. Erfahrungsfokussierte Beratung in der Praxis. (Hearing voices and recovery: Experience focused counselling in practice)*. Psychiatrieverlag.

Schnackenberg, J., Fleming, M., Walker, H. & Martin, C.R. (2018). Experience focussed counselling with voice hearers: Towards a trans-diagnostic key to understanding past and current distress – a thematic enquiry. *Community Mental Health Journal, 54*(7), 1071–1081.

Smith, D.B. (2007). *Muses, madmen, and prophets: Rethinking the history, science, and meaning of auditory hallucinations*. Penguin Press.

Tien, A.Y. (1991). Distributions of hallucinations in the population. *Social Psychiatry and Psychiatric Epidemiology, 26*(6), 287–292.

Waters, F. & Fernyhough, C. (2017). Hallucinations: A systematic review of points of similarity and difference across diagnostic classes. *Schizophrenia Bulletin, 43*(1), 32–43.

Woods, A. (2013). The voice-hearer. *Journal of Mental Health 22*, 263–270.

Woods, A. (2017). On shame and voice-hearing. *Medical Humanities, 43*(4), 251–256.

Part one

Hearing our voices

1 The Maastricht Approach: social and personal perspectives on hearing voices

Dirk Corstens

Marius Romme and Sandra Escher published three books about hearing voices: *Accepting Voices* (Romme & Escher, 1993), *Making Sense of Voices* (Romme & Escher, 2000) and *Living with Voices* (Romme et al., 2009). Essentially, these titles provide the outline of the Maastricht Approach. It is called 'Maastricht' because this is the city where we worked together, with others, to create a vibrant Hearing Voices Movement.

The titles of the books can serve as milestones of the approach. This is a recovery process both for voice hearers and for society too, as it allows the emancipation of voice hearers. The fundamental underpinning belief is that voice hearing is a natural and personal human experience. It does not belong to psychiatry. People can cope, or learn to cope, with their voices. At the same time, though, we recognise that hearing voices can often be a complex experience, with implications for the personal life of the voice hearer and those around them.

These implications, though, are culturally bound. In ancient cultures (the concept of the Self is quite modern), hearing voices was much more common than nowadays; it steered people's behaviour and had much more influence on daily life (Jaynes, 1986; Robbins, 2011). In receptive hearing-voices communities, such experiences are inclusive. Support is readily offered for the novice. In such societies, voice hearers connect with society via personal stories, education, political action, the media, social media and the internet; their citizens learn that hearing voices is a meaningful but sometimes difficult experience.

In the paranormal culture, hearing voices is considered a gift, an openness to the spiritual world. Not everybody can handle this, and they get support to help them deal with these entities and stay firmly on the ground. In several religions, hearing voices is seen as a negative force that should be banned; some use rituals in an attempt to send these demons away. But in other cultures, hearing voices is a sign that the person is in contact with the ancestors and regarded as a source of cultural wisdom.

In the traditional psychiatric professional community, though, hearing voices is seen as a sign of illness that should be cured. The eradication of hearing voices is preached, and almost any means is used to get rid of the phenomenon. From our social psychiatry perspective, the main interest is in voice hearers as a group, how they are marginalised in society and what support can be mobilised to help them.

So, in some cultures, these experiences are embraced, while in others hearing voices can lead to social rejection because it is regarded as a state of being out of control that is dangerous and needs to be halted. All these different perspectives have their consequences for the individual and for society.

When hearing voices is accepted as a human experience, personally and socially, and when it is approached as being a meaningful experience, people can live, or learn to live, with their voices and perhaps discover that hearing voices is an enriching experience. It may even benefit society.

It is from this perspective that I will describe the Maastricht Approach to hearing voices, which supports the voice hearer to gain mastery over their voices in a way that is accustomed to the person and their voices.

> *Learning point 1*
>
> Attitudes to and coping with hearing voices are culturally bound.
>
> - In what way does your own cultural background define how you cope with your voices? Have you explored how other people deal with their voices?
> - Have you talked to other people in your environment about your voices? How do their opinions influence how you cope with your voices?
> - Have you exchanged information with other voice hearers?
>
> (People offering support or working professionally with voice hearers can usefully ask themselves the same questions.)

Accepting voices

Social

Hearing the first-hand stories from other voice hearers who have acquired some mastery over their voices and related experiences is very important in the first stage of accepting the voices. There are celebrities who hear voices and lead successful lives. These stories normalise hearing voices. Socrates, for example, was convinced that 'world leaders' like himself heard a 'daimon' that inspired them to do great things. Psychiatric survivors' stories can also provide hope. Getting acquainted with the struggles others went through and how they dealt with them creates connection with other voice hearers. Acquiring hope is essential if someone is to learn to share their experiences. And starting to share your own experience, to tell your own story, to raise *your own voice,* can lead to acceptance by others. It gives others insight into your personal struggle and creates support because they can empathise with you. Journals, books, the media and social media are all sources of helpful information and very important for creating positive perspectives. Many voice hearers are marginalised as 'disturbed', 'a problem that should be solved', and voice hearers feel abandoned and alone with it. Self-help groups and hearing voices networks offer the chance to share experiences and feel you belong. Meetings and congresses for voice hearers and their allies are very powerful in connecting people, providing mutual support and creating friendships. Connections with other voice hearers is perhaps the root of recovery.

Personal

For many children, it is quite natural to have conversations with invisible friends or voices. Mostly the voices that children hear disappear as they grow older (Escher & Romme, 2013), but some voice-hearing experiences can continue and become negative over time. Accepting your voices is not an easy task and it doesn't always come easily. Initially, most voice hearers feel overwhelmed when they hear voices for the first time. Many try to fight their negative voices. Negative voices exert power, they seem to know every personal detail about you. They can distort your perspective of the world. These voice hearers don't want to hear their voices, as they seem to ruin their lives. The voices create intense fear and make them feel estranged. The voice hearers may feel extremely isolated as a consequence. What the negative voices say can be painful, weird, insulting, threatening or manipulative. You want to find explanations for these experiences, which are often found in a very fearful worldview in which the person feels threatened. If you are not able to share your experience of hearing voices, you are likely to think you're the only voice hearer in the world.

Accepting the voices means that you acknowledge they are real for you and that others should also acknowledge that you hear voices. Acceptance is not doing what they tell you to do; on the contrary, it means you refuse to be captured by them. Acceptance is to feel that they do somehow belong to you, that you can't get rid of them, and that you have to master your own emotions in relation to them. Acceptance is an awareness that you have to relate to them.

In this phase of accepting voices, writing about them, keeping a diary, negotiating with them, not reacting too personally to them but trying to listen to them for a short period each day are all productive ways of acknowledging the voices. Voices need to be heard but shouldn't be obeyed. You start to build up a relationship with them. You acknowledge that you have a relationship with them, whether you like it or not. Learning to ignore the voices is also paramount, because it is impossible to listen 24 hours a day to voices. You must learn to hear them – after all, hearing is one of your senses. Hearing, listening and not obeying are key to coping with the voices.

The Maastricht Hearing Voices Interview

The Maastricht Hearing Voices Interview is a powerful tool to learn how to cope with your voices. It creates some emotional distance and breaks through the avoidance of thinking about your experiences. Twelve questions are asked in the Maastricht Hearing Voices Interview:

1. The nature of the experience itself.
2. Characteristics of the voices.
3. The history of hearing voices.
4. What triggers the voices?
5. What do the voices say?
6. How do you explain the origin of the voices?
7. What impact do the voices have on your daily life?
8. Your relationship with the voices.
9. Your coping strategies.
10. Questions relating to your childhood (emotional neglect, attachment issues, bullying, physical and/or sexual abuse, and so forth).
11. Your medical history.
12. Your social network.

You can use the interview on your own, or it can be used by someone else asking you the questions. This doesn't need to be a professional.

This interview may have three goals:

- to obtain information about you and your history in order to structure the experience
- to make a personal 'construct' (see next step, 'Making sense')
- to find ways to help you cope better with the voices.

Personally, I like to bring into the interview stories I have heard from other voice hearers – stories that provide hope. You can find many such stories in the book *Living with Voices* (Romme et al., 2009). I find it gives hope and direction to the voice hearer, builds up a relationship and provides suggestions like time structuring and listening exercises.

> *Learning point 2*
>
> Accepting your voices starts with knowing what you are experiencing when you hear voices. The voices have a story to tell.
>
> - How many voices do you hear? Do they have names? Do they resemble people you know or have known? How do they interact with you and

with each other? When did they emerge in your life? What were the circumstances then? Write this down for yourself.
- Has anyone helped you to understand your voices?
- Do you accept your voices? How did you come to accept them? How do you cope with them?

Making sense of voices

Social

Non-voice hearers can't imagine what it is like to hear voices. They find it strange and frightening. Voices create anxiety in non-voice hearers too, and in professionals who haven't had these kinds of experiences. This explains a great deal of the animosity voice hearers encounter in society and in traditional psychiatric practice. What makes it even more difficult is that the experience is often kept private from others, through fear, shame or stigma. 'I don't think this person hears voices' is something I hear regularly in consultations with psychiatric colleagues. The only one who knows if they hear voices is the person themself. Voice hearers who talk out loud to their voices on the street are likely to be shunned by passers-by. Sometimes people talking to their voices create fear when their words have an aggressive undertone. All these anxious reactions hinder the person in making sense of the voices. Everybody in society should realise that these experiences make sense if you know the context – they have a personal emotional cause; they are connected to individual vulnerability and the individual's history. Voice hearers need to be supported to learn to speak out with their *own voice*. When voice hearers can make the connection between their voices and their personal life experiences, things often fall into place and they are better able to cope with their voices and manage them, as described below. Empathy and inclusion are the most important social means to recovery.

Personal

Research and personal experience of talking with voice hearers have shown us that there is often a strong relationship between the characteristics of the voices and what they say and the voice hearer's personal history. The question 'What has happened in your life?' is a very important one. In our research (Honig et al., 1998), 80% of the voice hearers told us they first heard voices when they were experiencing an emotionally overwhelming situation. The meaning of the voices is often erased, due to fear of the voices, or by a psychiatric 'diagnosis', or in an attempt to avoid re-experiencing trauma.

The voices themselves won't tell you straight away why they are bothering you. Working with the voice hearer, we try to make sense of the voices by answering two fundamental questions. We call this the *construct*, because we re-*construct* meaning together:

1. Who or what do the voices represent (actual people you know or have known, or particular emotions or assumptions)?
2. What underlying social-emotional problems do the voices represent?

To answer these two questions, we use the information that we have learned from the interview:

1. Identity of the voices.
2. Characteristics and content.
3. Triggers/impact.
4. History of the voices.
5. History before the voices.

Here is an example. It is anonymised. Judy is 39 years old, married with one son, and has lived for almost 10 years in sheltered accommodation. She was given the diagnosis of schizophrenia. She hears one voice.

Identity: One male voice, 42 years old.

Characteristics and content: Shouting, threatening, manipulating, commenting and commanding: 'You should kill yourself, if you don't do what I say you will die, you're a bad mother, you're stupid, the world would be better off without you.' The voice reminds her of her brother, who is three years older and who said similar things when they were young.

Triggers: Feelings of guilt, which make the voice more threatening.

History of the voice: The voice started when she was 13, just after her father came home drunk and hit her in the face.

History before the voice: Both mother and brother humiliated her repeatedly. She had to do the dirty housework and was kept home from school. She still can't properly read and write. Her father was fond of her and kind. He defended her against humiliating remarks made by her brother and mother. When her father hit her, her safe haven was destroyed. Her world became totally threatening.

The construct

Who does the voice represent? Her brother, who is three years older, said similar things to her when they were young.

What problems does the voice represent? They include a very negative self-image, not being assertive, not being able to express her needs, emotional neglect in her youth, being without support for a long time. Psychiatry is now her safe haven.

After a good conversation with her brother, with whom she got on quite well in adulthood, and starting a course to learn to read and write (she was also a fast learner), her voice had less impact on her. She started to have conversations with her voice and set limits to when she listened to him. She started to *own* her voice.

She left the sheltered home and moved into independent accommodation, tapered down her medication and improved her contact with her son.

Sometimes it is this easy to have such a good outcome. Most of the time it is more complicated, but when the voices make personal sense, this is a start of empowerment and gradual recovery.

In this way you can replace the illness label with a meaningful construct that directs recovery; a shift from disempowering symptoms of an illness to problems that it may be possible to resolve.

> *Learning point 3*
>
> Voices often have a personal meaning to the voice hearer. They may be linked with social and emotional issues – for example, you may find it difficult to deal with anger, or have a negative, disempowering view of yourself.
>
> - In what way do your voices relate to your life? Are there issues in your life that you are afraid of? Do the voices say things that confront you with things that you fear?
> - How can you own your voices? How can they contribute to your empowerment?

Living with voices

Social

In most recovery stories described in *Living with Voices* (Romme et al., 2009), people mention that the unconditional support of an ally was of most importance, not treatment or medication. Indeed, most of the 50 individuals in the book ultimately stopped taking medication. What really helped was having someone they could share their experiences with, who didn't reject them because of their experiences but instead believed in them. Recovery is a personal journey. It is about owning your own story, owning your own experiences and owning your voices.

Connecting with other voice hearers is also important for many voice hearers (Longden et al., 2018). It helps to share experiences, to be heard and to be listened to. Speaking out leads to understanding and insight. From a social perspective, it is important to offer these opportunities. Social stigma should be challenged. A society that considers hearing voices to be part of human experience will create a completely different starting point for voice hearers.

Personal

In a conversation with Jim, a voice hearer (also anonymised), I asked him what impact his voices had on his life at present. My psychiatric colleagues had given him the 'diagnosis' of schizophrenia; indeed, his 'symptoms' met the formal psychiatric diagnostic criteria. His hearing voices experience was complex. He heard a lot of different and changing voices; almost all were people he knew or had known. Jim is a skilled guitar player and teaches young people to play guitar. He told me that the main problem was that the voices criticised him when he was giving guitar lessons. The voices he heard when he was teaching were people who were connected with his guitar world: a teacher, a friend who also played guitar, a person who sold guitars and one of his guitar heroes. The voices were very critical and interrupted his teaching by making mean comments. They made him feel incompetent and lose concentration and confidence during the lessons. The people who his voices represented were not his enemies at all. They were all skilled and knowledgeable people. The voices were fed by his own feelings of insecurity.

I suggested to Jim that he could invite these voices to have a conversation with him about playing the guitar and teaching. 'I am sure they want you to become a good teacher,' I said. 'If you tell them that you feel insecure sometimes and want their help, things will change in your relationship with them. Voices generally exaggerate, otherwise you would not listen to them. If they are too kind, they won't attract your attention. Obviously, the way they tell you things about your teaching is not helping you at all. But if you make peace with them beforehand and accept their support, you will acknowledge their skills, and that possibly will change their attitude. It will help if they know that you want to learn from them. Next time, before you welcome your pupil, invite the voices in but ask them to keep silent during the lesson and tell them that you will talk to them after the lesson. If they keep silent during the lesson, fine. If they don't, tell them to wait until the lesson is over and ignore them. When you have finished the lesson and your pupil has left, evaluate with them how the lesson went. Ask them for tips. Don't get into a discussion with them, but listen to what they have to say, look at what you can use and ignore what isn't helpful. Being too personally involved in these conversations will not teach you much. Explore what they have to teach you and decide what you agree with. Don't obey the voices but look for what can be helpful. Organise a train-the-trainer session with them!'

This is the type of conversation we have with voice hearers. You cannot change your voices, and the voices cannot change you. But they can make you feel miserable. You can give the voices power; they can make you feel powerless. It is the relationship with your voices that you can change, and you can only do that when *you* change your emotional reactions to them. It is helpful if you embrace the message that the voices have for you. Our goal is to improve the relationship between the voices and the voice hearer. We think that best serves recovery.

When applying Voice Dialogue principles[1] (Stone & Stone, 1993; see Chapter 19) to working with voices, we learn that in essence voices are protective in intention, but often not in practice. In Voice Dialogue, the so-called Operating Ego consists of different Selves or sub-personalities. One of these is called the Inner

---

1. Voice Dialogue is an approach to working with different parts in a person. We have adopted this approach for use with people who hear voices, too

Critic. The Inner Critic develops in order to protect the child from criticism from their parents and significant others. So the Inner Critic says things like 'You should behave' or 'Don't be stupid', because the child is expecting this criticism from their parents or some other significant figure in their life and is pre-empting it. The Inner Critic will often completely lose its original purpose and start criticising the person all the time so it becomes destructive, rather than protective, as originally intended. In Voice Dialogue practice, we call the person who relates to the sub-personalities of the person the facilitator. The facilitator has conversations with all the Selves, including the Inner Critic. My advice is that the facilitator should ask simple questions such as 'What is your name? How old are you? When did you emerge in the life of the person? What is your role? How do you feel about the person? Is it hard work to help the person? What would happen if you were not there? Do you have recommendations for the person? How can they acknowledge you?' If the Self is addressed in this way, it will expose its intentions and the protective intention will emerge.

We do the same when talking with the voices (Corstens et al., 2012). The questions will often evoke a completely different picture of the voice; it will become clear why the voice is so angry, how the relationship with the voice can be improved, and how the voice can be acknowledged. We then promote similar conversations between the voice hearer and their voices, in order to improve the relationship.

Research review

There is a very small literature on this approach to understanding and working with people's voices. Here are some of the main studies, and I have added a reading list below.

Angela Woods (2013, p.263) reviews the meaning of the word 'voice hearer' and how it has changed in the past decades. In two articles (Longden et al., 2012; Corstens & Longden, 2013), Eleanor Longden and I, with other colleagues, explain how to make a construct and report our study demonstrating how making a construct made sense for 100 voice hearers who mostly had a long history of voice hearing and extensive contact with mental health services.

In another article (Corstens et al., 2014), we set an agenda for research from the perspective of the Hearing Voices Movement. In the journal *Psychosis: Psychological, social and integrative approaches*, Craig Steel and colleagues from the University of Reading describe a pilot project where making the construct and talking with voices was delivered as a treatment for 15 voice hearers (Steel et al., 2019). The results are similar to those achieved by cognitive behavioural therapy. And, most recently, Eleanor Longden and Tony Morrison at the University of Manchester are running a feasibility study for a randomised controlled trial (RCT) to compare this approach with treatment as usual (Longden et al., 2021a, 2021b).

Conclusion

In the Maastricht Approach, we strive for the emancipation of voice hearers. Voice hearers can share their experiences, be proud of their voices and, by joining groups and networks of voice hearers, discover that they are not alone, that they are part of the human race, and that their hearing voices is a natural experience, like being left-handed or having dyslexia. It is possible to cope with voices and discover that they have a personal meaning. Making sense of voices is essential to learn to solve the underlying problems and/or discover the creative potential of the voices. Living with voices is relating with voices, and the aim is to own them and make them part of your personal experience as a whole, just as dreaming is a part of you.

Mike, a Danish voice hearer who had originally been given a diagnosis of schizophrenia, wrote this testimony for me in 2018: 'I experienced voices from age four 'til I was 27 years old. This month it's five years since they left me, and I still often miss them! In the beginning they were my pals, but then around my teenage years (13) I stopped listening and started acting out, so that made us *frienemies*. They tried to help, but I did the opposite. In 2012 they became my pals once more. I had a voice dialogue with them and Dirk Corstens, and that changed everything for me. I started working and fighting with them instead of against them, and together this made me whole again! I have always viewed them as parts of me that were separated because of traumatic experiences. Today I live a good life with my girlfriend, who I have been with for almost five years, and I work with other people who experience voices or other things, and now I'm starting to attend college in August, so that later I can become a teacher. I was originally a forestry worker. Now I give lectures and talks about voice hearing and my experiences with it.'

Mike changed his relationship with his voices, and then he could continue his recovery journey. He recovered from life's adversities.

Recommended further reading

Deschrijver, M. (2018). *It's all in my head: A story about hearing voices*. The Choir Press.

McCarthy-Jones, S. (2012). *Hearing voices: The histories, causes and meanings of auditory hallucinations*. Cambridge University Press.

McCarthy-Jones, S. (2017). *Can't you hear them? The science and significance of hearing voices*. Jessica Kingsley Publishers.

References

Corstens, D. & Longden, E. (2013). The origins of voices: Links between life history and voice-hearing in a survey of 100 cases. *Psychosis: Psychological, social and integrative approaches, 5*(3), 270–285.

Corstens, D., Longden, E. & May, R. (2012). Talking with voices: Exploring what is expressed by the voices people hear. *Psychosis: Psychological, social and integrative approaches, 4*(2), 95–104.

Corstens, D., Longden, E., McCarthy-Jones, S., Waddingham, R. & Thomas, N. (2014). Emerging perspectives from the Hearing Voices Movement: Implications for research and practice. *Schizophrenia Bulletin, 40*(4), s285–294.

Escher, S. & Romme, M. (2013). *Children hearing voices*. PCCS Books.

Honig, A., Romme, M., Ensink, B., Escher, S., Pennings M. & De Vries, M. (1998). Auditory hallucinations: A comparison between patients and non-patients. *Journal of Nervous and Mental Disease, 186*(10), 646651.

Jaynes, J. (1986). Consciousness and the voices of the mind. *Canadian Psychology, 27*(2), 128–148.

Longden, E., Corstens D., Escher, A. & Romme, M. (2012). Hearing voices in biographical context: A framework to give meaning to voice-hearing experiences. *Psychosis: Psychological, social and integrative approaches, 4*(3), 224–234.

Longden, E., Corstens, D., Morrison, A.P., Larkin, A., Murphy, E., Holden, N., Steele, A., Branitsky, A. & Bowe, S. (2021b). A treatment protocol to guide the delivery of dialogical engagement with auditory hallucinations: Experience from the Talking with Voices pilot trial. *Psychology and Psychotherapy: Theory, research and practice.* https://doi.org/10.1111/papt.12331

Longden, E., Corstens, D., Pyle, M., Emsley, R., Peters, S., Chauhan, N., Dehmahdi, N. & Morrison, A.P. (2021a). Engaging dialogically with auditory hallucinations: Design, rationale and baseline sample characteristics of the Talking with Voices pilot trial. *Psychosis: Psychological, social and integrative approaches.* https://doi.org/10.1080/17522439.2021.1884740

Longden, E., Read, J. & Dillon, J. (2018). Assessing the impact and effectiveness of Hearing Voices Network self-help groups. *Community Mental Health Journal, 54*(2), 184–188.

Robbins, M. (2011). *The primordial mind in health and illness: A cross-cultural perspective.* Routledge.

Romme, M. & Escher, S. (1993). *Accepting voices.* Mind Publications.

Romme, M. &, Escher, S. (2000). *Making sense of voices: A guide for mental health professionals working with voice-hearers.* Mind Publications.

Romme, M., Escher, S., Dillon, J., Corstens, D. & Morris, M. (2009). *Living with voices: 50 stories of recovery.* PCCS Books.

Steel, C., Schnackenberg, J., Perry, H., Longden, E., Greenfield, E. & Corstens, D. (2019). Making sense of voices: A case series. *Psychosis: Psychological, social and integrative approaches, 11*(1), 3–15.

Stone, H. & Stone, S. (1993). *Embracing your Inner Critic.* Harper San Francisco.

Woods, A. (2013). The voice-hearer. *Journal of Mental Health, 22*(3), 263–270.

2 Hearing voices: why the words we use matter

Akiko Hart

'Language matters,' or so we assert in the critical mental health field. What we mean by this is perhaps less clear.

When I first joined the Hearing Voices team at Mind in Camden, I was tongue-tied. Everyone around me used words and expressions that were unfamiliar: people had *lived experience*, you *sat with* distress, you *held hope* for someone.

I was worried about saying the wrong thing, thoughtlessly upsetting someone or being judged for my ineptitude. There was a secret code, it seemed, and it took me a while to find my way around it. Now, I am fluent in critical mental health.

This perhaps illustrates some of the context around our language battles in mental health: as well as being a site of scientific, philosophical and political contest, it is also an identity signifier. Using the 'right' language can grant you access to certain circles; it can demonstrate that you share the same values as the wider group. Immediately, we might see that, however well-meaning the focus on 'language' can be, it comes with a set of often unspoken rules that can serve to unify but also to demarcate and exclude (Jones & Kelly, 2015).

The exhortation that 'language matters' is seemingly everywhere in mental health: from mental health campaigns aimed at the general public, such as Time to Change, campaigns focusing on the media (Kinderman & Cooke, 2018) and policy documents from professional bodies (Division of Clinical Psychology, 2015). The underlying assumption is that a change in language will bring about a change in practice (Richards, 2018).

To an outsider, the mental health community's preoccupation with language might seem baffling, perhaps even a distraction. Why can't people just agree, or agree enough? Surely what matters is less what something is called and more the quality of care an individual receives, or the budget allocated to mental health? To a linguist, our endless arguments about language can seem equally confusing. Many assert that what we mean by 'language' is in fact 'words', and what we are arguing about are theoretical frameworks of mental health and the values underpinning them (Galasiński, 2017a). It is, indeed, increasingly common for a conceptual reframing of mental health to be formulated as a linguistic call to arms to drop the language of disorder (Kinderman et al, 2013; A Disorder for Everyone!, n.d.).

When it comes to voices and related experiences, it is almost commonplace, although not always a reality, that individuals should have the right to speak about their experiences in the words they choose, and that we should use those words back to them. Difficulties arise when we, whether we are voice hearers, mental health professionals, academics, journalists or members of the public, speak about experiences more generally. In that context, there is an established and growing conversation around the merits of 'hearing voices' over 'hallucinations'. However this argument barely penetrates the academy, where 'auditory verbal hallucinations' (AVH) is the key search indicator in the clinical literature and required by high-impact-factor psychiatric journals. It is, therefore, the main term used by researchers, even ones sympathetic to the arguments against it. In fact, the terms 'AVH' and 'hearing voices' are often used interchangeably in the clinical literature (de Leede Smith & Barkus, 2013; Moskowitz & Corstens, 2007; McCarthy-Jones & Longden, 2013), and the use of 'hearing voices' does not preclude diagnostic framings (Luhrmann et al., 2015).

The argument around 'hearing voices' and 'hallucinations' also does not permeate the media, where the terms are also used interchangeably (Melley, 2018). On the one hand, finding the words that best fit one's experiences and that can be shared with others is, for many people, an everyday, personal endeavour. But it is also a conversation that has taken on a deeper political and professional significance on the fringes of the mental health sector, in activist, alternative and critical mental health circles. Still far from mainstream, it tends to be internally focused on other actors in mental health – in particular psychiatry, although there are growing moves to influence the wider public (Kinderman & Cooke, 2018).

The arguments for using 'hearing voices' instead of 'hallucinations' are as follows: i) the former uses everyday, neutral and ordinary language, instead of medical terminology, to signify that voice hearing is not a categorised symptom of a disorder or an illness but a human experience that exists on a dimensional scale; ii) 'hearing voices' is a political reclaiming of the experience; iii) it is a broader term that captures experiences that are not well represented by 'hallucinations'; iv) 'hearing voices' has something to say about the reality of the experience.

The first claim is that experiences denoted by 'auditory verbal hallucinations' or 'hallucinations' have traditionally been conceptualised within a medical framework as the symptom of a mental disorder, such as schizophrenia, acute psychotic disorder or borderline personality disorder, but are more helpfully understood as a broad and diverse human experience, on a spectrum, which can occur in a wide variety of clinical and non-clinical contexts. This deliberate move from 'hallucinations' to 'voices' and from 'patient' to 'voice hearer' was heralded in the work of the Hearing Voices Movement (Romme et al., 2009; Dillon et al, 2012; Dillon & May, 2002). It makes a number of ontological, epistemological and political claims about the experience in itself (and, therefore, its causes and possible treatment), wider conceptualisations of mental health, and the identity of the voice hearer (Woods, 2013).

> While 'auditory hallucinations' is the preferred jargon within psychiatric literature, the term 'hearing voices', which uses ordinary, non-pathologising language framed subjectively, has been reclaimed. This is part of a wider aim within the mental health user movement to decolonize medicalized language of human experience. (Dillon et al., 2012, p.311)

The counter-claim to 'it's just words' is that the words we use to describe and explain voice hearing are also political. They are highly charged, and can hurt, validate, empower and silence (Dillon et al., 2012; Waddingham, 2013; Healey, 2012). 'Hearing voices' and 'voice hearer' are not neutral signifiers but rather carry within them the implicit critique that the pathologisation of the experience by 20th- and 21st-century psychiatry and psychology has been harmful to the individuals concerned (Woods, 2013). Notwithstanding the complex history of 'hallucinations' beyond psychiatry (Telles-Correia et al., 2015), the word is now seen by many as a slur that invalidates the experience and discredits the individual. Thus, as well as a reframing, 'hearing voices' is also a reclaiming of the experience, and indexes wider conversations in the c/s/x movement[1] around where knowledge is produced, which expertise is valued and whose voices are heard:

> My focus on language is, sometimes, seen as an irritation to allies. I can be accused of being pedantic and missing the point. Does it matter if we sometimes slip into the language of illness when we all agree that these experiences are meaningful, personal and have value? Yes, it does. The language of illness was the language used by the thief who first stole a person's experience and replaced it with 'schizophrenia'. Every time we use words from this language, we inadvertently add our seal of approval to this thievery and make it that much harder for people to reclaim their experience as their own. Words have power. (Waddingham, 2013)

What preoccupies proponents of the term 'hearing voices' and their colleagues within broader fields such as Disability Studies and Mad Studies, is *who* is doing the naming (Shaw, 2016; Russo & Shulkes, 2016, p.33). Reclaiming 'hearing voices' as a meaningful and heterogenous experience that exists beyond the scope of mental illness might allow us to trouble narratives of madness and (ir)rationality, and foreground the 'voice hearer' as possessing insight and agency, so that they are considered to be the active producer of knowledge.

The third argument is that 'hearing voices' is a broader umbrella term than 'hallucinations', in that it encompasses hermeneutic frameworks that

---

1. Consumer/survivor/ex-patient movement

'hallucinations' struggles to accommodate, such as spiritual voices; indeed, it can welcome 'hallucinations' into its fold. Last, both terms have something to say about the reality of the experience. 'Hallucinations', in parallel with 'delusions', implies both in common parlance and in clinical settings that the experience, while perhaps real to the person experiencing it, is false or erroneous. 'Hearing voices' arguably makes no such judgement about the reality of the experience and, as well as leaving open greater possibilities as to the nature, agency and origin of the voices, creates bridges with other historical and cultural representations (Woods, 2013).

For the reasons outlined above, I use 'hearing voices', and argue for its adoption in my work and practice. However, I am also aware that the move towards 'hearing voices' brings new troubles. The argument that 'hearing voices' is more neutral than 'hallucinations' is tenuous, bypassing linguistic concerns around the neutrality of any words, as well as over-simplifying the demarcation between medical and non-medical language (Galasiński, 2017b, 2017c). Indeed, talking about 'distress' or 'hearing voices' is hardly neutral, as some argue (Kinderman & Cooke, 2018; Johnstone & Boyle, 2018, p.316): it can be a political, philosophical and sometimes ethical positioning against the 'medical model' – in itself, a contentious framing.

In this way, our allegiances and differences, our identities and relationships are reflected and enacted through the words we use. More generally, the focus on 'language', by which we usually mean lexical material, can disregard higher-order concerns, such as syntax, context and what is happening between you and me when we talk. I might say the 'wrong' words, but that might not matter if I treat you with respect. Or I might use the words you want me to, but I might mean something different by them. It can also serve to solidify hierarchies and marginalisation by privileging those voices and narratives that have access to these debates.

Which experiences are neglected through picking some words and not others? Is it possible or desirable to have umbrella terms to scoop up all experiences? 'Hearing voices' is often used as shorthand to mean hearing, seeing or sensing things that others don't – and, in effect, other sensory experiences are squeezed out. Research papers rarely talk about tactile or olfactory experiences, themselves just as powerful and meaningful as auditory ones. Equally, many people do not hear voices, but singing, music, sound, non-human voices, words, thoughts or presences. Indeed, 'hearing' or 'seeing' might not be the best descriptors for a host of experiences that rest on the hinterlands of perception. Throughout, the ineffable and the wordless are occluded.

The experience of 'hearing voices' is already reified in the public's mind as denoting negative, commanding voices. Our challenge is, perhaps, to resist top-down moves to impose 'better' terminology, and to open ourselves up to a more curious and critical stance. A first step might be to acknowledge the limitations and political costs of arguing about language in order to embrace an imperfect way of speaking about the experience of 'hearing voices' – one that reflects its deep heterogeneities, its inherent messiness, and the myriad ways in which people make sense of it.

> *Learning points*
> - How might our words impact on other people's experiences?
> - When we speak about our personal experiences, we can choose the words we use to best describe them. What are the challenges when talking about other people's experiences, and how best can we honour people's different perspectives?
> - Are any words 'neutral'?
> - Why do the words we choose to use matter?

References

A Disorder for Everyone! (n.d.). www.adisorder4everyone.com

de Leede Smith, S. & Barkus, E. (2013). A comprehensive review of auditory verbal hallucinations: Lifetime prevalence, correlates and mechanisms in healthy and clinical individuals. *Frontiers in Human Neuroscience, 16*(7), 367. doi: 10.3389/fnhum.2013.00367

Dillon, J. & May, R. (2002). Reclaiming experience. *Clinical Psychology, 17*, 25–27.

Dillon, J., Bullimore, P., Lampshire, D. & Chamberlin, J. (2012). The work of experience-based experts. In: J. Read & J. Dillon (Eds.), *Models of madness: Psychological, social and biological approaches to psychosis* (pp.305–319). Routledge.

Division of Clinical Psychology (2015). *Guidelines on language in relation to functional psychiatric diagnosis*. British Psychological Society.

Galasiński, D. (2017a). *Is it about language?* [Blog.] http://dariuszgalasinski.com/2017/12/21/language-2/

Galasiński, D. (2017b). *Vocabulary of disease?* [Blog.] http://dariuszgalasinski.com/2017/12/09/vocabulary/

Galasiński, D. (2017c). *On 'ordinary non-medical language'*. [Blog.] http://dariuszgalasinski.com/2017/12/11/ordinary/

Healey, K. (2012). *Hearing voices… A normal human experience*. Holistic Mental Health Conference, Toronto June 21–22. https://recoverynetworktoronto.files.wordpress.com/2012/06/hearing-voices-a-normal-human-experience-25jun20121.pdf

Johnstone, L. & Boyle, M., with Cromby, J., Dillon, J,. Harper, D., Kinderman, P., Longden, E., Pilgrim, D. & Read, J. (2018). *The Power Threat Meaning Framework: Towards the identification of patterns in emotional distress, unusual experiences and troubled or troubling behaviour as an alternative to functional psychiatric diagnosis*. British Psychological Society.

Jones, N. & Kelly, T. (2015). Inconvenient complications: On the heterogeneities of madness and their relationship to disability'. In: H. Spandler, J. Anderson & B. Sapey (Eds.), *Madness, distress and the politics of disablement* (pp.43–55). Policy Press.

Kinderman, P. & Cooke, A. (2018). *Mind your language! A guide to language about mental health and psychological wellbeing in the media and the creative arts*. https://livrepository.liverpool.ac.uk/3022118/2/mind%20your%20language%20v7.pdf

Kinderman, P., Read, J. & Moncrieff, J. (2013). Drop the language of disorder. *Evidence-Based Mental Health, 16*(1), 2–3.

Luhrmann, T., Padmavati, R., Tharoor, H. & Osei, A. (2015). Differences in voice-hearing experiences of people with psychosis in the USA, India and Ghana: interview-based study. *British Journal of Psychiatry, 206*(1), 41–44.

McCarthy-Jones, S. & Longden, E. (2013). The voices others cannot hear. *The Psychologist, 26*, 570–575.

Melley, J. (2018, June 8). The children who hear voices. *BBC News.* www.bbc.co.uk/news/health-44398292

Moskowitz, A. & Corstens, D. (2007). Auditory hallucinations: Psychotic symptom or dissociative experience?' *Journal of Psychological Trauma, 6*(2–3), 35–63.

Richards, V. (2018). The importance of language in mental health care. *Lancet Psychiatry, 5*(6), 460–461.

Romme, M., Escher, S., Dillon, J., Corstens, D. & Morris, M. (2009). *Living with voices: 50 stories of recovery.* PCCS Books.

Russo, J. & Shulkes, D. (2016). What we talk about when we talk about disability: Making sense of debates in the European user/survivor movement. In: H. Spandler, J. Anderson & B. Sapey (Eds.), *Madness, distress and the politics of disablement* (pp.27–42). Policy Press.

Shaw, C. (2016). Telling stories. *Philosophy, Psychiatry, & Psychology, 23*(3), 277–279.

Telles-Correia, D., Moreira, A.L. & Gonçalves, J.S. (2015). Hallucinations and related concepts – their conceptual background. *Frontiers in Psychology* 6, 991. doi: 10.3389/fpsyg.2015.00991

Waddingham, R. (2013, August 27). Symptom or experience? Does language matter? *Mad in America.* www.madinamerica.com/2013/08/does-language-matter/

Woods, A. (2013). The voice-hearer. *Journal of Mental Health, 22*(3), 263–270.

3 Hearing voices groups
Peter Bullimore

Background

I founded the Sheffield Hearing Voices group in 1996, with Sally Bramley. I am a voice hearer and Sally is an occupational therapist. At the time, I had been a patient for 10 years, going in and out of psychiatric hospitals.

My psychosis started as a result of childhood sexual abuse. My babysitter would come round on a Friday evening and put on horror films. I was quite a nervous child and I didn't want to watch the films, but she would make me. She'd turn the lights out so it was dark, and she would keep giving me glasses of fizzy drinks. Eventually I'd say that I wanted to go to the toilet, but I would be too frightened to go upstairs, so I would wet myself. When my parents came home, the television was off and the lights were on, and the babysitter would say, 'I told him to go to the toilet and he took no notice.' At such a young age, I thought that, if they believed that, they would believe anything. That was when the abuse really started. It was sexual and physical abuse, and downright disgusting. This went on from the age of five until I was nearly 13, but I was too frightened to tell anybody.

When I turned seven, I became very paranoid, thinking that the entire world knew what was happening but no one was prepared to help me. So, I became very socially isolated and started to hear voices. As I got older, the abuse escalated, getting more intense and severe. When I was being abused at the age of 12, there were times when I would get aroused, but I just couldn't understand why, because I hated the abuse. When that happened, the voices would return to criticise me. One voice became 10 voices, then 10 voices became 20 voices, and they were very destructive and violent. It got to the point where I hit my best friend because I thought that my head was going to explode. I was carrying this secret around that I just couldn't tell anyone, and it really affected my behaviour. We had an electric lawnmower and one day my mum was cleaning the blades. The voices urged me to turn it on, which I did, and I nearly cut her fingers off.

The lowest point turned out to be a turning point on reflection. Just before my 13th birthday, the babysitter came round and had full sex with me. I was so worried that she could be pregnant. Eventually I said to my parents that I didn't want this woman to come round anymore, and they agreed. The abuse stopped and the voices went away, lying repressed and buried until I was 19 years old.

Transition towards illness

The problem was that I never told anyone about the voices or the abuse. I got married at a young age and became a father, but I never told my wife what I was going through. We had three children, and then I lost my job. It was during the recession, and I couldn't find work. The house was threatened with repossession, and I had no idea how we were going to survive. Eventually I found work manufacturing fire surrounds. It was a good job, but I was working seven days a week and was still not able to repay any of the money we owed. Under these stresses and pressures, the voices came back. I remember the first one. It was a Friday evening; I'd just got paid, and I was walking into Sheffield town centre when I heard a really loud, dominant voice. It kept saying, 'You are Mickey McAvoy, you're worth millions!' He was one of the ringleaders in the 1983 Brink's-Mat robbery at Heathrow, and I foolishly believed what this voice was telling me. So, I walked into the first pub I found and bought everybody a drink, then another. When I went home, I was in real trouble as I had no money left. But I couldn't explain why I had done it and my wife thought that I was crazy.

Crisis point

I had nowhere to turn to and it was becoming a living hell. My wife encouraged me to see a GP who just said that I was stressed and gave me beta blockers. But I had a really bad period of insomnia and hadn't slept properly for days. It was the early hours of Sunday morning, and I was lying on the settee in the front room when I had an out-of-body experience. I couldn't get back into my body and I thought that I was dead. Eventually I started to cry uncontrollably, which is something I had learnt as a child that you don't do, as it's a sign of weakness. My wife kept asking me what was wrong, and I said to her, 'Why did you let me die on my own, after all I've done for you?' She couldn't understand what I was saying and encouraged me not to go to work the next day. But I ignored her and went. There was a problem on a job and this man was shouting down the phone at me, so I told him to f*** off. I was told, 'You can't speak to people like that!', which was the final straw. I hit the man in the office over the head with the telephone and walked out. I went home and just curled up in a chair. I didn't wash. I didn't shave, and I didn't eat or drink properly. I was just locked in this fearful world of voices, paranoia and depression.

Contact with services and treatment

Eventually the doctor came and said that he thought that I should go into hospital. At this time, I was very ignorant about mental health, so I thought that they'd put me on a general ward with nurses fussing round for a few weeks. But that night my dad drove me to the local psychiatric unit. The experience was a real eye-opener. The hospital was absolutely filthy. There were double mattresses on single beds and people lying in the corridors. It was horrible. Eventually a doctor came to see me and said she was going to give me a rectal examination. I had no idea why this was necessary, but it was like the abuse was happening all over again and part of the paranoid plot. I ran down the corridor and was stopped by this male nurse who said that, if I tried to leave, they would section me. I realise now that this is coercion and is actually illegal. But not knowing that at the time, I stayed and was sectioned for the first of many times over 10 years. During this first admission, I couldn't look in the mirror because I couldn't see myself. I only saw a demon. The figure had long hair, a beard and had black marks round the eyes. On reflection, that was me! I was taking a combination of 25 drugs a day, so I had gone black round the eyes. But the voices were still there. This was my life for nearly 10 years.

Contact with mental health professionals

Then I got a new occupational therapist, who was amazing. She never saw me as just my diagnosis, but instead she always looked beyond the label to see me. When you're in the mental health system, you tend to put everyone on a pedestal as your confidence and self-esteem is so low. She addressed that by telling me a bit about herself and the stresses and traumas she'd had in her life. I thought, 'Wow, this woman does understand and she has got feelings and emotions.' She asked me why I isolated myself on a Friday and found out that I was abused on that day. I couldn't cope, but she helped me work through it. I also got a new psychiatrist, who was great – young and enthusiastic. He wasn't bothered about an appointment system and had an 'open door policy', which I really liked. He started to reduce my drugs, so things were picking up.

My wife's social worker told me about a hearing voices group at Sheffield Mind and encouraged me to go. At this point, I was the archetypal 'schizophrenic' – I didn't wash or shave and was scruffy. There were 10 other people at this group, but it struck me that they were all smart and presentable. I thought they couldn't be 'schizos' as, if they were, they would be scruffy like me! But then they started to share their experiences. I realised that was where I belonged and that I could take off the mask that I'd been wearing for years. They asked me if I wanted to go to a workshop but I didn't know what a workshop was. I turned up wondering where's the workbench; what are we going to make? But three people from the Hearing Voices Network shared their experiences of recovery and what really struck me was how the content of their voices was related to life events. I suddenly thought that perhaps there was another explanation for all of this. I was still on heavy medication, but the seed had been sown that this organisation existed. This was the start of my recovery.

In 1998 I had been the victim of an unprovoked attack that required me to have 14 stitches in my face. When I was leaving court after the trial of my attacker, my keyworker, Sally Bramley, told me that I had to start to take control of my life, as I had endured the trial and not had any major setbacks through hearing my voices. Later that afternoon, Sally said that the hearing voices group in Sheffield had closed down and challenged me to start another one. Initially, I was very reluctant but, with her help and encouragement, I agreed. Sally arranged a room at a local day centre and we decided the meetings would take place on Thursday afternoons between 14.00 and 15.00. At the first meeting, six people from the day centre attended, and we set the ground rules. Then we designed a flyer to advertise the group and did a blanket mail out. We targeted psychiatric hospitals, community teams, drug and alcohol units, accident and emergency departments, day centres, probation services, hostels and libraries.

The numbers grew but there was resistance from some psychiatrists to let clients attend. So I spent time visiting community psychiatric teams and explaining the aims of the group. The group aimed to provide education, and not therapy. We were not attacking psychiatry; indeed, we were trying to be collaborative with clinicians and service providers. We made an effort not to alienate services, and workers started to enquire if their clients could attend. As a result of our persistence and determination, the group grew in numbers. But then it slowly dwindled away and I decided to find out why this had happened. I got someone to do an external evaluation. The researcher asked people why they didn't attend anymore, and the feedback was that the group was good but the time and day needed to be changed. The members preferred Monday mornings, as so many of them had been isolated over the weekend.

The new group took place from 10.30 am until 11.30 am every Monday. The numbers rapidly increased over the years, and professionals and workers began to take a great interest in the group. As of today, the group has 85 members. The main reason for its success has been the continuity and commitment of the group's facilitators. They do not exclude anyone. The group is made interesting and varied by bringing in outside speakers. The group has entered its 23rd year and is the longest-running hearing voices group in the world. It is seen as an important part of the mental health community, as it has developed into a network that delivers teaching internationally around the world. Some of the group's members deliver the teaching and training.

There are now more than 180 hearing voices groups in the UK alone, and many others worldwide. There are hearing voices networks in 35 countries. It is the fastest-growing user movement in the world and comprises not just people with lived experiences of hearing voices but many health professionals from many different disciplines.

The key principles of the hearing voices approach

The key principles of the hearing voices approach are:

- Accept that hearing voices (and related experiences) are valid human experiences.
- Respect each person's framework of understanding and beliefs about their experiences.
- Foster and enable the safety and wellbeing of all.

- Promote hope.
- Create safe spaces to share experiences and network for deeper connections.
- Believe in each person's resilience and capacity to take control of their experiences and recover.
- Work collaboratively and inclusively with other services to develop knowledge and use holistic approaches to recovery.
- Foster and support self-determination and self-empowerment.
- Encourage service providers, families and friends to join and connect with voice hearers as allies.

Voice hearers have told how adopting the key principles of the hearing voices network approach changed their understanding of their experiences and improved their quality of life. Here are some comments I have heard from voice hearers:

> I am able to see an episode beginning and use approaches that Pete shared with me to manage it better.
>
> I feel like I've discovered myself as a human being and not a monster. It helped to speak to someone who has had similar experiences.
>
> Gave me hope as you know you are talking to someone who really understands.
>
> Helped me talk about my problems and open up… I have become more self-accepting.
>
> Helped me change how I view my experiences. Instead of putting me into a box, it empowers me.
>
> Instead of a symptom of an illness, I saw the voices as part of me… I could define them as I want.
>
> Before it was all about how to get through each hour and day, but now I understand more about why I'm affected by these things.

Learning point 1
- It is important to see the voice hearer as a person with agency.
- It may not be possible to eradicate the voices, but people can learn techniques for negotiating with their voices.
- But first we have to understand the significance of the voices to the person.

Hearing voices is normal

The most important question we should ask someone when they come into psychiatric services is 'What has happened to you?', not 'What is wrong with you?'

– the more likely question to be asked. Research has found that, if we don't ask this question, it takes on average 16 years for someone to disclose (Read et al., 2007).

Mainstream biological psychiatry traditionally regards the phenomenon of voice hearing as a 'delusion', a 'symptom' of 'psychosis' or 'schizophrenia'. It is commonly assumed that what the voices say is meaningless and that the experience does not have any significance for the voice hearer.

Furthermore, it is traditionally believed that talking to someone about the voices they hear is 'colluding' with the 'delusion' and likely to reinforce it. In line with the mainstream biomedical model of psychiatry, antipsychotic medication remains the first-line treatment offered to voice hearers in the mental health system, with the aim of eliminating the voice(s) (Romme & Escher, 1993).

However, many people with a diagnosis of schizophrenia still hear voices, despite taking the medication. These drugs also often produce severe, disabling effects, which can affect a person's quality of life and physical health (Moncrieff, 2020).

Marius Romme and Sandra Escher's collaborative research with voice hearers (1993) laid the foundations for the Hearing Voices Approach and significantly changed the way that the phenomenon of voice hearing is understood and responded to today. Their research demonstrated that hearing voices is a natural phenomenon in human experience that is actually quite common; indeed, many people hear voices and never think to remark on it or find it a problem, and it needs to be accepted and supported (Beavan et al., 2011).

In addition, research has shown that there is a relationship between past or recent traumatic or intensely emotional events (for example, accident, divorce, death of a loved one, sexual or physical abuse, love affairs, pregnancy and birth) and the onset of voice hearing (Beavan et al., 2011; Read & Fraser, 1998; Hammersley et al., 2008; Read et al., 2009; Read & Bentall, 2012; Varese et al., 2012). Some researchers suggest that as many as 70% of adults and 85% of children (Escher et al., 2004; Romme & Escher, 2010; Millham & Easton, 1998; Beavan et al., 2011; Watkins, 2008; McCarthy-Jones, 2012) link their voice hearing to the experience of a difficult life event.

Romme and Escher's suggestions for changing entrenched perceptions of voice hearing are that professionals should attempt to accept patients' experiences of their voices.

> What this research shows is that we must accept that the voices exist. We must also accept that we cannot change the voices. They are not curable, just as you cannot cure left-handedness – human variations are not open to cure – only to coping. Therefore to assist people to cope we should not give them therapy that does not work. We should let people decide for themselves what helps or not. It takes time for people to accept that hearing voices is something that belongs to them. (Romme, in Baker, 2009, p.26)

There are some psychiatrists and psychologists who now work with people in a more open way, using talking therapies to explore the meaning of the voices.

Although this is not yet the norm in mainstream psychiatry, an increasing number of health professionals are beginning to understand that the key to understanding voice hearing and associated beliefs or so-called delusions (such as paranoia, for example) is to normalise these experiences. A more holistic approach is now being used to help a person make sense of their experiences of paranoia, unusual beliefs, problematic thoughts and hearing voices.

The important information that we have discovered is that when we encourage voice hearers to adopt these approaches, we find that the voices themselves are not the problem. Instead, it is the fear and the paranoia created by the voices that is the problem, which is often based on what the voices say. When we understand the real message of the voices from a metaphorical perspective, based on the person's narrative, it enables us to work with the person to normalise their experiences and learn ways to live with and manage them.

We use the Maastricht Interview for hearing voices (Romme & Escher, 2000), which is a semi-structured questionnaire and aims to open up discussions about the nature and content of the voices, such as who and what do they represent (see Chapter 1).

The topics covered in the Maastricht Interview include:

- the nature of the experience
- the voice characteristics
- the history of voice hearing
- voice triggers
- the content of the voices
- explanations for the origins of the voices
- the impact of the voices on life
- the relationship with the voices
- cognitive, behavioural and physiological coping strategies
- childhood experiences
- medical history
- social network.

Workers who have undertaken the Maastricht Interview training have told us:

> [I am now] able to see patient's voice hearing from a different perspective – fresh optimism about how to help them.
>
> Having worked with someone for five years with voices, I have felt useless most of the time because I've not known how to help.
>
> I feel it re-generated the realisation of how people's difficulties emerge/link. Normalisation of the phenomena instead of adopting the illness model – very good.

> Reinforced the resilience of people that do hear voices.
>
> Helped me understand how complex the nature of trauma can be, and how it affects people in many ways.

I also founded the National Paranoia Network, built on the same principles, which I set up with Terence McLaughlin, a psychologist, in 2004 in Sheffield, UK, and run with Kate Crawford and Shaun Hunt. Paranoia is another so-called symptom of psychosis. Our aim is to raise awareness of how disabling paranoia and what we prefer to call unusual beliefs (rather than delusions) can be and to break down social taboos. The network runs training sessions globally for professional bodies and all interested parties on how to understand a person's paranoia and beliefs to help them make sense of them.

Conclusion

In this chapter, I have challenged the validity of the diagnosis of schizophrenia and highlighted how suffering traumatic experiences, such as sexual, physical and emotional abuse can cause a person to hear voices. I have also shown how hearing voices is a common human experience and how a person can learn to understand the message of their voices, make sense of them and live a fulfilling life. It also shows the positive outcomes between a voice hearer and worker when they discuss the person's experience using the voice hearer's frame of reference.

References

Baker, P. (2009). *The voice inside: A practical guide for and about people who hear voices*. P&P Press.

Beavan, V., Read, J. & Cartwright, C. (2011). The prevalence of voice-hearers in the general population: A literature review. *Journal of Mental Health 20*(3), 281–292.

Escher, S., Morris, M., Buiks, A., Delespaul, P., van Os, J. & Romme, M. (2004). Determinants of outcome in the pathways through care for children hearing voices. *International Journal of Social Welfare, 13*(3), 208–222.

Hammersley, P., Read, J., Woodall, S. & Dillon, J. (2008). Childhood trauma and psychosis: The genie is out of the bottle. *Journal of Psychological Trauma*, 6(2–3), 7–20.

McCarthy-Jones, S. (2012). *Hearing voices: The histories, causes and meanings of auditory verbal hallucinations*. Cambridge University Press.

Millham, A. & Easton, S. (1998). Prevalence of auditory hallucinations in nurses in mental health. *Journal of Psychiatric and Mental Health Nursing, 5*(2), 95–99.

Moncrieff, J. (2020). *A straight talking introduction to psychiatric drugs* (2nd ed.). PCCS Books.

Read, J. & Bentall, R. (2012). Negative childhood experiences and mental health: theoretical, clinical and primary prevention implications. *British Journal of Psychiatry, 200*(2), 89–91.

Read, J. & Fraser, A. (1998). Abuse histories of psychiatric inpatients: to ask or not to ask? *Psychiatric Services, 49*(3), 355–359.

Read, J., Bentall, R. & Fosse, R. (2009). Time to abandon the bio-bio-bio-model of psychosis: Exploring the epigenetic and psychological mechanisms by which adverse life events lead to psychotic symptoms. *Epidemiologia e Psichiatria Sociale, 18*(4), 299–310.

Read, J., Hammersley, P. & Rudegeair, T. (2007). Why, when and how to ask about childhood abuse. *Advances in Psychiatric Treatment, 13*(2), 10 –110.

Romme, M. & Escher, S. (1993). *Accepting voices*. Mind Publications.

Romme, M. & Escher, S. (2000). *Making sense of voices: A guide for mental health professionals working with voice-hearers*. Mind Publications.

Romme, M. & Escher, S. (2010). Personal history and hearing voices. In: F. Laroi & A. Aleman (Eds.), *Hallucinations. A guide to treatment and management* (pp.233–256). Oxford University Press.

Varese, F., Smeets, F., Drukker, M., Lieverse, R., Lataster, T., Viechtbauer, W., Read, J., van Os, J. & Bentall, R.P. (2012). Childhood adversities increase the risk of psychosis: A meta-analysis of patient-control, prospective- and cross-sectional cohort studies. *Schizophrenia Bulletin, 38*(4), 661–671.

Watkins, J. (2008). *Hearing voices: A common human experience*. Michelle Anderson Pty Ltd.

4   Facilitating hearing voices groups
Sasha Priddy and Charlotte Howard

Within the realm of mainstream psychiatry, hearing voices groups (HVGs) can offer a powerful alternative to dominant practices around the experience of voice hearing. In contrast to biopsychosocial and biomedical frameworks, HVGs aim to facilitate a process of exploration and personal meaning-making through creating spaces that enable empowerment, emancipation and liberation. For many, these spaces offer a restorative forum for peer support, where diversity of experience and identity are welcomed and respected, rather than silenced.

We both have personal experience of facilitating and engaging in HVGs. As such, in the spirit of the groups' ethos, we would like to begin this chapter from a position of human connection, through sharing our first encounter with our own HVG. In this chapter, we hope to continue cascading out the ripples of solidarity that we have experienced from being part of an HVG and to encourage you, the reader, to seek out opportunities to grow and support the HVG community through facilitating your own hearing voices group.

Sasha: the importance of shedding your 'professional self'

I first entered the world of inpatient mental health settings as a psychology student on a placement year. The first hospital I worked in was situated in a picturesque location, set against an area of woodland and just a stone's throw from the local beach. Unfortunately, my experiences of the internal world of the hospital did not match this idyllic exterior. As a fresh-faced student, I had no idea of what to expect on entering the doors of the hospital. I can remember feeling stunned and shaken by what constituted 'normal' life there. Although the hospital was run by many well-intended members of staff from a variety of professional backgrounds, the hostility of the environment could not be ignored. I quickly became familiar with its schedule of restrictive practices, where fresh-air was rationed, timetabled activities were mandatory, caffeine was prohibited, medication was regular, and restraints were not uncommon. It was within this regimented, frightening and powerful context that I first encountered an HVG, and I came to see it as an oasis and antidote to some of the more unsavoury practices embedded within psychiatric services.

Charlotte: the opportunity to share your 'personal self'

I first came across HVGs when I moved to a personality disorder rehabilitation unit after spending a prolonged period in an acute ward and in a psychiatric intensive care unit. Throughout my time in services, I had felt that hearing voices was stigmatised and a subject not usually talked about. I attended my first HVG and was pleased that there was a forum that discussed voices and noises in a relaxed, open and non-judgemental way.

I have gained a lot from the group that I attended and it has stayed with me throughout my life in the community, away from inpatient psychiatric services. I learned that I was not alone in my experiences with voices and that not everyone holds the stereotypical views that are common in society. The group allowed me to explore my voices in a safe environment and helped me to verbalise my experiences without judgement. I felt safe with the other members and will forever be grateful to the facilitators of the group for providing me with a setting where I could discover myself, which other, general groups had not previously given. I feel privileged to have been part of other service users' journeys to developing understanding of their own voices.

The origins of the Hearing Voices Movement

The origins of the Hearing Voices Movement (HVM) can be traced back to the 1980s and are rooted in a collaboration between a psychiatrist, Marius Romme, his client, Patsy Hague, and a researcher, Sandra Escher. Their research into the experience of voice hearing questioned the dominant 'illness' narrative by demonstrating that many people who hear voices do not come into contact with psychiatric services or necessarily require 'treatment' (Corstens et al., 2014). This research proved to be a catalyst for the development of the emancipatory Hearing Voices Movement, which acknowledges the importance of understanding voice hearing in the context of a person's past and present life (Corstens et al., 2014). Accordingly, the HVM advocates a position of accepting and sense-making, where voices are not seen as an 'aberrant symptom of schizophrenia to be endured, but a complex, significant and meaningful reaction to be explored' (Longden, 2013). The Hearing Voices Network (HVN), which embodies the principles of the HVM, provides a peer-focused framework for the creating of safe spaces in which these values can be enacted – namely, HVGs.

What are hearing voices groups?

HVGs use a peer support format, allowing members to support each other and connect through their lived experience. In line with the principles of the HVM, HVGs do not promote or exclude any explanation of voice hearing. Rather, HVGs provide a forum for open exploration of 'unusual' sensory experiences, where people can explore their voice-hearing experiences without fearing that they are exposing themselves to potential judgement, censorship or threats to their autonomy. In HVGs, members are encouraged to develop their own relationship with their voices and their meaning, rather than automatically cast these experiences aside as 'psychotic'. For some people, hearing voices can initially be confusing, chaotic, unpredictable and distressing, and so the voices are regarded by many mental health services as a 'problem' to be eradicated. However, the HVM positions all these experiences as meaningful attempts to survive maddening experiences and environments. As such, the underlying purpose of HVGs is to empower the person to explore their voice-hearing experience in whatever way is meaningful for them. This may include exploring spiritual, cultural, historical, social, paranormal and any other beliefs or factors that feel significant to their experience.

Facilitation and membership: a symbiotic process

The non-prescriptive nature of HVGs means that the content and structure of these spaces are largely shaped by, and therefore receptive to, the needs of group members, through a collaborative, grassroots process. As such, the role of a 'facilitator' should be taken very literally. Their primary role is not to 'lead' the group, but to facilitate others' ability to contribute to the space. Providing this facilitation involves an awareness of the barriers to group participation. For many people who hear voices, engaging with mental health services is associated with experiences of being implicitly or explicitly undermined through challenges to their autonomy, control and dignity. For these reasons, some groups choose to adopt a 'closed' membership approach, in which only people who identify as experiencing voices or 'unusual' sensory experiences are invited to attend. These groups might be preferred as they allow people to regain ownership over their experiences without feeling they are being observed by a 'professional' bystander. However, some settings and services may not be able or willing to allow closed groups to take place. In these settings, where professionals insist on attending, it is imperative that their involvement does not detract from the HVM values or lead to a tokenistic space.

In all circumstances, it is preferable to have two facilitators present, as this can have both practical and relational benefits in ensuring a safe and containing space. Ideally, at least one facilitator will have personal experience of voice hearing, or at the very least have lived experience of psychiatric services, although we recognise that this will not always be possible. Reflections and disclosures from the facilitator are welcomed whenever this is relevant and comfortable, to actively dissolve any form of 'us and them' divide. In our opinion, the formation of these relationships plays the most significant role in facilitating opportunities for liberation within HVGs, particularly in contexts in which people are likely to experience being 'done to'.

Practically shaping the space

Practical elements of the group also serve to create the group identity. The location, time, name, environment and other factors all influence the group experience. In secure settings, these factors may signal an even more powerful message, as the group attempts to create a pocket of liberation within systems that can feel oppressive. Therefore, attention must be given to the psychological safety of the physical space. For example, in a secure mental health setting, it would be necessary to consider whether the room where the group is to meet is used for other functions that may be associated with difficult or disempowering experiences for group members. It is also important to assess whether the location offers the required privacy. Facilitators should try to find a space that both meets the practical requirements (as to size, availability and so on), and considers process issues. For example, the walls should be thick enough to prevent group discussions being overheard and protect against conversations in neighbouring rooms contaminating the group's space.

Clear start and finish times should be agreed, to provide containment and consistency. When establishing the length of the meeting, time should be allowed for conversations to 'warm up' and 'wind down', as well as for each group member to feel able to meaningfully contribute. Some groups may choose to develop a structure in which members partake in particular rituals: reading an introductory values statement, inviting members to participate in a 'check-in' and 'check-out', or having mid-point breaks, for example. This can support consistency and shared facilitation of the group.

Most groups choose to use the 'HVG' title, but it is important to consider whether the group name represents the group identity and whom it wishes to welcome. In our own group, some people experienced noises, rather than distinct voices, so we renamed it the 'Voices and Noises Group', to be more explicitly representative and inclusive.

Learning point 1

What is being communicated through your own HVG space? If you are already part of a HVG, these questions might be something to consider with other group members:

- Is the room associated with any other experiences for group members?
- Does the room offer adequate privacy, so group members feel able to speak freely?
- Can you offer the space consistently (i.e. same location and time)?
- In what ways is the space welcoming?
- In what ways could the space prohibit participation?

What resources are available to you to ensure that group members feel welcome (i.e. tea/coffee facilities or an introductory handbook/leaflet)?

Tools and resources

For any HVG, we would suggest that a toolbox of resources is developed, which will evolve over time with the changing group membership. This is both a practical and a symbolic process, whereby the knowledge of group members is retained within the group through their contributions. We would suggest the toolbox should include the following items to aid exploration, provide information and offer structure:

- *A values statement* – created by group members to communicate the purpose and values of their group. HVGs that adopt an 'open' group membership might find this particularly helpful to welcome new members and introduce the core values of the group.
- *Group expectations* – collaboratively agreeing ground rules ensures that group members identify expectations, rules and boundaries that create a safe and welcoming space.
- *A group structure* – group members can choose to take on the role of 'meeting keeper', guiding the group in accordance with the agreed structure.
- *Sensory items* – these can be used for grounding exercises or self-soothing exercises.
- *Books and videos* – the HVN website[1] lists a number of resources, including relevant literature, leaflets and videos that can be loaned out or viewed/read together.
- *Items to invite conversation* – as a group, we developed 'question cards' (see Table 4.1). People could choose a card to answer before sharing it with the room.
- *Transition book/legacy document* – for messages and stories from group members, to create a repository of shared wisdom and hope between members past, present and future (see Table 4.2).

Within-group processes: facilitating safe exploration

For any person attending their first HVG, the opportunity to discuss the detail and meaning behind their experiences may feel like uncharted territory. Previous attempts to engage in such conversations elsewhere may have caused confusion, induced feelings of shame and initiated an expectation that their voices will be judged negatively. Facilitators must endeavour to attune themselves to the pace of group members: some will feel confident in sharing and exploring their voices, others will feel uncertain and need to develop trust in the process. So, silence and conversation must be equally valued, which requires the facilitator to feel comfortable with holding the silence when needed.

The 'Three Phases of Voice Hearing' (Romme & Escher, 1989) offers a useful framework for facilitators to sensitively consider the different processes

---

1. See www.hearing-voices.org

Table 4.1: Conversation cards to explore voices

Has hearing voices brought anything positive to your life?	Have you noticed that your voice(s) are present when you feel certain emotions?	Do you and your voice(s) have respect for each other?
Do you have any beliefs that others think are unusual, but are related to the voice(s) you hear?	How do you describe your relationship with your voice(s)? Is it positive, negative, neutral or something else?	Do you and your voice have an equal relationship?
Can you relate to the feelings that you think your voice is expressing?	Could you change your response to the voice, in terms of how you behave or what you say? What impact might this have?	Does your voice threaten to do things? How could you test out whether your voice has the power to carry out these threats?
What do you need to look after yourself? How does this help when you're finding things difficult?	Do you think there is anything that triggers your voices? Have you thought about avoiding these? Or finding ways to manage the triggers?	What feelings might your voice be trying to communicate to you? How would you like someone to respond to you if you felt that way? Can you give your voice that response?
Is there anything you've learned through your experience of voice hearing that might help others?	When you hear a voice, how do you feel?	Are these ways that you can respectfully disagree with your voices, when needed?

Table 4.2: A transitions book message

To all the past, present and future members of the Voices & Noises group.

I feel privileged to have been a part of this group with you all! The courage, kindness, and openness and hope that I have seen here has been inspirational. I will remember the willingness to be vulnerable, the sensitivity to that vulnerability and the wonderfully diverse understandings you have all offered to your own and others' experiences.

But I think the most important thing I have seen here is the ability to laugh, smile and find joy together – and how this can even be done in the more difficult and darker times. I hope this group will continue to offer all these things and wish you the very best.

Sasha

that group members might be experiencing in relation to their voices. This theoretical model proposes three broad phases to the voice-hearing experience: the 'startling' phase ('What is happening to me?'), the 'organisation' phase ('I'm trying to understand my voices') and the 'stabilisation' phase ('I hear voices and I can cope with it') (Hearing Voice Network Aotearoa, 2014). Keeping these phases in mind can help facilitators pace exploration. For example, when people are in the startling phase, the facilitator might want to consider how to ensure the group can demonstrate that it is a safe space where experiences can be shared without judgement. Learning point 2 below suggests some initial questions that might help to establish trust through a fundamental acknowledgement that the voices are real. If people are in the later organisational phase, the conversation might be opened up to explore the meaning of the voices and facilitate understanding between people's contexts and their voices' content or origins. The bringing together of people at different stages of their experience of voice hearing is an invaluable aspect of the group, allowing members to use the wisdom they have gathered on their journeys to support others.

> *Learning point 2*
>
> Questions such as those in the Maastricht Interview (Romme & Escher, 2000) can be used to facilitate the safe exploration of a group member's voice-hearing experience, such as:
>
> - What does the voice say?
> - When do you hear it most?
> - Does its tone of voice change?
> - How does the voice seem to feel when you talk about it?
>
> Over time, these questions might move on to explore the meaning of the voice, through asking things such as:
>
> - Why do you think the voice is more present in those moments?
> - What might the voice be communicating to you?
> - In what ways is the voice helpful?

Supervision: sustaining the spirit of the HVM in ourselves and others

Facilitators of the group may want to consider having supervision specifically for HVGs, in addition to their regular supervision. This should not be used to discuss group members' disclosures but as a space to revisit whether facilitators are adhering to and promoting the ethos of the HVM within the group. An approach outlined by Reynolds (2014) offers a taste of what this supervision space might look like for people concerned with social justice and human rights, such as those advocating a hearing voices approach. Reynolds (2014) proposes a 'supervision of solidarity' that places ethical justice-doing at the core of the process. This approach is not intended specifically for facilitators involved in HVGs, but we would argue that this ethically-orientated supervision style lends itself to the human rights and social justice values embedded within the HVM.

Looking beyond HVGs: changing the narrative

As discussed throughout this chapter, HVG groups can offer safe and soothing spaces within toxic systems. However, we must be mindful to not allow this to lead to complacency. Powerful systems, services and people may intentionally, or unintentionally, repurpose grassroots activism to neutralise, dismantle and assimilate its identity into old systems. As such, introducing HVGs into psychiatric services can involve walking a delicate tightrope 'between exclusion and colonisation' (Russo & Beresford, 2015). To maintain this delicate balance, we suggest that facilitators should actively apply the values of the HVM to work and to conversations outside the HVG, such as workshops or training sessions.

Many mental health professionals will endorse the idea that we need to move away from 'What is wrong with you?' to 'What has happened to you?' when thinking about human distress (Longden, 2013), but perhaps this doesn't go far enough. Higgs (2020) suggests that we need to actively consider 'What is *still* happening to you?' In this spirit, we hope that you will join us in recognising that being an HVG facilitator can, and must, extend beyond the four walls of your group meetings. It is through a true commitment to this role that we can seek to meaningfully contribute to the emancipation of voice hearers, through advocating for their liberation from oppressive systems.

> **Establishing a hearing voices group: key considerations**
>
> 1. All group members should be involved in shaping their own HVG.
> 2. Pay attention to the physical space – e.g. consider whether the room is practical and safe.
> 3. Facilitators should aim for group facilitation, rather than direct 'leadership' – i.e. the group is led by personal wisdoms, not 'expertise'.
> 4. Develop ground rules/group expectations about what is necessary for the group to feel safe.
> 5. Group structure – co-create a group structure to form a loose framework for sessions.
> 6. Invite and accept a range of beliefs about voices – group members should feel able to understand their voices in any way that is meaningful and helpful for them.
> 7. Develop a resource box together that can be routinely accessed, shared and used throughout the sessions (see 'Tools and resources' above).

References

Corstens, D., Longden, E, McCarthy-Jones, S., Waddingham, R. & Thomas, N. (2014). Emerging perspectives from the Hearing Voices Movement: Implications for research and practice. *Schizophrenia Bulletin, 40*(4), 285–294.

Hearing Voices Network Aotearoa (2014). *Three phases of voice hearing.* [Online]. Hearing Voices Network Aotearoa. www.hearingvoices.org.nz/attachments/article/89/Three%20Phases%20of%20 Voice%20Hearing.pdf

Higgs, R. (2020). Reconceptualizing psychosis: The hearing voices movement and social approaches to health. *Health and Human Rights Journal, 21*(2).

Longden, E. (2013). *Learning from the voices in my head.* TED Books.

Reynolds, V. (2014). Centering ethics in group supervision: fostering cultures of critique and structuring safety. *The International Journal of Narrative Therapy and Community Work, 1*, 1–13.

Romme, M.A. J. & Escher, A.D.M.A.C. (1989). Hearing voices. *Schizophrenia Bulletin, 15*(2), 209–216.

Romme, M. & Escher, S. (2000). *Making sense of voices: A guide for professionals who work with voice hearers.* Mind Publications.

Russo, J. & Beresford, P. (2015). Between exclusion and colonisation: Seeking a place for mad people's knowledge in academia. *Disability & Society, 30*(1), 153–157.

5 Painting has helped me to cope with my voices

Reshma Valliappan

People have asked me if my 'schizophrenia' has gone away. I have said 'no'. People have asked me if I still have my symptoms – the voices, the visual hallucinations, the delusions and paranoia, the inability to care for myself and to comprehend things. I have said 'no'. People have assumed that I am no longer 'schizophrenic'. This is because the definition of recovery comes from a system that has for a long time promoted the disappearance of 'symptoms'. Mental health professionals think that we are doing well if we stop hearing voices. This makes me think I am not doing well if I begin hearing voices again – something must be wrong with me again.

I was grateful to meet my psychiatrist because he saw me as a person, rather than a collection of symptoms that needed to be treated. He allowed space for discussion, and even at times allowed me to argue with him. Owing to the rapport and trust that he built with me, I felt that I could easily confide in him about the 'symptoms' that I was experiencing. This bonding is necessary for someone with 'schizophrenia', especially when our minds have strayed away from the emotional and mental security we may have had with our family members. To be given some level of security (that is, a safe mental, physical, emotional, religious and spiritual space) with respect to our mind and body is really important, particularly when there is a power inequality in our relationship with the mental health professional who has been put on a pedestal at the same level as God. Every person on earth perceives medical practitioners in this light, because the life of their loved one lies entirely in the hands of medical science. The faith that families have in this medical 'science' is all they have left. In many cultures, including mine, faith and answers are also found in god-men, voodoo priests or tantriks.[1] My dad is a scientist, so he believed in medical science and that I would

---

1. Tantra is a non-traditional Hindu path towards achieving enlightenment without having to renunciate worldly desires. The practice combines chants, hymns, sexual movements or acts, dance and alchemical methods to prosper, gain wealth, protect or even harm another. Someone who practises Tantra is referred to as a tantrik. The majority of self-proclaimed tantriks are feared for practising black magic but are also consulted for exorcism, as they are believed to be spiritually stronger in handling negative energies than other paths. However, almost all tantriks that offer these services by knocking on doors or by advertising themselves are scams.

be helped by psychiatrists, hospitals and pharmacists. My mum, on the other hand, encouraged me to visit ashrams of locally acclaimed gurus, miracle-performing godmen, and to take part in rituals, including bathing ceremonies.

Neither approach helped. I still heard voices, even with the 14 pills that I had to take each day. I also saw visions, even though evil attachments had been swept away from me with brooms. I gained 28 kilograms. I'd wake up to a pillow soaked in saliva, my muscles stiff, my body bloated and feet like those of an elephant due to severe water retention. This only added to my unhappiness. Depression became a secondary condition, caused by the medications and the 'schizophrenia' diagnosis.

My dad had given up all hope of helping me by then, as I was telling my family daily that I wanted to kill myself. He was on the verge of killing all of us and himself, because there was no support or help available from others. Neighbours thought that I was being treated for drug addiction, and so stayed away. Some family members and friends were suggesting the most ridiculous of cures, which included getting me married, as they thought that sexual intercourse could cure me. Other suggestions of ways to help me included locking me up and exorcising me, my room and the entire house. We were told that I was cursed. All of these 'cures' were tried and tested to some extent. My dad also asked my psychiatrist if ECT would help me. Fortunately, my doctor said, 'No. It would only make things worse.'

> *Learning point 1*
> - Have you ever felt that you are just viewed as 'symptoms' of an illness? Are your emotions, such as anger and sadness, also seen as 'symptoms'?
> - Do you get angry when your feelings and thoughts are not validated or even acknowledged?
> - How many people with 'schizophrenia' do you think are allowed to freely share their thoughts with others?
> - Do you believe in faith-healing and witch-doctors? How do different cultures and religions understand voice hearing differently?

Then, one day, I stopped taking my medications. I had done this before, only this time I had stayed on the medications for quite a long time and had found that they offered me not one single ounce of happiness, acceptance and independence in my own mind and in my life. How was it that I was taking 14 pills a day, yet I was still hearing voices and seeing distressing visions of people? When my psychiatrist asked me about the voices and the visions, I told him, 'Doctor, it's horrible. It's like my mind is getting raped.'

'What do you mean by that?' he asked me.

'It's like I'm watching things being done to me, but I can't do anything about it this time, not even physically, because of what my body has become.'

My psychiatrist understood what I had said. My body had developed many different kinds of physical issues that disabled it. How could a person survive the mind and body both losing their strength?

Before my body had these disabilities, I could react and respond to my mind and to the 'symptoms'. This ability to respond or react gave me some level of control. This is a natural trait of being human, which I lost due to taking the medications. But when I stopped taking my medications this time round, no one could notice the difference, as my reactions had been entirely numbed by the cocktail of medications I had had in my system for so long. I felt stupid. I could hardly read a sentence, which was a big contrast – I used to love reading, and sometimes had five books on the go at once. I also used to solve crossword puzzles over breakfast and have conversations at the same time.

The voices convinced me that my food was poisoned, so I flushed it down the toilet with my medications, or I wrapped the food up and threw it into a sanitary napkin disposal bag. There were times when I got caught, because my mother knew that I didn't have my menstrual cycle that week. I learnt to regurgitate my food and pills and flush them down the loo.

But then came that day where this voice said, 'Get up. Paint. You lazy oaf!' I was only half awake. I could not tell if I was dreaming or if I was back to hearing my voices louder than ever. Ignoring the voice's command, I shut my eyes.

'I SAID GET UP AND PAINT!' the voice commanded, and it kept on, getting louder and louder, until it was yelling: 'GET UP AND PAINT! GET UP AND PAINT!' This continued for half an hour until I gave in, as there was no winning with the voices. I knew that it was useless to try to sleep when the voices were this loud.

So I got out of bed and walked into my room to look for my paints. The voice pointed out, 'Look, right there. Use the study table. Take out the brushes. Clean them. Get water. Take the blue. Then white. Then orange. Draw a circle.' I followed in the way that a student would follow if she were attending an art class for the first time. The voice kept telling me what to do. I painted almost as if I was in a trance, my body just a conduit for this energy that was passing through me. After an hour of painting, I walked into the kitchen and helped myself to a glass of water. This was something that I could not do before. I sat calmly at the table and asked my mum for food. She was taken by surprise, as I normally did not utter any word or ask for anything. My mum went out to my dad, who was in the garden, and told him what I had said. Dad went up to my room and said to my sister, 'Girl, what was your *didi* doing?'[2] My sister looked up at my dad, and then took a look at my study table, and said, 'Painting.'

It has been 16 years since I was commanded to paint and picked up that brush (in 2004). The voice that I hear commanding me to paint has continued all of these years. The first time that I ever heard a voice was a month before my 15th birthday. I heard the voice when I ran away from home in 1995. Each time that I am overwhelmed by family issues and relationships, I have severe 'meltdowns', to

---

2. *Didi* is a Hindi word meaning elder sister.

the point where I want to kill myself. The voice will not stop until I give in to it. I have to cancel everything I am doing, such as study and appointments. Everything has to be put to one side, including self-care and grooming. The only thing that I am able to do when I am hearing the voice is feed my cat when it meows for food.

> *Learning point 2*
> - Have you found an activity that helps you to cope with your voices? What is this activity? Why does it help?
> - Have other people noticed that an activity has helped you?

Figure 5.1: I hear voices because I am a good listener

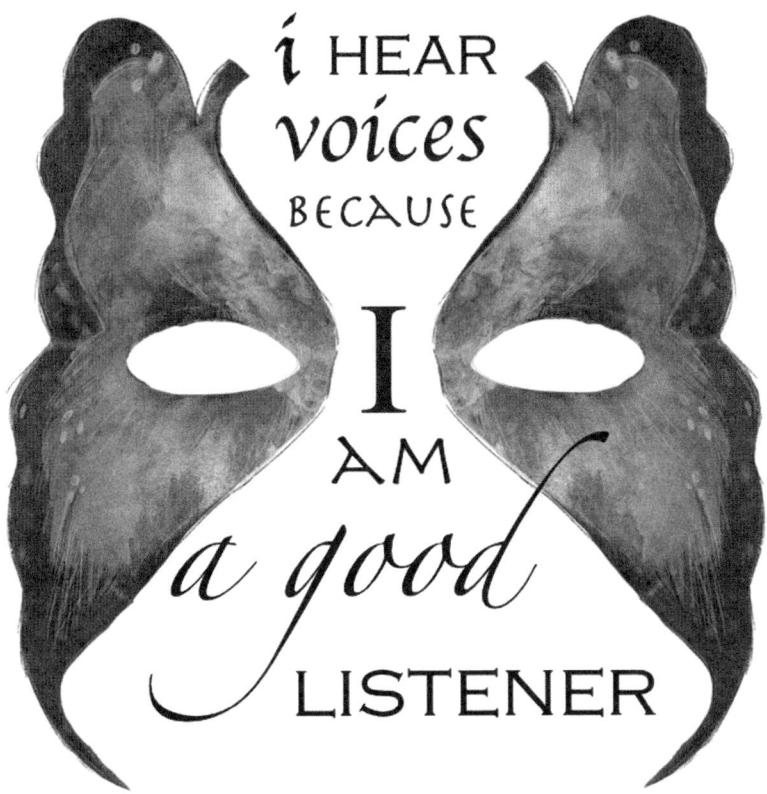

I have now had 27 years to make sense of my internal and external voices, and it has been a long journey of discovery. During this time, I completed three Master's degrees, published articles, authored my memoir, travelled for mental health-related work, gave lectures, conducted workshops and classes, provided peer support for others and carers, and had a craniotomy for a brain tumour that left me with sleep disorders and scar epilepsy. I have dealt with many family crises, including relatives being burned in gas explosions, my dad having three heart attacks and my mum battling breast cancer. In addition, I have faced a lot more life issues, including attempted suicide and difficult political situations. I am recognised as an Ashoka Fellow social changemaker,[3] and I have developed creative tools to enable self-healing, teaching and financial independence. It is important for me to mention these difficulties because I have experienced the added challenge of being a woman living in India's patriarchal society.

Painting has a central role in my life. Its effects are similar to those of meditation. Painting for me is contemplative meditation. There is no denying its therapeutic value in today's world. The process of creating art demands a high level of patience, which is challenging for most people. I learned how to be patient when I used to wait up to four hours in an outpatient department in a hospital for an appointment with a consultant psychiatrist. While I was in this state of paranoia, there was an expectation from those around me that I should remain calm. I could hear the voices all around me. A commanding voice kept repeating to me, 'You will go back and paint.' Most people listen to meditation coaches repeating 'affirmations' that help them to reprogramme their minds during sleep. It is said that the subconscious mind, when it is reprogrammed, can achieve wonders, and almost cause a switch in the person's consciousness. It is not far-fetched for me to say that my mind underwent its own subconscious switching; it didn't need me to plug in an earphone and pay a mindfulness coach for help. In one of my papers, I have suggested that 'perhaps the only difference between my schizophrenic mind and that of others is that I dream with my eyes open' (Valliappan, 2011). Therefore, the characters from my subconscious mind tend to mix with the characters and people in my real or everyday consciousness, and as a result I experience a confused reality.

Many artists tend to suffer periods of frustration and physical exhaustion, owing to having to be patient at many levels, and this is not only during the process of creating a drawing or painting. There are many different elements to juggle when painting. I need to be patient when I work with different materials. I have to try out different ideas and then feel inspired to produce an artwork. I decide whether to choose to paint for myself or for business. If I choose to do paintings for clients, I need to master the basics of marketing, accounting, design and so forth. The physical exhaustion caused by painting forces me to lie down and pass out into a deep sleep. My body and mind have to rest.

Painting did a lot more for me. It exhausted my body and mind, and then kick-started a process of self-healing and connection with others; it gave me a career to focus on, which benefitted my health. The financial investment in my art career cost as much as regular medical treatment would have cost. My mind created its own security. I developed the confidence to meet others, particularly those who are interested in my art, and this helped me to gain a better acceptance of myself. I realised that, if these people were interested in my art, they were interested in me.

---

3. Ashoka Fellows are social innovators who are recognised for their ability to transform communities, influence policies and law and create necessary change.

It took time for me to become disciplined with my art, because I am prone to laziness. Knowing that my art is a natural part of life and not merely a 'symptom' creeping in gave me some comfort. The process of building a career as an artist has taught me many things.

Knowing that there will be days or months where there won't be sales of my paintings means that I have to plan other sources of income. This has taught me to let go of a lot of self-talk within. It has taught me to learn to let go in life. Every painting that I create is like my own baby. It has a voice that made it. I have had to let go of each painting.

I found it difficult to deal with negative and critical comments that people made about my paintings. Often these comments were made by people who knew nothing about art. These negative comments were no different from the voices in my head. I had no choice but to hear the voices in my head. But I had a choice not to hear the voices of real people criticising my art. I simply needed to find out how and when to switch off. Eventually I came to notice that 80% of the voices inside my head were the voices of real people that remained in my subconscious. There were people in my head that I could not recognise, and that scared me, because no one told me such a thing was possible unless you had 'schizophrenia'.

As I painted, I would see visions of the person, which could be a specific situation or set of circumstances about them that haunted me. Telling the real person whom I connected to the vision was a waste of energy and time, because often people don't want to revisit their wrongdoings or the pain that they have caused, and sometimes the person isn't in your life any longer. This is the reality of life. Our traumas or pain stay on, even if the person isn't in our life any longer. We cannot force them to help us deal with the pain; we simply have to work with it alone. With music, I could consciously begin to work with my issues of past, present and future anxieties. Paintings that were created without music were different too. And hence, my art does not have just one style. My paintings might appear as works that are created by many different people, and not from a single person alone. The majority of artists can be spotted by their unique individual style that makes their works easily recognisable. But I paint from many different spaces.

Having established art as my career – as opposed to it just being a therapeutic process – I have to step out to buy supplies, visit framers, engage with buyers and get things done in order to make a living. There are days when I can't do these things, and I know that I will not have money for the next month. Learning to be okay with a loss of time is constantly challenging. This challenge is something that all artists face, and it is not related to my 'schizophrenia'. Every artist struggles with their own ups and downs, family issues and days when they don't paint and don't have work. I understood this once I interacted with other artists on social media platforms. When I saw that our occupational troubles were the same, I could move away from the position where I believed that everything was to do with my 'schizophrenia' or finding the voices too difficult to deal with. My voices change over time. When I spot someone on a social platform, I tell myself that I would like to get to know them better. My social anxiety stops me from making that attempt sometimes. But my self-talk has now turned into a voice repeating itself, 'Call him. Call her. Say hi. Just get to know them. Make friends. It is okay.'

When I was diagnosed with 'schizophrenia', there was nothing that helped. No one could show me the way. No one had any helpful advice to offer me. Would I get better? Would I be the same person? Would I look this bad with these horrible body issues? Would I ever have friends?

'Schizophrenia' happened and got in the way. 'Schizophrenia' forced me to choose differently. The voices formed to make me more aware of things. They've not been wrong. They gave me a beautiful tool for my journey and they still do. All I had to do was listen. Schizophrenia is 'the way'. My way.

Relapse isn't a 'thing' that happens. It is created. There is no escape to life, and there is no escaping relapsing. It is not actually relapsing, but about taking a step back, or sometimes two or more, to catch a glance at my painting and see if I have missed out on a stroke or a colour. I have to watch my painting from a distance and think it through. Does it need to be worked on or is it finished?

I paint because, if I hadn't, I would have had to fall back on those medications. Today I paint, because I know how to.

> *Learning point 3*
> - Why do you think that my art helps me?
> - How do you think my art helps me explore the voices in my paintings?
> - Does any activity help you to express yourself and step outside to connect with other people?

Reference

Valliappan, R. (2011). The art within madness. *Samyukta: A Journal of Women's Studies, IX(2)*, 66–83.

6 Voices: victim to victor
Ron Coleman

When I walked into my first hearing voices group some 30 years ago, little did I realise the effect that this group would have on the rest of my life. In this chapter I will explore the importance of self-help groups, structuring time, voice profiling, voice dialogue, understanding the personal narrative and the role of finding emotional innocence in the recovery process. I will use my own story as a means to explain each of them. The route that allows one to move beyond being a victim is not straightforward. My own recovery has had more twists and turns than any other event in my life.

Self-help

When I went into my first hearing voices group, I was greeted by a woman called Anne, who asked me 'if I heard voices'. I replied that I did, to which she simply said: 'They are real.' These three words have remained the cornerstone of my beliefs about recovery. Up until I heard them, I believed that I was powerless and could do nothing for myself, because my voices were hallucinations that I had no control over. If the voices were real, however, then I could do something about them. I no longer needed to wait for the magic pill that might cure me. I could start to do things for myself.

The first thing I decided to do was join the self-help group. I consider myself lucky that the Manchester group was truly about helping yourself. My teachers in the group were all going through the same struggle as I was. It was in the hearing voices group that I learned that it was possible to enter into conversations with my voices and to negotiate with them. It was in the group that I learned to have conversations with other people. I also began to have conversations with myself. Most importantly, it was in the group that I learned to be confident in the conversations that I was having.

The format of the group was simple. In the first hour we would take it in turns to say how our week had been. People often focused on their relationship with their voices. We then would have a cup of tea. In the second hour, we talked about our voices and how we managed them, with an emphasis on taking back power from the voices. We never talked about getting rid of the voices. We talked about living with our voices.

In the group I learned that I had to take responsibility for the things that were mine. As time went on, I also learned that meant taking responsibility not only for my actions but also for my emotions. I would argue that self-help groups are the foundation stones of recovery for voice hearers.

Structured time

It was in the group that I first heard about structuring time with my voices. The idea of having time that was essentially voice free was both exhilarating and frightening. Indeed, if truth be told, initially I did not believe it was possible. Some members of the group were already using this technique, and so, over coffee, I asked them to teach me. The way it works is as follows:

1. Start to have a conversation with your voices, one at a time at the outset (if you hear more than one). It is important to ask each voice its name, if you do not already know it.

2. If the voice gives you their name, you should always use it when addressing the voice. If the voice refuses to give you a name, then ask why. Or if you are working with someone, get them to ask the voice its name. If the voice still refuses to give an answer, then give the voice a name. Personally, I like the name 'no name', as I found that using it gave me greater power. I have noticed that the voices often don't like being given this name and will very soon give you their name, or at least what they want to be called in that moment.

3. Once you have given names to all of the voices that you hear,[1] move into a conversation about time-sharing, negotiating either collectively with all the voices or with one voice at a time. Explain your need to have your own space, but also acknowledge that the voices need to spend time with you. It is important that trust is built during these conversations. It took me a full year of trying this approach before my voices would leave me alone during the working day. If I broke my side of the bargain and didn't spend one hour every evening with the voices, then they would start to interfere in my daily life.

4. Start with small steps. I began with negotiating with the voices to go away for one minute, then two minutes, then four minutes, then eight minutes, and so on, until I reached my goal of not hearing the voices during the day.

As you can see, the structure belongs to you, not the voices. The fact that it belongs to you means that you get to know your voices better and better.

---

1. If a person hears hundreds of voices, work with the dominant voices, and ideally no more than six voices at a time.

> *Learning point 1*
> - Have you tried structuring time-sharing with your voice(s)?
> - Have you tried giving your voice(s) name(s)?

Voice profiles and the importance of story

As you get to know your voices, you begin to realise that they all have defining characteristics. In the early days of profiling, we would ask whether the voices were male or female, positive or negative, abusive or non-abusive, commanding or advisory. We also asked about what the voices said. As time went on, we learned to be more flexible and the profiles became much more varied and detailed. However, one question was especially significant: 'What age is the voice, and is it significant?' – because voice profiles cannot be understood without knowing their context, and the context is provided through the narrative (the story) that each voice has to tell. The following example will hopefully help you understand this important relationship between voice profile, voice story and voice impact. It also shows the ongoing need to be open to trying out new things and to learn from processes already tried out.

This story is true, although names and places have been changed to protect the person's identity. 'Jenny' has also given permission for her story to be shared.

Jenny's parents divorced when she was a child. She lived with her mother and had no contact with her father. Her mother met a new partner, whom Jenny liked initially. When her mother married him, Jenny found herself with a stepfather. Everything was good at the beginning, but it wasn't long before her stepfather began to take an interest in Jenny; not as a daughter, but as an object that he could abuse. This continued for about two years before Jenny told her grandmother what was happening. The grandmother told Jenny's mother, who refused to believe it. In frustration, the grandmother finally took Jenny to live with her. Her grandmother did not go to the authorities for fear that she too would lose Jenny, and Jenny did not fault her grandmother for this. Indeed, she felt her grandmother had done a good job in bringing her up. Jenny married when she was in her late teens and got divorced in her mid-20s. She had two children during the marriage. Her grandmother died when Jenny was 32, which left her feeling very alone, since she did not talk to her mother, who was still married to Jenny's abuser.

Jenny started hearing an occasional voice when she was in her late teens, but thought nothing of it. During the break-up of her marriage, her voices became much worse, and it was at this time that she came to the attention of psychiatric services. She ended up being given a diagnosis of paranoid schizophrenia and was put on various neuroleptics, none of which did anything to stop the voices.

Jenny was prone to self-harming and spent a lot of her hospital admissions detained on section. At the point where she joined our group, she had finally managed to bring her self-injury under control, although she had not stopped completely.

She found it helpful to join a self-help group. She identified four voices. The first was male, very negative, always abusive and commanding. This voice would tell her that everything was her fault, that she deserved everything that happened to her, and that she was a slut. This voice she knew was the voice of her stepfather. The second voice was a contrast to the first voice in every way: it was female, very positive, never hostile, and everything it said was soothing and helpful. This voice would tell Jenny that things would be okay, and that she (the voice) would protect her. Jenny knew this to be the voice of her grandmother. The third voice was the voice of a female child, who would do nothing but scream all the time. In some ways this was the most difficult voice for Jenny, in that the screaming never made any sense. It was only after some time that Jenny identified it as her own voice when she was being abused. The fourth voice was a male voice that was a mixture of everything. This voice was positive and negative, abusive and non-abusive, advisory and commanding. We called it her neutral voice, and she knew it to be the voice of her ex-husband.

Table 6.1: Jenny's voice profile

Gender	Positive/Negative	Abusive/Non-abusive	Commanding/Advisory	Known/Name	Content
Male	Negative	Abusive	Commanding	Abuser	Princess
Female	Positive	Non-abusive	Advisory	Grandmother	Be okay
Female child	Screamed	All	The	Time	
Male	Both	Both	Both	Both	All over the place

Once we had a life history and a voice profile, Jenny was able to relate the voices to her life experience, and she decided that her real problem was not actually the voices but the fact that she had been sexually abused and that this issue had never been properly resolved. The voice impact profile adds depth to the voice profile in Figure 6.1 by exploring the impact that the voices had in Jenny's life. This brings a richness that enhances the person's story. It also gives the person working with them a number of entry points for helping them to form their developing story. In my opinion, it also helps the client take control and lead the process much earlier.

Table 6.2: Jenny's voice impact profile

Gender	Relationship	Intensity	Influence	Name	Purpose/Function
Male	Negative	High	High	Abuser	Maintains Jenny's victim status

Female	Positive	Low	Medium	Grandmother	Creates security
Female child	Negative	High	High	Jenny as a child	Creates helplessness
Male	Both	Medium	Medium	Ex-husband	Creates confusion

So for example, when I first started working with Jenny, I encouraged her to confront the abuser, using voice dialogue. Later, however, having completed the voice impact profile, Jenny agreed to explore the purpose or function of the abusive voice. I asked her which had been more helpful.

Ron: In the voice impact profile, Jenny, you have identified the function of the first male voice as being to maintain your victim status. Can you explain to me what that means to you?

Jenny: Well, I guess what I am saying is that my victim persona was very much influenced by the intensity of my stepfather's role in my life, especially when I was younger and felt I had no control over his response to me. [Pause] Looking back, I would say that I was continually in victim mode.

Ron: I know that I am asking you to reflect on what happened many years ago, and that this might be distressing, so if you want to stop just say so.

Jenny: No, I'm okay about it.

Ron: That's great. When we worked together in the past, we started our voice dialoguing with the voice of the abuser and that caused a lot of distress for you. What if, instead of dialoguing with the abuser's voice, we were to explore its function – that is, the victim status that you identified? For example, you always talked about being a victim as if that is something that is your fault, and, like me, you had to work through this journey of emotional innocence in order to establish this victim status not as a negative about you but as being directly related to what had happened to you. What has always concerned me about that process for you was that, even after you went through the distress involved in finding yourself innocent, the voice of the abuser was still powerful and still retained the ability to impact on you through the child's response.

Jenny: Yes, getting rid of my victim status was done through massive pain, but it was worth it.

Ron: What if, instead of trying to talk with the abuser, we had explored your victim status. Do you think that would have made a difference to your level of distress?

Jenny: Honestly, Ron, I don't know for sure, but I think that this may have been a bit easier.

Although Jenny could not say for definite, it is my contention that using this approach would have been less stressful for her and may have reduced the amount of time that we worked together. It also shows that learning about voices and emotions is an ongoing process for all of us and that there are not always easy ways forward. In any case, Jenny did manage to find a way to recovery in no small part as a result of our work together, resulting in her managing to leave the mental health services.

Finding emotional innocence

Like Jenny, I was subjected to childhood sexual abuse and one of the voices that I heard was the voice of my abuser, who was a Catholic priest. The impact that this voice had on me was initially twofold: it was my dominant voice, but it also dominated my life, in that I felt powerless when the priest's voice was speaking to me (see Figure 6.1). Second, my response to this voice, which was to self-harm (see Figure 6.2), appeared to any onlooker who didn't know my story to be completely mad.

The biggest problem around self-harm and other behaviours, such as heavy alcohol or drug use, anger, non-engagement with workers or shouting at your voices, is that they are often seen by everyone, including the voice hearer themselves, as an indication that they (the voice hearer) are the problem. This is often the case when the person is a survivor of childhood sexual abuse and they blame themselves for what has happened. Indeed, my feeling of blame was so intense and my feeling of guilt so great that I often could do nothing. There came a point in my journey when I knew that I would have to deal with the voice of the priest or simply just give up and die. I needed to stop feeling guilty all of the time and rediscover my innocence.

In mental health, professionals often work with people at a very intellectual level. This can be found in work with survivors too. For example, when we are talking to someone who has been abused, they are likely to tell us it is their fault. We will probably say something like this: 'But you were only 10 when this happened, and the person who did it to you was an adult. Can you understand that you were in an impossible situation, and that the adult had all the power? Therefore, it cannot be your fault.'

When this was said to me, I replied: 'Yes, I can see what you're saying, but it is still my fault.' In other words, intellectually I could understand the argument, but my emotions still screamed at me that it was my fault. I came to the conclusion, therefore, that intellectual innocence is not enough when dealing with the guilt and shame that surround childhood sexual abuse (and, indeed, adult sexual abuse). What I needed was somehow to find emotional innocence. In order to do this, I first needed to understand how my guilt was constructed. Instinctively, I knew that guilt is not linear, and that it has many layers. I also knew that guilt is individual, and that everyone would have to identify their own layers of guilt.

Personally, I found three layers of guilt that together were keeping me in the position of victim. I called these three layers simple guilt, complex guilt and profound guilt. In order to find emotional innocence, I knew that I would have to explore and understand each layer.

> *Learning point 2*
> - Do you experience any feelings of guilt? Is this guilt linked to your voice-hearing experiences?
> - What are your strategies for coping with this guilt?

Simple guilt

My simple guilt was rooted in the voice of the Catholic priest. The voice would tell me that I had led him into sin, what happened was my fault and that I deserved to burn in hell. This became almost a mantra, and I would repeat it to myself. So, of course, I blamed myself. I would also respond by burning myself, which to any observers, including mental health workers, made me seem really mad – or, as the system called it, 'floridly psychotic'. I was often given a hard time by staff, who regarded my self-harm as a behaviour issue and treated me accordingly. In fact, instead of trying to manage the perceived problem of my 'self-harming behaviour', they should have been exploring how I viewed the problem.

My reality was very different from their perceptions. My method of self-harm had its basis in my religious beliefs as a Roman Catholic. I had been taught that when I died I would go to a place called Purgatory, where I would be cleansed by fire. I believed that the sins I had committed in making the priest sin were so bad that they needed to be cleansed while I was still alive, hence the burning. So, burning myself was a response to the guilt that I felt, which was in turn a response to what the priest had said. The real problem here was not my behaviour but the failure of workers to ask the right questions. If they had asked the right questions and had been able to connect my story with my behaviour and my emotions, the outcome might have been different. This did not happen, and I continued to believe that it was my fault. This guilt became my constant companion.

If this had been my only guilt, I believe that I could have worked through it very quickly. The difficulty was that this was just my first guilt.

Complex guilt

My second guilt (complex guilt) focused around my sexual orientation. I spent years wondering whether I was straight, gay or bisexual at a time when homophobia was much worse than it is today. This was in the 1960s and 1970s, when gay-bashing was seen as normal. For much of this time, I felt very alone, as I had no one to talk to about it. I couldn't really talk to my mates, who were all part of the same rugby team I played in. In those days, you would never talk to your parents about your sexuality, for fear of being rejected by your family. Therefore, I did not talk to anyone, and I became convinced that I was strange.

My behavioural response to this was to find ways to prove that I was a 'real man', and for many years I would tumble into bed with anyone, hoping that one day it would be the right person, and yet I would wake up the next morning feeling both guilty and ashamed. I failed to find the person I was looking for, and this ensured that the problems that I had around my sexual identity continued. I went round and round a cycle that went something like this: 'I do not know whether I'm straight, gay or bisexual. I believe I led the priest into sin. Therefore, I must be gay or bisexual.' In other words, my initial guilt fed on my second guilt, which then re-fed my first guilt, and so on. It is this cycle that creates the complexity. Just to complicate matters more, I was also dealing with the next layer of guilt, the profound guilt.

Profound guilt

Profound guilt is often the hidden guilt. The guilt is about something so disgusting, so foul, that it cannot normally be named. Indeed, many survivors call this guilt 'the secret'. For a long time, many people believed that the secret was the fact that we had been abused and we had not been able to disclose it. But, if this was the case, surely people would begin their recovery journeys once they had disclosed the abuse? Since this does not appear to happen, it is easily assumed that either the secret is not important or the abuse itself is not the secret. The latter is my truth. My secret was not the abuse; it was the knowledge held by an internal voice that I heard that would say things to me like, 'You are a pervert'. Despite what I said to people about my abuse, I had derived pleasure from my abuse, and this was why I kept going back to it time and time again. This internal voice has never been an external voice, yet it was probably as powerful as the priest's voice. It was the voice that ensured that I could not move from intellectual innocence to emotional innocence. It was the main reason that I did not talk about my abuse, because if I talked about my abuse, my sins (guilt) would be laid bare to the world.

I was 38 years old when someone finally gave me the answer to my guilt. The person I was seeing was a psychologist, and she told me that, if you are sexually stimulated, then you respond, whether you want to or not. It's a simple physiological fact. Honestly, at the age of 38, I did not know this, and I have since discovered that many other survivors do not know it. Once I had the information, I was able to deconstruct my abuse and finally find myself innocent.

In a note of caution, I would say that finding myself innocent came with a price, as I had to come to terms with the fact that I had spent more than 20 years of my life blaming myself for something for which I had no responsibility. I had also wasted more than 10 years of my life in psychiatric systems as the victim, yet in my moment of victory, I was in fact at my most vulnerable. If my abuser had been in the room, I most probably would have tried to kill him. The other thing that I thought about at that time was killing myself. I guess that what I am saying is that the moment of victory can be dangerous.

> ### *Learning point 3*
> - Have your voices changed over time?
> - What strategies do you have for coping with frightening voices?

Recently, my family started to notice that I was becoming forgetful. Eventually I went to see my doctor, who referred me to a memory clinic, after which I was given a label of minor cognitive disorder. This has since changed to a working diagnosis of Lewy body dementia (for more on this, see Chapter 21). I have started to develop my own programme for dealing with this. The voices I have heard for years have been joined by new voices, and also visual experiences, which can be positive or negative experiences. My years in the Hearing Voices Movement is once again serving me well, because even when I see things that are frightening or hear the new voices talk in a menacing way, I do not fear them; I know I can exist as a Victim or live as a Victor.

7 The things they say
Aimee Wilson

The hardest thing about hearing voices is attempting to make sense of the experience. How can anyone help you to cope with voices when you can't understand them yourself?

I remember feeling mind-numbing, overwhelming panic when I first heard a voice. I'd been told horror stories about how people who heard voices were 'crazy' or 'mental' and were locked away in the local psychiatric hospital, where they'd be given electric-shock treatment. So, that's how I felt when I was leaving work one day and, all of a sudden, I heard a strange male voice telling me that I was useless and should kill myself. I'd never heard his voice before, but for some reason it felt like I'd known him all my life. He didn't sound like anyone I knew, and he wasn't saying anything that people had said before, yet it was almost as though he was saying the things that I thought about myself. When he called me 'useless' and told me that I deserved to die because all the bad things in my life had been my fault, I wondered whether he was echoing my deepest, darkest thoughts.

It is almost impossible to find any kind of comfort when, the moment you hear voices, you're immediately facing your first dilemma: do you tell someone about it?

When I made my first suicide attempt, two years after the abuse, no one knew what had happened to me or that I was hearing voices. So, when the psychiatrist and social workers assessed me in A&E, they were baffled as to what could have motivated me to swallow so many tablets. There was no history of depression and nothing seemed to have triggered it. I was detained under Section 2 of the Mental Health Act and admitted to psychiatric hospital, where for the first time I met other people who heard voices too. I wasn't the only person in the world to be experiencing this! I wasn't alone. But with this realisation came the worry that, 'Yes, other people can hear voices, but they are all in hospital, so they must be mentally ill. Does this mean I am crazy?' I didn't know then that people could experience voices in different ways, and that their voices could mean something different to each person. I thought that it meant that I would never leave the hospital. I was so terrified about telling a professional that, when I finally did, I was surprised to be asked if the voice had a name, as though it were 'normal'. I didn't consider that, for mental health professionals, finding out that someone is hearing voices is probably a daily occurrence.

> *Learning point 1*
> - Have you been asked about what voices you hear?
> - Did it help to share your experience of hearing voices with a mental health professional?

During those first few years of hearing voices, the only silence that I managed to get was when I did what the voices were commanding me to do. They'd tell me to self-harm or to engage in other dangerous behaviour, and because they were in my head, there was literally no escape. I couldn't just go into another room or take a walk. The voices were everywhere. It took me a few years to be able to describe how I heard the voices, because professionals would always ask if they sounded to me like people talking to me ordinarily, like them. I couldn't find a way to convey my experience to anyone else. The best I could come up with was to tell them that hearing voices was like listening to music through headphones – the sound goes in through your ears, but seems to fill up your entire head. So, if silencing the voices meant self-harming or attempting suicide, then I was prepared to do it in order to have a few moments of peace and quiet.

When I did self-harm or take an overdose, professionals would be confused. They labelled me as being an 'attention-seeker' for doing these things and then seeking help. I had to learn to explain that I was doing what the voices were telling me to do, so that the voices would stop., I didn't want to hurt myself, and I didn't want to die. Learning to explain this to people who had – most likely – never heard voices like mine was incredibly hard. I could barely understand what was happening myself, so I found it really exhausting to try to explain it to others. It was so frustrating to see my behaviours affect others, yet I was unable to explain the reasoning behind my actions. I believed that each of the voices I could hear had their own personality, and my behaviour and attitude reflected this. If the angriest voice was the loudest, then I was furious. If the childish voice was loud, then I was playful and energetic. If the sly voice was taking over my head, then I could be secretive and untrustworthy.

> *Learning point 2*
> - Have you ever self-harmed? Did you self-harm in response to hearing voices?
> - How did mental health professionals react when they found out that you had self-harmed?

Explaining my behavioural responses to the voices was made harder by the fact that the usual response when I talked about them was silence or concern. People are generally scared of things that they don't understand, so they make assumptions, and they use these as a foundation on which to build a stigmatised view of the voice hearer. I found that the police (on the whole) assumed that someone who hears voices should be sectioned under the Mental Health Act and hospitalised; they are frightened by it. Unfortunately, the media's portrayal of voice hearers is often that they are violent, aggressive and unhinged. They sensationalise it to get more readers. They seem to believe that no one wants to hear about a person who is living and functioning who hears voices. Through my blog,[1] however, I've discovered that there's actually an interest out there to learn more about the lives of voice hearers, and an eagerness to understand the experience. Maybe it's because people are curious. Certainly, the constant barrage of tweets, posts, photos, statuses and check-ins on social media suggest we should put our life out there for the world to see. There is, I think, a keen eagerness to learn more.

It took me a few years to learn where my voices come from, and even longer to understand why they were there. While the mental health professionals were clear with me that I didn't have some sort of psychosis or schizophrenia, they also didn't explain exactly what my diagnosis of borderline personality disorder meant in terms of hearing voices. As I am quite an anxious and easily scared person, it was terrifying to have something inside of me that I didn't understand, and I worried that the reason no one was explaining it to me was because they didn't understand it either. I felt completely alone: not only was I the only person hearing these voices, but no one could make sense of them either. At that point, I was too mentally unwell to find the ability to understand them myself, and I wanted to be told what they meant. I finally began to understand more when I started dialectical behaviour therapy and trauma therapy, which explained to me about how I had sub-consciously split myself into different parts, and that these parts were the voices talking to me, as though they were separate beings.

Learning point 3
- Do you think other people understand voice hearing?
- What do you think is the most common image among the public and in the media of someone who hears voices?

I found it hard to understand how I had different 'parts'. I had always wondered why I found it hard to remember anything from my childhood and early teens, until a psychologist explained that I had separated my life into two sections: 'before the abuse' and 'after the abuse' that I had suffered when I was 15. I could comprehend this. It was difficult to understand because, obviously, the decision to split my life

---

1. www.imnotdisordered.co.uk

into these two different parts had not been a conscious one, but, at the same time, I knew why my mind or body would make such a decision. My mind was trying to protect itself from becoming overwhelmed by memories; whether they were 'good' or 'bad', they were still memories of my early birthdays, Christmases, trips to the park, moving house, learning to read and write and so on. To remember all of that, as well as the abuse, was just too much. It felt as if my mind was a bowl and someone was filling it with water until it spilled over the sides. I came to understand my voices as being separate pieces of myself. Each of the three voices I heard had a different personality and a different attitude to life. There was Albert, who was always angry, Annie, who was sly, and Henry, who was childish.

When the abuse physically ended, I was left with a lot of emotions; in particular, I was overwhelmed by uncontrollable anger. It felt as though I was angry with everyone and everything, where there was no limit to the anger. The anger was just there all of the time, and there was nothing I could do about it. Annie's personality felt so much a part of me that I really struggled to accept it, because Annie was so manipulative and sneaky and I didn't want to acknowledge that I had that in me. I think there comes a time, though, in everyone's life where we finally learn about the parts of us that we have denied and parts that we have felt ashamed or guilty about, knowing that they were there.

Henry's childishness seemed to make much more sense, as I connected this to the abuse. I lost a lot of childhood memories when I separated my life into the two parts. It made sense that there was a part of me who still wanted to indulge in the childish ways that Henry seemed so fond of.

I think that a big misconception around voices – and it's definitely one that I held – is that a person has to have a psychiatric diagnosis like psychosis or schizophrenia to experience them. In fact, voices can be manifestations of lots of different things, and the sooner we recognise this, the sooner we can move forward in understanding them and getting rid of the stigma that surrounds them.

8   Journey to recovery
Clifford O'Connor

On my journey to recovery, caring support was necessary. It takes a special type of person, one who is wise, caring and compassionate, to decode emotional distress. It isn't always obvious where to find these people. The private mental health hospital that I visited assessed my funds as insufficient for their treatment plan. It was an unexpected and expensive assessment of my situation. I visited a hypnotherapist, who diverted blood to my feet to prove that hypnotherapy works, before transforming my childhood emotions with timeline therapy. Elsewhere, I was asked to put on a skullcap with electrodes and was reassured that my brain was functioning normally. I even had pins stuck into me to relieve my stress. I read many self-help books and then decided that I needed to face my anxiety with a 'flooding technique'. So, I immersed myself in fear. Eventually, I received effective support from NHS clinical psychotherapy, both for my presenting problems and later for handling the voices that I went on to hear.

Initially, 'voice hearing' was a distressing experience. Sometimes, it still is. I viewed my new, additional, internal voice as hostile, invisible, powerful and external. I didn't recognise the voice as being part of me. It was saying things that I would never normally say, in a voice that was completely different to mine. Its tone was unpleasant, and the voice had an intense energy to it. It said things that made me uncomfortable.

So, the Maastricht Interview (see Chapter 1), implemented by a caring clinical psychotherapist, was incredibly useful, because it left me feeling empowered. The therapist created a vague construct for my medical file, because we were both new to the process. I realised that my invisible enemy could be faced, described and made visible. It took ages to develop a useful working description of the voice. The most important step was to identify a single voice that kept saying 'We think...' By claiming to be plural, the voice seemed more powerful. Accepting ownership of that voice was also important. It stopped me from blaming external sources.

I was surprised when my therapist suggested joining a self-help support group to further the progress we were making. This was a group of voice hearers who were all anxious like me. We were all gathered together to discuss or listen to our unusual experiences. It was the last place that I expected to find answers. I was no longer confident in group settings, even when I attended relaxed social meetings. The small-group setting made me realise that I wasn't alone with these experiences.

Attending weekly group meetings helped me to recover my confidence. Hearing myself talking to the small group was important, because I reconnected with my natural voice. It became a break from listening to my hostile voice.

After learning techniques for managing my voice, I became ready to accept ownership of it. I discovered that the voice was connected with my thinking. Just by thinking (internally), I could change the words being spoken (the content). I also learnt to call up my natural voice with a meditation technique. I learnt that, if I accepted and cared for a hostile voice, it became more tolerable.

Sharing and applying knowledge gained by experience captures the spirit of the international peer support movement. It is a movement that is inspirational and valuable to people who perceive difficult thoughts or emotions via voices. Together we can dare to warn of pitfalls, like dangerous medications, and expertly support and guide each other towards useful recovery strategies. I have benefitted from peer support, and I remain grateful to the professionals who facilitated my recovery.

It wasn't long before I was co-chairing these meetings. I grew in confidence, as I was able to explore the mysteries of adversity alongside brave, caring, compassionate voice hearers who provided role models for survival. Everyone was treated as equals, and we took turns to politely listen to each person (if they wanted to speak). Even people's voices were welcome to express themselves. Together we grew in confidence, and, when the group seemed too small, I reminded everyone of the larger national and international network of peer support that was available.

It was a great privilege both to learn about how to cope with voices and to facilitate and chair the group to the benefit of others. But I also needed to learn how to make sure that some of the issues that group members brought to the group would not be burdening me unduly. I also found that I wanted to have a space where I could explore this experience of hearing voices even further – beyond the initial drive to learn how to cope with them.

Learning point 1

- Are you alone with your experience, or do you benefit from having support?
- Some people find meaning in their voices when they consider them in the context of their lives and consequently make good use of these insights to improve on how they go about living their lives. What do you think about that?

- Have you explored the meaning(s) of your voice(s)? If you have, did this include the possibility of thinking about a possible metaphorical or symbolic meaning, which some people find helpful?
- Have you considered whether there may be other issues in your life that need resolving that may have preceded you experiencing voices? Have you had helpful support for these issues or found your own ways?
- Are there any problems that hinder your progress? What are you going to do about any of those identified hindrances?

Avoiding pitfalls

If you want to come out of an ongoing negative cycle of being on medication, then it may be helpful for you to know that not everyone believes that medications are effective (in fact, I have never met anyone who felt them to be very effective at all), and some even contend that they are known to maintain discomfort, or may even cause harm, such as sudden unexplained death or indiscriminate effects on the brain (Breggin & Cohen, 2007; Moncrieff, 2020; see also your medication leaflet). If you feel you want to know more about the pros and cons of medication, you may want to read more about it in Chapter 15 in this book.

I personally escaped the medication horror by gradually reducing my prescribed dose. From speaking to other people, I do understand that this needs to be done very carefully and slowly (Breggin & Cohen, 2007; Timimi, 2021). Then, I managed without psychiatric support. Peter Breggin and David Cohen's book (2007) *Your Drug May Be Your Problem* was a useful source of encouragement. Psychiatrists and researchers debate the value of medication, but the side effects can have a negative impact on the voice hearer.

Alternative patient-empowering approaches are safer and make more sense to me. I took back responsibility for managing my mental health. Medication became my metaphor for disruptive external influences.

Many people wrongly assume that mental health difficulties are the result of alcohol or drug abuse, but in my experience that is seldom the case. That said, I know of one patient who masked his difficulties with alcohol because he preferred to be thought of as an alcoholic rather than mentally ill. People have used alcohol to try to suppress the voices, but this method just creates secondary problems and side effects that are similar to some of the difficulties caused by prescribed medications. These methods of coping may contribute to the stigma around hearing voices.

Learning point 2
- Assess the effects of engaging with professionals. Do they champion recovery or hopelessness?

- Explore who is responsible for your health once you seek outside assistance. Why is it that, when a patient has had 'a long history of mental illness', it is the patient who is seen as having failed, not the professionals? Explore the pros and cons of assistance and the points of interest. For example, pro – professionals are expected to be ethical and have successful outcomes; con – they may not have much time for you or may be feeling overwhelmed by their workload. Their language may be beyond comprehension.
- Draw out positive aspects of your brief encounters – the ones that you can benefit from. Identify pitfalls and hindrances. Hopefully you'll feel more in control and able to usefully assess the service you are getting. Professional relationships can be challenging. Hopefully your assessment will highlight more benefits than issues.

Accepting ownership

It is important to recognise that stress-induced voice hearing can be a coping response for complex experiences such as physical or emotional trauma, which may also express itself physically, psychologically and emotionally. Voice hearing may indicate that there are ongoing unresolved difficulties. For that reason, some survivors of mental distress worry about eliminating the voice-hearing safety valve. Let us assume that the voices have developed for a good reason.

Even so, I needed to exert some control. Hearing voices is unbearable otherwise. With a sense of control, it became easier to suppose that my voices might be understood. When you can tune in or out at will, it becomes possible to explore the voices and understand them, and perhaps to stop hearing them altogether, by making them redundant.

I realised that medical treatment wasn't going to improve my experience of my voices. So, I looked for alternatives. I found it very helpful to regularly listen to pleasant and calmly expressed talks, for example in the form of podcasts by various people on topics such as compassion and meditating. This was helpful in terms of both the useful and soothing content and also the calm and caring tone of the voice. I felt that I could tune into an external friendly voice and ignore the internal undermining voice. Some boring talks even helped me fall asleep. I recaptured responsibility for my sleep patterns, and later for my thinking, speech and behaviour.

The importance of managing my mood slowly dawned on me. I read a book edited by the psychiatrist Marius Romme and colleagues (2009), *Living With Voices: 50 stories of recovery*, which included descriptions of how other voice hearers recovered. It was inspiring. Other stories left me feeling sad.

When I was at my lowest, I was being encouraged to end my own life by a voice that I heard as if through a speaker in the wall. At that point, I found what helped me not follow through was focusing on a simple, genuine, friendly smile on a book cover of a calm and internationally well-known spiritual figure – the Dalai Lama (2000). Suddenly the book, and the person's relaxed posture, made perfect sense. Learning about numerous meditations and teachings also really helped. I learned over time that undermining voices are very common. But, with courage, these voices can be regarded with compassion, and that this can help disarm them.

Tailored meditations form the foundations for many coping practices. Constant repetition of a simple phrase or word – a mantra – can also help. I sometimes use the word 'me'. Me-me-me-me-me-me-me-me. It might seem self-centred, but it helps me to connect with my normal internal voice. Another technique is speaking or singing out loud.

'Disco' is a technique that I developed to control the words a voice can say. If I'm tired of the voice being nasty, then I have learned how to get this voice to actually say the lyrics of a song called 'Disco' in my head. The words are very affirming and delightful. The voice then sings the words to that song. I feel it would even be possible to get the voice to read affirmations or sing my praises. This technique can even enhance the content of what the voice says. It is empowering to have control of what the voices say as, for that to work, I believe the voice must be an extension of my thinking and not external. I now think of voice hearing as communication with and the manifestation of my subconscious.

'Make an appointment with the voices' was a technique suggested by my therapist. I choose a time and a place when it is acceptable for the subconscious to have its say. During this time, I tune in to what the voice is saying and pay attention to it. At other times, I gently remind the voice to wait for the appointed time. My voice respects the boundaries when I assert them and I can enforce these boundaries by techniques such as concentrating on a painting tutorial, listening to a podcast, and so forth. This routine has made my life much easier. I can work all day uninterrupted and then tune in (at appointed times) when I'm ready to explore the voice.

'Mindfulness' is popular in psychology as a starting point for identifying emotions and feelings and labelling them. I use it to focus attention on my voice. I find that, if a voice is constantly ignored when it has something to say, it will get more difficult to manage. If I tune in regularly to the voice, it behaves more reasonably. I have learnt to witness what is being said rather than react to it. Very often voices use metaphorical language. It is a mistake to take the voices' message literally. This mistake is regularly made by professionals and other people. That is why it is difficult to talk about the experience.

Not taking everything literally but learning to 'translate' or 'interpret' a voice was something that I found particularly helpful. Fortunately, it was something that I am used to from other areas of my life, as I have a limited working knowledge of German – I had relatives in Germany and was often asked to translate a conversation for people who couldn't follow it. In the same way, I learned that voices could also be interpreted. I was listening to a hostile nasty voice, and I didn't understand the underlying metaphor or what it represented. So, I 'interpreted' what the voice was saying into the opposite meaning. Instantly this transformed the message and our relationship. Translation is necessary if the voice content is unpleasant. It can sometimes be interesting working out the opposite of what the voice is saying.

The number of voices we hear is also significant. If we remember that voices tend to be messengers, or signals, of emotional questions that need to be addressed in one's life, then it also makes sense that passively relying exclusively on medication might even increase the number of voices people hear. This is the same as what happens when a person develops a migraine or a headache because they have got too much stress going on in their lives; simply taking a painkiller is not really the answer. Until the person changes what is causing their stress levels, they will continue to have physical difficulties, such as a headache. Simply continuing to take a painkiller may even be quite harmful in the medium and long run. It also does not help with learning better management of the stress situation.

Certainly, based on my own experience of reflecting and from speaking to other voice hearers, it does seem to be the case that an over-reliance on medication is more likely to increase the difficulty people have with their voices and possibly even the number of voices. This makes sense to me because the problems just keep stacking up and don't get understood or resolved. I have a natural internal thinking voice and a link to my subconscious via the additional voice. If any other voices appear, then I consider them to be just my additional voice acting out a different role. This balances the numbers equally. Taking such a stance helps me to avoid feeling overwhelmed by the experience. I feel very fortunate that I learned about other ways of approaching the voice-hearing experience, other than passively relating to them, very early on in my experience. I feel that allowed me to address things earlier in my life than I might have otherwise.

Finally, I also learned from a fellow voice hearer the helpful use of doodles. She suggested drawing a circle. Imagine that is you. Now draw the voice(s). We tried the technique in a peer support session. We mapped my voice experience in simple circle doodles. I drew two circles. One was almost filled with an internal circle nearly as large as itself. The second had a smaller circle inside it. When the internal circle is large, the voice is taking up too much time and attention. When the internal circle is small, the voice is a minor factor in my life. This is a helpful way to measure the intensity of my experience. I also realised that 'time' was an issue (recovering quickly). There is no stigma or embarrassment in displaying a seemingly random doodle of circles. I was amazed at the variety of doodles that were displayed in the group. The exercise was more useful than the more usual approach of selecting which boxes to tick on a form. It was more personal and acceptable to share.

For many years, I worked part-time as a peer support worker for the NHS. I have supported many emotionally disturbed people and have helped professionals guide patients towards finding peace. I received good reviews for my work with the NHS, and I am grateful for that. I also learned how life enriching hearing voices can be when managed effectively.

Learning point 3

- Can you accept ownership and responsibility for managing your voice(s)?
- What coping strategies could you develop?
- Why might compassionately acknowledging a voice be better than suppressing it?
- If you draw a circle that represents you, then how big within that circle would your voice(s) be?
- Can you see past the literal content of the voice(s) and work out the meaning of the voice(s)?
- What do you think a voice might represent?

References

Breggin, P.R. & Cohen, D. (2007). *Your drug may be your problem: How and why to stop taking psychiatric medications.* Da Capo Press

Dalai Lama. (2000). *The Dalai Lama's book of transformation.* Harper Collins.

Moncrieff, J. (2020). *A straight talking introduction to psychiatric drugs* (2nd ed.). PCCS Books.

Romme, M., Escher, S., Dillon J., Corstens, D. & Morris, M. (2009). *Living with voices: 50 stories of recovery.* PCCS Books.

Timimi, S. (2021). *A straight talking introduction to children's mental health problems* (2nd ed.). PCCS Books.

9 Hearing voices in grief
Jacqueline Hayes

I wasn't very surprised when I heard my mum speak to me after she died. I heard her a lot when she was alive! By that, I mean in every sense of hearing – including hearing her call me to her when she needed something and we were in separate cities. Vygotsky noticed how infants use the speech of their caregivers to regulate their actions: first as 'private speech' – the things that toddlers say to themselves; then internalised as 'inner speech'. He offered a direct theory of how interaction that is shared becomes thought that is private (Vygotsky, 1934/1987).

There are other early theorists that I imagine would not have been too surprised either. The American sociologist George Herbert Mead thought that we respond to ourselves through an internalised, 'generalised other' (Mead, 1934). For the British psychoanalyst Donald Winnicott, we are born out of our interactions with others (Winnicott, 1971). Influenced by the early relational psychoanalysts and scholars like Mead, Carl Rogers, who developed the person-centred approach to counselling, theorised that our self-concepts are moulded by the regard of others (Rogers, 1959).

This chapter introduces the reader to voice hearing in the context of the death of a significant other. It is based on my learnings as a researcher, psychotherapist and someone who hears voices. In the words that follow, I use 'in grief' and 'in bereavement' interchangeably to refer to the fact of someone's actual, physical death and its aftermath for the surviving person (which may continue for months, years or an entire lifetime). However, it is just as relevant to talk of grief and loss in other circumstances – the end of a relationship, the loss of a community through the impact of government austerity measures, the grief of an infant whose needs are not being met by caregivers – and many other voices may, of course, relate to these and other kinds of grief.

Voice hearing in grief

There is very little writing that is exclusively about voice hearing in grief.[1] Instead, these experiences tend to be studied as part of a group of phenomena that often happen to grieving people, such as visions, smells, touch and 'feelings' of the presence of the deceased person. These are sometimes referred to as hallucinations, but often by other terms such as a 'sense of presence' (Steffen & Coyle, 2011) or 'post-death encounters' (Troyer, 2014).

In my research, I have called them 'experiences of continued presence' – a bit clunky, I admit, but my aim is a deliberate distancing from the assumptions involved in the term 'hallucination' (i.e. that it is a false perception) and to emphasise instead the experiential qualities reported by the bereaved. I have wanted to leave open assumptions about causality, as I respect both spiritual and non-spiritual frames of reference.

Survey research suggests that experiencing continued presence is very common. Estimates range between 30% and 60% of the bereaved (Castelnovo et al., 2015), in mostly European samples. Hearing voices in grief occurs somewhere in the range of 9% to 30%, depending on which study you look at (Kamp et al., 2020). That is really a lot of people, if you think that everyone at some point in their life will experience bereavement. One of the things that I have examined (Hayes, 2011; Hayes & Leudar, 2016) is what this experience is like. I found huge variation in the language used by the voices. Consider the following examples:[2]

> 'You're a loser, don't even bother carrying on.' (Matt)
>
> 'It's alright dear, it's me.' (Esme)
>
> 'I love you.' (Inge)

Even without the context attached to hearing these words, we can already see that there is a wide range of meaning – from the insult that Matt hears to the declaration of love heard by Inge. We can already make some sense of these examples, even before we know who it is that is speaking or what the situation is. Taking this a step further, using the example of Inge:

Inge: I will tell him about, everything that's going on and the only thing, we had a thing we used to say to each other, like, I will say 'I love you' and he would say 'I love you' and I would say, 'Will we be together forever?' and he would say, 'Yes' and I would say 'Do you promise?' and he would say 'Yes'… that's the only thing he still says back. He says that still.

We now understand that Inge hears this voice as part of a conversation with her loved one. She initiates it and the voice answers her, just as the person did when

---

1. See Hayes, 2011, chapters 4 and 5, as an exception to this rule.
2. All names used in this chapter are pseudonyms.

he was living. Equipped with more details of her life story and relationship history, we can then understand that the voice is that of her late boyfriend, whose death at a tragically young age in an accident while abroad plunged Inge into a fierce and all-consuming grief. The voice, when it happens now, is not simply good or bad; it is bittersweet, bringing into focus all of this: the love, the cruel and abrupt loss of their 'forever', his presence, his gaping absence.

Many voices in grief are of this ambivalent nature, although some are also straightforwardly helpful, in the same way that many other voices are. I found examples of voices helping the bereaved with practical problems they were facing by giving them instructions or information when they needed it (Hayes & Leudar, 2016). Some of this help, however, was focused on the relationship to the deceased itself.

Unfinished business

There are times when hearing a voice helps someone to resolve a conflict or resentment between themselves and the deceased. Aggie, for example, whose boyfriend had also died at a very young age, heard his voice after his death apologising to her for breaking up with her in the six months before he died. They had been reconciled shortly before his death, but had not discussed the problems that had happened between them. Hearing his voice since helped her cross a gulf in her understanding of their relationship, allowing her to soothe a ferocious combination of pain, anger, guilt and confusion.

Other voices I came across (Hayes, 2011; Hayes & Leudar, 2016; Hayes & Steffen, 2018) highlighted family conflicts or secrets, but without always offering resolution. Julie's story illustrates this. She began hearing her mother's voice shortly after her death. At first, it called her name; not her preferred name, but the name she was known by in the family. The voice then began to insult her, calling her denigrating, sexist terms like 'slag' and saying destructive things ('Take all your tablets'). Julie revealed that, as an adult, she had discovered a family secret that had dominated the atmosphere of her childhood: her father had been having a relationship with another woman and, on top of that, had named Julie after this lover. The ongoing infidelity, and the meaning of her name, had never been openly discussed in the family, remaining a shameful secret. Julie had attempted to distance herself from this by taking a different variation of her full name, but the voice continued to use the name she rejected. By using the name alongside the insults, the voice functioned to continue to identify her with her mother's rival and the threat to the family structure. Julie said that, although her mother, when alive, had never spoken to her with such violence and hostility, she nevertheless had felt continually rejected by her throughout her life. This was an unspoken undercurrent to the relationship, exacerbated by the position of her older brother as 'the favourite' (see Hayes, 2011, Chapter 4).

Hearing a voice in grief, for Julie, magnified the rejection she felt from her mother, crystallising it in abusive words – words that Julie felt continually distracted by and trampled on by. This is just one example of how hearing voices in grief can highlight important unfinished business with the deceased, even, as with voices in non-grief circumstances, if it does not always offer an immediately obvious way to resolve it.

> ### Learning point 1
>
> The qualities of the voices heard in grief usually fit the relationship in the past when the deceased was alive. A kind and helpful grandmother will continue to help, a boyfriend will continue to show his love, and a critical parent will continue to undermine. The most challenging voices in grief can sometimes continue and magnify the painful elements of the relationship with the deceased.
>
> Have you heard the voice of someone who has died? If so:
>
> - What was it that you heard them say?
> - What kind of effect did this have on you, both at the time, and looking back now?

Sources of distress

Many, perhaps most of the voices heard in grief are not distressing. There are, however, as Julie's story illustrates, times when the experience can be incredibly challenging. In research (e.g. Hayes & Leudar, 2016; Hayes & Steffen, 2018; Sabucedo et al., 2021), we have tried to identify some of the sources of distress. One of the most important is when a voice is continuing the most oppressive and hostile elements of a relationship.

A second source relates to the here-and-now situation in which the voice is heard. Does the voice facilitate the hearer to achieve a task or distract them and undermine what they are engaged in? For example, a person may hear a voice while at work that affects their concentration in a meeting and becomes an untimely reminder of pain.[3] A feeling of absence that is sometimes felt most fiercely at times when there is a presence of the deceased can be another source of difficulty, especially when the bereaved person feels ill equipped to cope with such raw grief (Hayes & Leudar, 2016).

However, sometimes hearing a voice in grief can have helpful immediate consequences and be a source of comfort, yet become an anxiety when the hearer considers how others may view this. Such worries are reported time and time again in research, and it is to this taboo that we now turn.

---

3. Feelings of grief are rarely convenient in their timing.

> ### Learning point 2
> Sources of distress may be when a voice in grief continues difficult aspects of the relationship with the person who has died, interferes with action rather than facilitating it, foregrounds the absence of the deceased and the bereaved person cannot cope with the grief at this time, or is viewed in terms of societal taboo.
>
> - If you have heard a voice of someone who has died have you told anyone about this? If you were to tell someone, what kind of a response would you want?
> - If you have not heard such a voice, thinking over the last month or so, have you spoken to another person about a relationship difficulty or a secret? What, if anything, helped you in the way they responded to you? Was there anything that led you to feel more ashamed or isolated?

Mourning, voices and taboo

Hearing voices is a stigmatised experience in our society. So too is grief. Darian Leader has drawn attention to the erosion in industrialised societies of the rituals that make grief public. Instead, the experience is often forced inwards, and underground (Leader, 2008). This impoverishment of public space for grief is even more pronounced as I write during the Covid-19 pandemic – a period of social distancing, when many bereaved people are unable even to gather for a funeral, which is one of the few rituals around death that survive in UK society.

Coupled with this, I believe we are currently suffering a crisis of emotional differentiation. By this, I mean that the complexity of our emotional lives very often becomes reduced to polar positives and negatives. We make sense of ourselves and each other within a context, and part of our current context is a culture of constant evaluation. We buy something online and are asked to rate the buying experience, and then to rate what we have bought before we have even used it. Schools, teachers and five-year-old pupils are rated. Therapies are rated. Some therapies ask us to identify goals for the therapy when we might be highly confused about our lives and our direction, or to identify and measure the extent of our 'negative' thoughts and beliefs. I'm not saying all of this is dysfunctional, or not pragmatic, or does not sometimes redress power imbalances, if used with care. I found it quite useful to see ratings when I was choosing a vacuum cleaner, and often wonder why tenants are not asked to rate landlords. But what I have noticed is that, within this evaluative culture, when it is over-extended to encompass our personal experiences and relationships with others, it does not help us to tolerate discomfort and notice ambivalence.

In everyday speech, thoughts and feelings are often spoken of as positive or negative, ironing out their varied functions in different contexts. For example, anger, often described as 'negative', particularly in women, can be very functional if we are using it to protect ourselves from danger or harm. You may wonder why I say this here: the reason is, grief and culture intersect. When it comes to grieving,[4] there is often a pressure to 'focus on the positive', 'remember the good times', and 'not to speak ill of the dead', so any ambivalence that might be felt towards the deceased gets pushed away and repressed. This is especially the case when a person thinks of themselves too rigidly as a 'positive person' and doesn't allow emotions they consider 'negative' to enter their awareness. Where, though, do all of these feelings and experiences go when there is a collective denial of them? How can we mourn (as we will all need to, even if those who are 'lucky' enough will not do this until later in their lives) when we blunt so many of our feelings and regard them as unpalatable for ourselves and others? What happens when there isn't a language for the changing presence and absence of the deepest connections, within and without us? Where do these truths become voiced?

For those experiencing challenging voices in grief, there is a compound stigma operating, with the potential to trap us in an isolated misery. The most consistent finding in research about experiencing presence is the privacy of the experience – and this privacy is deliberate. Rees' (1971) influential survey of widows in the Welsh countryside found that 72% had never disclosed their experiences to anyone else, for fear of being judged, ridiculed or ignored. The bereaved have mentioned this since in several studies (Grimby, 1993; Hayes, 2011; Steffen & Coyle, 2011). Very recently, Pablo Sabucedo surveyed therapy practitioners in the UK and Spain about working psychotherapeutically with unwanted and ambivalent presences of the deceased (Sabucedo et al., 2021), and 48% of them mentioned, without any prompting, that societal stigma contributes to the distress of their patients/clients. The bereaved voice hearer becomes afraid of how others might view them if they disclose their experience, and this contributes to their suffering.

Working with the healing potential

Given what research tells us about the ingredients of distress (see learning point 2), when hearing a voice in grief, societal as well as individual remedies are required. But what can a counsellor do to help someone who is challenged by the voice they are hearing in grief?

One path is to explore the meaning for the voice hearer of their previous relationship with the deceased. The bereaved's feelings are very likely to be complex and fraught with ambivalence (for example, a mix of loss and relief, or pining for the person and feeling rage towards them simultaneously), and therapy may

---

4. Climate grief is a good example of this. We are shown overwhelmingly by the scientific community that we are damaging our planet, but the loss and anger this generates are constantly repressed in most of us, and so cannot be used to fuel action and change.

involve focusing on any significant unfinished business that is burdening them. Regarding these voices in grief as portals into formative relational realities allows the possibility for release of important learning and growth.

If a client is unwilling or unable to explore the past relationship at a moment in time, then another route may be to try to change the response to the deceased in the here-and-now. For example, if a person hears undermining comments, what do they think of them, and what would they like to say back? They may never before have been invited or able to explore this, because the previous dynamic between the bereaved and the deceased has become cemented.[5]

These kinds of conversations may well occur naturally in the course of an empathic and holding therapeutic process, and are best done at the pace and level of tolerance of a client (Hayes & Steffen, 2018). However, there are particular techniques that may also be useful for facilitating this dialogue, such as the 'empty chair' method in Gestalt and emotion-focused therapies (see Elliott et al., 2004), writing letters to the deceased, and making pieces of art about the relationship, such as photography or a cartoon. If group support is available, a psychodrama or sociodrama could be created. It is best to be cautious, however, with the more vivid and structured techniques, as some clients may find bringing the deceased 'back to life' in this way too distressing or frightening at that time. It is important too to remember that, in practice, much may be achieved without bringing the unwanted voice centre-stage. The simple need to talk through the various emotions and experiences involved in the grieving and voice-hearing process with an interested and accepting listener is all too frequently unmet.[6]

Learning point 3

If you are being challenged by hearing the voice of a deceased person, you could consider the following questions:

- What did this person mean to you when they were alive?
- What do they mean to you now?

Freud said that when we mourn, we mourn not only for the person but also for who we were to them.

- What aspects of yourself could you be grieving? These may not be obvious or necessarily desirable traits or identities, but they will feel very familiar.

---

5. This will resonate with relating therapy (Hayward et al., 2009) and voice dialogue (Corstens et al., 2012), which appear to also have roots in Gestalt and other humanistic relational therapies.

6. For more guidance on working with both welcome and unwelcome experiences of the deceased, see Hayes and Steffen (2018).

Connection to 'relatives'

It may not surprise the reader to know that hearing voices in grief has many features in common with hearing voices in other circumstances, even though these topics are rarely studied and discussed together in research.

As with bereavement voices, non-bereavement voices usually say things that are meaningful to the hearer in a certain context. The voice might, for example, refer to the immediate environment the person is in, or aspects of their past experience. Furthermore, with all voices, the hearer may have choices in how they respond to the force of the language they hear (see Leudar et al., 1997; Hayes, 2011) – either diluting it, or strengthening it.[7] This has been observed by Leudar and Thomas (2000) in the voices of patients with a psychiatric diagnosis as well as non-patients, and by Hayes (2011) and Hayes and Steffen (2018) in grief voices. For example, if a voice issues an order or command to the hearer to do something (which happens with bereavement and non-bereavement voices), the hearer rarely automatically follows the instruction without considering its value and consequences (Leudar & Thomas, 2000; Hayes, 2011).

One important difference between bereavement and other kinds of voices, however, is the starkness with which a voice in grief is linked to significant events and others in a person's life. The voices heard in grief are rarely anonymous.[8] This provides the bereaved voice hearer with an immediate opening for making sense of their experience – the relationship with the deceased and the loss. In the case of non-bereavement voices, the links to the hearer's life may not always be so immediately apparent; they may be indirect or even symbolic. For example, many voice hearers may hear voices that say the same kinds of things to them that a critical parent, bully or abuser has said in the past, without sounding like the person's voice. The links to the hearer's life experience may need some excavating. The concept of 'continuing relationships' can be useful in thinking about all kinds of voices, not only those confined to grief. For example, a voice heard by a young person may continue a relationship with a school bully from their last school.

Conclusion

Hearing voices in grief highlights the fundamentally relational nature of our being. Like non-bereavement voices, and thinking in general, some of it is constructive and helpful and some of it is not. Some voice hearing needs to be worked with in order to figure out its meaning and significance.

---

7. This refers to the *pragmatic force* or, in other words, what the voice 'does' with words. This could include insulting, commanding, complimenting, apologising.

8. Or at least, very rarely *reported* as so. Anecdotally, Pablo Sabucedo, one of my PhD students, recently interviewed someone who heard anonymous-sounding voices that she later understood to be a message from the deceased. One could imagine that such experiences may also be fairly common – why wouldn't anonymous voices, which can comment on a range of life experiences, also have something to say about an event as important as the death of someone close?

When problems and challenges arise with hearing voices in grief, so often the problem gets situated within the person. But voice hearing in grief is so clearly located within a relationship: something two people have created together, both the mess and the beauty. Some of the problems are more about social issues; we perhaps need to create a more 'grief literate' community (Breen et al., 2020) so that death is no longer a taboo subject and a range of grief responses are not pathologised.

Connected with this, I believe we are currently suffering from an impoverishment of emotional differentiation, with complexity often reduced to positives and negatives. In order to understand and if necessary help with hearing voices in grief, we need to use subtler concepts of relationships: they are rarely simply good or bad; there is much ambivalence in almost all. Perhaps we need to look at our language use and move away from emotionally blunting terms that can limit our understanding of ourselves and push complex realities underground.

Acknowledgements

I am so grateful to everyone who has shared their stories with me over the years.

References

Breen, L.J., Kawashima, D., Joy, K., Cadell, S., Roth, D., Chow, A. & Macdonald, M.E. (2020). Grief literacy: A call to action for compassionate communities. *Death Studies*, 1–9. doi: 10.1080/07481187.2020.1739780.

Castelnovo, A., Cavallotti, S., Gambini, O. & D'Agostino, A. (2015). Post-bereavement hallucinatory experiences: A critical overview of population and clinical studies. *Journal of Affective Disorders*, *186*, 266–274.

Corstens, D., Longden, E. & May, R. (2012). Talking with voices: Exploring what is expressed by the voices people hear. *Psychosis, 4*(2), 95–104.

Elliott, R., Watson, J.C., Goldman, R.N. & Greenberg, L.S. (2004). *Learning emotion-focused therapy: The process-experiential approach to change*. American Psychological Association.

Grimby, A. (1993). Bereavement among elderly people: Grief reactions, post-bereavement hallucinations and quality of life. *Acta Psychiatrica Scandinavica, 87*(1), 72–80.

Hayes, J. (2011). *Experiencing the presence of the deceased: Symptoms, spirits, or ordinary life?* University of Manchester.

Hayes, J., & Leudar, I. (2016). Experiences of continued presence: On the practical consequences of 'hallucinations' in bereavement. *Psychology and Psychotherapy: Theory, research and practice, 89*(2), 194–210.

Hayes, J. & Steffen, E.M. (2018). Working with welcome and unwelcome presence in grief. In: D. Klass & E.M. Steffen (Eds.), *Continuing bonds in bereavement: New directions for research and practice* (pp.163–175). Routledge.

Hayward, M., Overton, J., Dorey, T. & Denney, J. (2009). Relating therapy for people who hear voices: A case series. *Clinical Psychology & Psychotherapy: An international journal of theory & practice, 16*(3), 216–227.

Kamp, K., Steffen, E.M., Alderson-Day, B., Allen, P., Austad, A., Hayes, J., Laroi, F., Ratcliffe, M. & Sabucedo, P. (2020). *Sensory and quasi-sensory experiences of the deceased in bereavement: An interdisciplinary and integrative review.* (In review).

Leader, D. (2008). *The new black: Mourning, melancholia and depression.* Penguin.

Leudar, I. & Thomas, P. (2000). *Voices of reason, voices of insanity: Studies of verbal hallucinations.* Psychology Press.

Leudar, I., Thomas, P., McNally, D. & Glinski, A. (1997). What voices can do with words: Pragmatics of verbal hallucinations. *Psychological Medicine, 27*(4), 885–898. doi: 10.1017/s0033291797005138.

Mead, G.H. (1934). *Mind, self and society (Vol. III).* University of Chicago Press.

Rees, W.D. (1971). The hallucinations of widowhood. *British Medical Journal, 4*(5778), 37–41.

Rogers, C.R. (1959). *A theory of therapy, personality, and interpersonal relationships: As developed in the client-centered framework* (Vol. 3, pp.184–-256). McGraw-Hill.

Sabucedo, P., Evans, C., Gaitanidis, A. & Hayes, J. (2021). When experiences of presence go awry: A survey on psychotherapy practice with the ambivalent-to-distressing 'hallucination' of the deceased. *Psychology and Psychotherapy: Theory, research and practice, 94*(S2), 464–480.

Steffen, E. & Coyle, A. (2011). Sense of presence experiences and meaning-making in bereavement: A qualitative analysis. *Death Studies, 35*(7), 579–609.

Troyer, J.M. (2014). Older widowers and postdeath encounters: A qualitative investigation. *Death Studies, 38*(10), 637–647.

Vygotsky, L.S. (1934/1987). Thinking and speech. In R.W. Rieber & A.S. Carton (Eds.), *The collected works of L.S. Vygotsky (Vol. 1): Problems of general psychology* (pp.39–285). Plenum Press.

Winnicott, D.W. (1971). *Playing and reality.* Penguin Books.

10 Spirituality, religion and voices
Christopher C.H. Cook

The experience of hearing a voice in the absence of any speaker raises questions that are spiritually and psychologically significant. The scientist may be able to provide convincing explanations of how such voices arise. The clinician may offer effective (or ineffective) strategies for managing them. A priest or pastor may believe that they have insights into their demonic or divine origin. The question still arises as to what they mean to the person who hears them. How can voices make sense, spiritually, religiously, or in any other ultimately meaningful way?

While weekly church attendance has declined in Western society over the last one hundred years or more, people increasingly describe themselves as 'spiritual but not religious'. Worldwide, the great majority of people still identify as religious, even if this is individually defined or refers to a variety of different religions. This is not the place to debate the differences between spirituality and religion; both are contested concepts and both are difficult to define precisely. Both are concerned with relationship with the transcendent (whether or not defined in theistic (relating to the existence of God or gods) terms). Many people identify as both spiritual and religious. However, at risk of over-simplifying, spirituality is often characterised as offering more of an emphasis on subjective and inner experience; religion is correspondingly more widely understood as concerned with shared practices and beliefs in relation to the sacred.[1] In practice, the concepts overlap. Spirituality has its social dimension and religion has its concerns with the inner life.

Voice hearing will be taken here to refer to what psychologists and psychiatrists might define as auditory verbal hallucinations – that is, voices heard in the absence of any objectively present speaker. However, this should not be taken to mean that the voices are 'not real'. Usually, they are experienced as very real, but the subjective nature of such experiences varies widely. Some are heard more inwardly, resembling the inner voices that form the basis for conscious thought for most people. Some

---

1. For further discussion, see Vaillant (2008), Cook (2013) and Mercadante (2014).

are heard externally, out loud, and more closely resemble voices heard when talking with a visibly and physically present conversation partner. Almost always, voice hearing is concerned with voices experienced as coming from a speaker other than the self, raising the question of exactly who the speaker is.[2]

> *Learning point 1*
>
> Before you read any further, you may like to consider the following questions:
>
> - Have your voices been spiritually meaningful for you?
> - How have other people (pastor, priest, health professional…) helped you to find spiritual or religious meaning in your voices? How have they been unhelpful?
> - When you hear voices, who is speaking?

Scientific research

Great advances have been made in the scientific understanding of voice hearing over the past 20–30 years. While voices are usually associated with psychiatric diagnoses, it is now known that they often occur where there is no evidence of psychopathology. The main difference between voices heard in the context of a diagnosed psychiatric illness and those that are not is that the former are much more likely to be experienced and related to by the voice hearer and those around them as negative, critical and otherwise unpleasant. This does not mean that we know that the voices are actually 'intending' to be negative, critical and unpleasant. Voices heard in the context of prayer or worship are often experienced and/or related to in a very positive way. Unfortunately, there has been little scientific research on such voices, but some important studies have been undertaken, notably by Tanya Luhrmann, mainly working within Christian congregations (Luhrmann, 2012).[3]

Voices share many of the characteristics of inner thoughts, and one of several theories is that they arise as a result of misattribution of such thoughts to an external source. However, it is also clear that any perception is a complex phenomenon, within which expectations and predictions of what might be expected form a significant part. Culture, life history, religious practices and traditions, among other factors, thus all contribute to the way in which we perceive and interpret the world around us. In ambiguous, complex or other psychologically unpredictable circumstances, people may be more or less predisposed to hearing voices (or seeing visions) in the absence of any perceivable external speaker. According to Luhrmann's research, proclivity (a tendency) to states of mental absorption, notably

---

2. I have provided a fuller introduction to the topic in the Introduction in Cook (2018).
3. For a fuller review of the research than is provided here, see Cook (2018) and Fernyhough (2016).

during prayer or worship, may be a particular factor that makes such phenomena more likely. However, it is not just the individual tendency that is important.

Within Christian circles, voices and visions seem to be more frequent in some traditions than others. It has been suggested, for example, that Protestants hear voices and Catholics see visions. This is almost certainly an oversimplification, and many religious experiences of voices also include visual or other sensory elements in addition to the voice. However, there seems to be some truth to the idea that expectation plays a part. In general, and perhaps with some exceptions, Hindus do not have visions of the Virgin Mary and Christians do not hear the voice of Krishna. Frequency of voice-hearing experiences also appears to vary within the same religious tradition across different geographical and cultural contexts.

It has been suggested that the frequency of religious hallucinations is declining in the secular Western world, but the evidence for this is unclear and a recent overview of research suggests that there is no overall downward trend (Cook, 2015). There does appear to be fluctuation across time, which may be for a variety of reasons. Religious voices would seem to be infrequent in countries where few people describe themselves as religious, such as China, but research designs have not been consistent or precise in defining what makes a voice spiritual/religious. In a country where spiritual/religious frames of reference are rarely used, it is not surprising that voices are rarely identified as spiritual/religious.

Spirituality untethered

The concept of spirituality as something to be distinguished from religion has arisen in a secular Western context. While religious spiritualities are still both important and common, a spiritual marketplace has developed within which the traditional faiths compete with newer spiritualities, unbounded by doctrine, institution or external authority (Roof, 1999). Such spiritualities include New Age, feminist and eco-, among many others. They tend to be concerned with feelings, inwardness and the quest for self-discovery or self-actualisation.

Voices encountered in the context of such a spirituality do not have the advantage of scripture, tradition or doctrine as interpretive tools. On the other hand, there is the possibility of drawing on elements of multiple different faith traditions and the opportunity to self-define the meaning and significance of such experiences. The voices themselves may also offer self-interpretation. Thus, for example, when trying to work out whether her voices are of divine origin, Skye Thomas (a voice hearer and author) reports (she generally denotes her voices in capitals):

> I'll tell you honestly, I like to call THEM guardian angels. It's the most politically correct answer. Most of the books THEY sent me were about connecting with your guardian angels… THEY want me to tell you to research communications and real life relationships with angels, not the ancient religious beliefs or hierarchies or archangels or patron saints or any of that stuff. None of that means anything to THEM. (Thomas, 2004, pp.75–76)

Thomas expresses a wish to try to understand her voices in relationship to God, but the voices resist this:

> THEY say THEY don't need a God in charge because THEY are all interconnected and share a common vision and have universal love that is non-individualistic. Each is separate, but part of one energy source of love and compassion. (Thomas, 2004, p.76)

Thomas's experience is related by way of an autobiographical account, and provides an example of one woman trying to make sense of the voices that she has heard. Other voice-hearing experiences initiate, or become a part of, a wider community experience of listening to the voices within. Thus, the Findhorn community (a spiritually minded community in Scotland with a focus on ecological living) arose as a result of the voice-hearing experiences of its founder, Eileen Caddy. Initially focused around attention to an inner voice that Caddy then relayed to others, there was eventually (at the instigation of the voice) a shift to all members of the community paying attention to their own experience of the voice within.[4]

Religion

Almost all of the world's major faith traditions provide scriptural and traditional examples of experiences that might sound like voice hearing. It is not uncommonly asserted that founders of religions, such as Moses, Jesus or Mohammed, were voice hearers. Similarly, St Paul (formerly known as Saul) is recorded in the Christian New Testament as hearing a voice on the road to Damascus:

> 'Saul, Saul, why do you persecute me?' He asked, 'Who are you, Lord?' The reply came, 'I am Jesus, whom you are persecuting. But get up and enter the city, and you will be told what you are to do.' (Acts 9, 4–6)[5]

Such experiences seem not to have been common for Paul (or for Jesus), but they apparently occurred frequently for Moses and for Mohammed. In both cases, we should be wary of jumping to conclusions. We cannot interview Paul or Moses and ask them what their experiences of voices were like. We do not know what kinds of experiences they had, only what the voice is recorded as having said. We therefore cannot say that they were voice hearers with any degree of confidence that their experiences in any way resembled modern-day voice hearing. On the other hand, we also cannot rule out the possibility that their voices were exactly the same. Given the wide variety of contemporary experiences referred to as voice hearing, it is entirely possible that they were similar to at least some of them.

Scriptural stories (that is, sacred stories held to be authoritative within religious traditions) of the hearing of voices provide models, or patterns, against which contemporary experiences may be compared. Whether Moses or St Paul

---

4. See further discussion in Cook (2018), pp.26–29.
5. Biblical quotations are from the New Revised Standard Version.

were voice hearers or not, the biblical stories about them provide both a precedent and a point of comparison for contemporary experiences of voice hearing within Jewish, Christian or other religious contexts.

There seem to be a relatively small number of patterns for voice hearing that recur relatively frequently. Within the Christian tradition, these include the conversion of St Paul and the temptation of St Anthony (an influential 3rd–4th-century Christian monk from Egypt). There is also a more conversational pattern of dialogical communication with God or other spiritual beings. It is less clear what the biblical or historical prototype for this is, but Margery Kempe, in the 14th century, provides a good example in the medieval Catholic Church. Tanya Luhrmann's research in the Vineyard churches in the USA (2012) offers a well-documented contemporary example in the context of evangelical charismatic Christianity.

It is interesting that Christians describing conversion experiences similar to St Paul's sometimes point out that they were not familiar with the story of St Paul prior to their own conversion experience. This suggests in itself an awareness that, at moments of crisis, voice-hearing experiences may follow familiar religious patterns. On the other hand, the accounts of St Paul's experience, as recorded in the book of Acts, follow a simple fundamental pattern. At a point of crisis, a voice addresses Paul by name and initiates a change of heart and life. Such a pattern is not unique to religious conversion experiences and may be associated with change of vocation or crises of other kinds. Famously, according to tradition, the voice from the crucifix in San Damiano initiated St Francis's (the founder of a religious order called the Franciscans) vocation to rebuild Christ's church. The words were unique to St Francis, but the pattern of a voice associated with a crisis and a change of heart is fundamentally similar to that found in the story of St Paul.

For St Paul and St Francis, the voice appears to have been an almost unique, once-in-a-lifetime experience. For Margery Kempe, as recorded in her *Book*, the voices appear to have continued frequently throughout her life:

> Sometimes our Lady spoke to her mind; sometimes St Peter, sometimes St Paul, sometimes St Katherine, or whatever saint in heaven she was devoted to, appeared to her soul and taught her how she should love our Lord and how she should please him. These conversations were so sweet, so holy and so devout, that often this creature could not bear it, but fell down and twisted and wrenched her body about, and made remarkable faces and gestures, with vehement sobbings and great abundance of tears… (Windeatt, 1994, p.75)

Opinion was divided among Margery's contemporaries as to whether or not these were genuine spiritual experiences, but the controversy seems to have revolved more around Margery's flamboyant and emotional presentation of them, rather than about the fundamental premise. The possibility of experiencing converse with God or the saints seems not to have been in doubt. Similarly, in the contemporary context, in specific churches of a particular tradition across the world, such as those studied by Luhrmann in North America, while there may be discussion about whether or not individual voices were actually from God, the fundamental premise that God sometimes speaks to people in prayer is affirmed. In this way, the experience is both normalised and given a positive connotation.[6]

As indicated at the beginning of this chapter, one of the main features distinguishing voices associated with psychiatric diagnosis from those not associated with such diagnoses is that the latter are generally experienced and related to as more positive and are consequently associated with less negative emotions. An example of a distressing experience of relating to voices in a Christian context is provided by Jo Barber:

> One day when I was sitting in church I heard what I thought was the voice of the devil calling me. I was petrified. It was very insistent. I do not know why I thought it was the devil; it just was, and I just knew. He was threatening to control me and said that I did not belong to Christ. I sat there for a while paralyzed with fright, and finally left the church without speaking to anyone, in a very distressed state. (Barber, 2016, p.123)

Barber goes on to give a moving account of clergy and mental health professionals who variously were or were not helpful in their attempts to help her in the wake of this experience. Eventually, her recovery involved a mixture of spiritual and psychological factors which together helped to bring her to a place of spiritual and religious wellbeing.

Learning point 2

Depending on your own background, you may relate to voices as spiritually or religiously significant, or perhaps as having no connection at all with faith or spirituality. Other people you know (or work with) may come from very different backgrounds than you. You may like to consider the following questions in relation to your own experiences, or those of other people whom you know.

- Do you identify as spiritual or religious, or perhaps both or neither?
- Is there anything explicitly religious in what your voices say?
- Are voices, visions or other religious experiences common in your spiritual/faith or cultural community? If so, in what ways are your voices similar or different to those that others hear?
- Are your voices similar to any that appear in the scriptures, spiritual or cultural writings or traditions that you are familiar with? In what way are your voices different to these voices?
- How do your voices make you feel – emotionally or spiritually?

---

6. For further discussion of the voices of St Paul, St Francis and Margery Kempe, Tanya Luhrmann's research and the broader field of voices in spiritual and religious context, see Cook (2018).

Spiritual and religious coping

As Barber's story illustrates, spirituality and religion both provide important coping resources in times of stress, illness or adversity. Similarly, they may provide helpful resources upon which to draw when voices are experienced as unpleasant, critical, intrusive or otherwise difficult to manage. The voice(s) may or may not be directly spiritual/religious in nature. (In any case, as has already been said, it is highly debatable as to what counts as a 'spiritual' or 'religious' voice.) Prayer, meditation (such as mindfulness), silence, music, devotional reading and other spiritual practices may all have a part to play. Sadly, there has been very little research to guide what might be helpful or unhelpful, and much may depend on trial and error. Having a psychologically well-informed spiritual director (a person who you consider you could learn from spiritually along your way), or a spiritually aware counsellor, may be helpful in providing an opportunity to discuss different approaches with another person. New approaches, such as the ones introduced in this book, may provide an opportunity for spiritual as well as personal or psychological growth.

> *Learning point 3*
>
> People have very different experiences of voice hearing, and come from very different spiritual/religious backgrounds. For some, there is a positive relationship between their voices and their spirituality. For others the two are in conflict.
>
> - How do your spiritual/religious tradition and beliefs help you to make sense of your voices?
> - How do your spiritual/religious beliefs help you to cope with any unpleasant, untrue, or unsettling things that your voices might say?
> - Does your faith/spirituality make it more difficult – in any way – to cope with (or make sense of) your voices?
> - Experiment with some new spiritual practices – prayer, music, meditation or devotional reading. How do these help you to make sense of what your voices say – or to cope better with any unpleasant things that they say?
> - How does any psychological help that you receive (or give to others) help to build or undermine spirituality and/or faith?

Revelatory voices

For some people, voices are more than just voices. They may be identified as spiritually or religiously significant figures, such as angels, spirits, saints, demons or even God. They may have significant things to say about past events or life or the wider world. Mental health professionals have too often dismissed the content of what voices say as unimportant. Conversely, it is easy to place too much importance on what they say, even to the extent of feeling compelled to obey them or believe them or share their message with others.

Religious traditions within which the voices of angels or demons play a part can reinforce this sense of their importance, but tradition has only handed down the voices that were agreed to be important. We do not know how many other figures in the past had similar experiences that were thought not to have been worth recording and passing on. This may be because they were widely thought to be unhelpful and best ignored, or it may be because the voice had things to say that were significant primarily to the individual who heard them and not to others.

There would not seem to be any good reason to assume that voices are beyond criticism or that they should automatically be dismissed as having nothing important to say. Voices may reveal things that are important – to the individual who hears them, to others, or to the wider community. They may even be a way in which God speaks to people, although this will ultimately be a matter of faith that some will accept and others will not.[7] Whether or not any particular thing that the voices say is important is a matter for careful and critical discernment. Family, friends, carers, professionals, spiritual advisors and others all have a part to play in this process.

Conclusion

Voices can be spiritually or religiously significant. Voices play a significant part in the stories of faith that have been handed down within spiritual and religious traditions. They are significant in people's life stories, whether in a purely individual way or in the context of a community of faith. Spirituality and religion have an important part to play for some people in managing their voices well.

Acknowledgements

I am grateful to the Wellcome Trust for the generous financial support I received from them in support of my part in the Hearing the Voice project at Durham University (grant number 108720/Z/15/Z).

---

7. For theological exploration of the possibility that voices may be revelatory, see Cook (2018, pp.199–225).

References

Barber, J. (2016). My story: A spiritual narrative. In C.C.H. Cook, A. Powell, & A. Sims (Eds.), *Spirituality and narrative in psychiatric practice: Stories of mind and soul* (pp.121–131). RCPsych Press.

Cook, C.C.H. (2013). Transcendence, immanence and mental health. In C.C.H. Cook (Ed.), *Spirituality, theology and mental health* (pp. 141–159). SCM Press.

Cook, C.C.H. (2015). Religious psychopathology: The prevalence of religious content of delusions and hallucinations in mental disorder. *International Journal of Social Psychiatry, 61*, 404–425.

Cook, C.C.H. (2018). *Hearing voices, demonic and divine: Scientific and theological perspectives.* Routledge.

Fernyhough, C. (2016). *The voices within: The history and science of how we talk to ourselves.* Profile.

Luhrmann, T.M. (2012). *When God talks back.* Knopf.

Mercadante, L. (2014). *Belief without borders: Inside the minds of the spiritual but not religious.* Oxford University Press.

Roof, W.C. (1999). *Spiritual marketplace: Baby boomers and the remaking of American religion.* Princeton University Press.

Thomas, S. (2004). *Voices: Divinity or insanity?* Purple Pixie.

Vaillant, G.E. (2008). *Spiritual evolution: A scientific defense of faith.* Broadway.

Windeatt, B.A. (Ed.). (1994). *The Book of Margery Kempe.* Penguin.

11 Voice hearing and cannabis: a harm-reduction approach

Rufus May and Kate Quinn

Cannabis is regarded in mainstream circles as being bad for your mental health, and specifically linked to experiences associated with a diagnosis of psychosis, including hearing voices. However, there is a debate about how bad it really is. Here, we look at some of the evidence for these arguments and voice hearers' own experiences of using cannabis. We recommend a harm-minimisation approach to cannabis. This means weighing up the benefits and drawbacks of cannabis use for each individual; finding ways to avoid using it if it seems damaging; using it moderately if the benefits outweigh the disadvantages, and building up other ways of achieving the positive effects cannabis may be providing.

The perspectives we collected from voice hearers for the purpose of writing this chapter were volunteered to us from a number of sources, including hearing-voices groups and social media. This was not part of a research study or our work in services and we acknowledge these perspectives may not be representative of voice hearers more generally. The people who contributed consented for their quotes to be included and they have been anonymised, using pseudonyms. The examples are intended to be illustrative and to encourage reflection.

What the research tells us

The possible link between smoking cannabis and developing 'psychosis' has been investigated by researchers for many years. There are many reasons why people may hear voices, but for the purpose of this chapter we have summarised the work that looks at psychosis more generally, as very few studies focus specifically on voice hearing. There is a well-established link between using cannabis and developing psychosis. Indeed, there have been so many studies in this area that a number of meta-analyses have been completed, which is a way of analysing the data in lots of papers and looking at the combined findings of many studies. For example, two meta-analyses that suggest this (Marconi et al., 2016; Large et al., 2011) both found that people who used cannabis in their teenage years had an increased risk of psychosis. This research seems to show that people who use cannabis are more likely to develop psychosis, and that people who are vulnerable to developing psychosis may be even more likely to become 'psychotic' if they smoke cannabis.

It has been more difficult to establish whether this link is causal: researchers are less sure if it is the cannabis itself that causes the psychosis or if other factors may also be involved. For example, some researchers have suggested that demographic differences between people who do and do not use cannabis might account for some of the link between cannabis use and psychosis (e.g. Sevy et al., 2010; Wade, 2005). Attempts to analyse the causal link, such as by Arseneault and colleagues (2004), suggest that there may be some people who are already at risk of developing psychosis for whom a particular kind of cannabis use during a critical age period (smoking lots of 'skunk' cannabis from a young age) does appear to cause the development of psychosis. They conclude:

> At the population level, elimination of cannabis use would reduce the incidence of schizophrenia by approximately 8%, assuming a causal relationship. Cannabis use appears to be neither a sufficient nor a necessary cause for psychosis. It is a component cause, part of a complex constellation of factors leading to psychosis. (p.110)

While such research does suggest that is it likely that cannabis use can contribute to the development of psychosis, it does not often mention voice hearing specifically; nor does it comment on the possible benefits or harm of cannabis for people who already hear voices, which we will discuss later.

There are two active ingredients in cannabis: tetrahydrocannabinol (THC) and cannabidiol (CBD). These seem to cancel each other out in terms of risk of psychosis: THC appears to be associated with psychosis and CBD has been found to have anti-psychotic properties, and has even shown promise as a treatment for psychosis (e.g. Leweke et al., 2012). Therefore, there is some evidence that cannabis with high CBD and low THC may be less harmful in relation to psychosis (England et al., 2017) and that people who use cannabis with higher CBD report fewer psychosis experiences than those who use higher THC cannabis (Schubart et al., 2011). Cannabis known as 'skunk' tends to have a relatively high THC content and low CBD, and there is evidence that its THC strength has increased over the years (Potter et al., 2008).

> *Learning point 1*
>
> If voice hearers are concerned that using cannabis is having negative effects, it might be worth reducing or avoiding the use of high THC cannabis and seeing if it makes any difference:

- Do you know the THC strength of the cannabis you use?
- Can you try cannabis that is more likely to have a higher CBD to THC ratio?

Possible benefits of cannabis for voices

Despite the evidence that smoking weed may not always be helpful for people who hear voices, some report positive effects of cannabis use, and this can become an arena of conflict between people who hear voices and those who support them, both within mental health services and at home. We have met a lot of relatives of people who smoke cannabis who complain that they feel that the drug has come between them and their loved one. This may be for a number of reasons – the person's behaviour, a sense of lack of connection with them or a general disapproval of the use of cannabis because it is illegal. Some families have taken a harm-minimisation approach, coming from a non-judgemental stance. For example, one of the parents we spoke to asked their teenage son not to smoke when they met up for dinner in the week as it seemed to affect his communication and ability to connect with them, but they were fine with him smoking with his friends at the weekend. Their son agreed to this request.

Learning point 2
- Are the people around you okay with you using cannabis? How do their attitudes affect you?
- Are you able to discuss and negotiate your cannabis use with family and friends so it doesn't affect your relationships negatively?

Personal experience of using cannabis

Some of the voice hearers we spoke to who use cannabis talked about certain benefits they find from cannabis. From talking to voice hearers who use cannabis, we have noticed that people who use it more often tend to report more benefits:

Helen: I started smoking cannabis several years after I began hearing voices (at age 21), on the advice of another service user. I find it incredibly helpful, with almost no side effects. I don't think it has any impact on the voices themselves, but what it does do is massively decrease the fear and distress associated with what they are saying to me. The only time I have experienced any adverse effects was one time in hospital, when I had to buy from a different person than normal (due to being in hospital) and, although I smoked a usual amount, I suspect it was a lot higher in THC and I became acutely paranoid. Otherwise, I have experienced no adverse effects, and I would use cannabis more frequently if I was able (and if not illegal, and if I didn't work in a health setting and the consequences of being caught in possession were not so high).

Clara: I find it helpful, as long as the THC-to-CBD ratio isn't too high. It helps me talk with my voices and tie in some of the difficult things they're feeling with some difficulties in my life that I had not seen before. Certain strains can help me sleep as well. If there's not much CBD and too much THC, though, it can make me feel very scared.

Sean: It has been something I have used for ages to help with sleep. Nothing else seems to work in the same way, and I have had problems with sleep for many years. I have tried medications and alcohol, as well as psychological techniques, but none have been as effective as cannabis. I am able to restrict my use to just smoking weed for sleep management. I don't feel that I need to use cannabis at other times. It does not seem to make my voices worse or better. The benefits seem to outweigh the risks for me.

Other people described more mixed experiences.

Melanie: I have found smoking some weed calms my anxiety and the voices, or possibly just makes the voices tolerable. But there have been times when I have gotten too stoned and made the voices worse and me paranoid. And I only indulge at home; if I am somewhere else, no matter how little I partake, it just causes paranoia.

Daniel: When I smoke less, I have more get up and go. However, I see using weed as part of my spiritual approach to life… I enjoy the relaxant effects, despite it having an overall effect of sapping my energy.

The research studies suggest that people experiencing 'psychosis' use cannabis mainly to cope with difficult feelings, but also for a host of other reasons (Green et al., 2004), which appears to be consistent with what we were told by the people we spoke to. Gregg and colleagues (2009) carried out research with people diagnosed with schizophrenia and found that there were three different ways that they used alcohol and drugs generally (including cannabis). First, they used it to chill out and connect with people; second, to manage difficult mental experiences, and third, to feel more creative and enhance their sense of self. For example, one person described how 'it calms me down, I can write poetry and things'. Another of their research participants described how it 'opens your mind. I can have a joint and sit down and draw'. In a personal communication, Gregg told us that she found that people diagnosed with schizophrenia report similar reasons for the specific use of cannabis (the reported study considered drug use more generally).

Unfortunately, the use of cannabis as a coping strategy can increase the risk of dependence in some cases (e.g. Spencer et al., 2002). For example, Jason told us:

The reason I don't smoke it is, if I do, I get very addicted and end up smoking it every day, and I know that slows me down and makes me more lazy about life. I am finding it good to go to a hearing voices group now, and I am learning about other ways to chill out and feel good about myself.

> *Learning point 3*
>
> If you have used cannabis, look back and try to work out when you have found it helpful and when you have found it unhelpful.
>
> - Have there been times when you have smoked more, or less, or not at all?
> - What have you noticed about these occasions in relation to how you feel, physically and mentally?

When cannabis might not be helpful

We heard from people who had made a decision that cannabis did not suit them and had decided to avoid it.

Sam: I smoked it when I was 16 and 17, but when I had some stressful life experiences, weed started to make me feel paranoid. I heard other people talking in the street and it seemed that they were talking about me, and saying I was a threat to them and that they wanted to get rid of me. After a few of these experiences where I heard voices even after the effects of the weed had worn off, I decided to stop smoking it. It helped to meet other people who had made a similar decision. Before that, I played down the problems with getting stoned, and focused on the idea that it helped me to connect with others. But meeting others like me who felt weed disagreed with them helped me let go of trying to make it work for me.

Sarah: I'm a 36-year-old woman who has been a voice hearer for the past four years. When I was in my early 20s, I went on a trip to New York City and tried marijuana for the first time. I immediately started experiencing an extreme amount of paranoia and an anxiety attack (I thought that my friends were there to take advantage of me and had given me something else, not marijuana). A sense of numbness started running throughout my body; at times it felt like things were crawling on me. I decided to sleep it off, and when I closed my eyes I had very bizarre visions. I returned to Vancouver, Canada, convinced that what I had tried in NYC must have been laced with something else and was not pure marijuana. My friends told me that, if I were to try it in the comfort of my own home, surrounded by people I know, I might have a different experience. So, I tried it one more time and the same thing happened. My bizarre experiences landed me in the hospital that night. So, I decided to never try marijuana again since it was not a pleasant experience for me. Fast forward years later, and I went through a very stressful time finishing graduate school and, shortly after, I had a psychotic breakdown, going through very similar experiences as when I tried marijuana. I had extreme paranoia and anxiety, and heard loud voices on top of it. I believe that if I were to try marijuana during this time, my voice-hearing experience would get intensified.

> *Learning point 4*
>
> If you find cannabis use unhelpful for your voices and/or mental health more generally, there may be other coping strategies you could use that would provide the benefits you seek from using cannabis, such as ways to manage anxiety. Some of the other chapters in this book (for example, Chapter 31 on 'Mindfulness and hearing voices') may offer some ideas.

Harm minimisation and cannabis

Cannabis use is extremely common in the UK and there is a greater acceptance towards it, especially when it is used for medicinal purposes. At the time of writing, the government is exploring changing the law so that medical cannabis can be prescribed for certain physical conditions. Also, CBD oil can now be bought legally as a relaxant and is recommended by its manufacturers for managing a range of health conditions, including anxiety. Harm minimisation is an alternative to trying to stop people smoking cannabis because of generalised concerns about its negative mental health effects. A harm minimisation approach means adopting an accepting attitude and trying to help people find ways of using cannabis so it doesn't lead to negative effects, either on their health or on their relationships with others and life generally.

Many people have told us how giving up cannabis use altogether has led to an improvement in their quality of life. It seems that some of us are more sensitive to the hallucinogenic properties of cannabis and the way it can enhance some dissociative experiences. If this describes you, it may be wise to stop using cannabis altogether. However, others may be able to build up other ways to relax and feel connected so they can continue to smoke cannabis that is lower in THC content, in safe, supportive surroundings so as to enhance the positive effects of the drug and minimise the more negative effects.

Release, a national charity that specialises in advising on drugs and drugs law, suggests the following ways to reduce the harm from using cannabis (Table 11.1)

Table 11.1: Harm reduction tips for cannabis use[1]

• Cut down or stop using tobacco as a mixing agent with the cannabis.
• Do not hold the smoke deeply in your lungs. This increases how much tar goes into your lungs and doesn't get you more stoned.
• Avoid inhaling deeply, for the same reason as above. You will be subjecting your lungs to more tar and other waste without getting you any more stoned.
• Regularly clean your pipe or bong. Avoid using plastic bottles or long pipes as this can produce fumes that are more likely to be toxic.
• You can use a vaporiser to protect your lungs from lung cancer. This will mean you inhale a lot less tar and carcinogens.
• Create time where you are not stoned to do important daily things in life – shopping, cleaning, tidying, exercise and so on.
• There are known benefits of cutting down. They can include reducing your tolerance so you can get stoned using less weed and so have more motivation and energy. Many people also describe improvements in memory and organisational skills and feeling physically healthier. However, some people report feeling worse, especially if they find cannabis useful for managing pain or other difficulties.

Table 11.2: Cutting down tips[2]

• Reduce or cut out tobacco.
• Use less cannabis per joint or pipe etc.
• Increase time between joints.
• Reduce your tobacco use.
• Reduce your caffeine use as caffeine counteracts the effects of cannabis and may lead you to want to take more cannabis to compensate. Consuming large amounts of caffeine may also lead to sleep problems.
• Increase physical exercise and/or other meaningful activities that don't involve getting stoned.
• Avoid compensating for the absence of cannabis by increasing your alcohol use.
• Reduce very gradually (e.g. 25% each week), as this will avoid more severe withdrawal problems such as disrupted sleep, low mood and loss of appetite.

---

1. Adapted from www.release.org.uk/drugs/cannabis/harm-reduction
2. Adapted from www.globaldrugsurvey.com

If you want to stop completely, be aware that you may experience side effects as the body adjusts to the absence of cannabis in the system. You may experience difficulties with sleeping, irritability, aggression, restlessness and low mood. For most people, these pass after four to 10 days, so persist. Remember, your body is having to adjust to a new normal; adverse reactions don't mean you need the cannabis and can't exist without it; you simply need to allow your body to regain a healthy equilibrium.

> *Learning point 5*
>
> If you would like to reduce your cannabis use, consider what activities you could engage in that might give you some of the benefits that cannabis use gives you (e.g. exercise, mindfulness, relaxation exercises, yoga, music, dance, walks in nature and so on). Are there ways to build up such activities before or as you try to reduce your cannabis use?

Conclusion

There is still heated debate about how bad cannabis is for people's mental health. The research shows that it is associated with a greater risk of psychosis, including voice hearing, particularly if young people use it intensely in their teenage years. However, others contest the gravity of this risk. We found that, while some people who hear or have heard voices find that it is useful to avoid cannabis, others say it can be a useful resource and helps them live with their voices. A harm minimisation approach to cannabis use is recommended, where individuals are supported to make informed decisions about whether or not they use cannabis and how they use it.

References

Arseneault, L., Cannon, M., Witton, J. & Murray, R.M. (2004). Causal association between cannabis and psychosis: Examination of the evidence. *British Journal of Psychiatry, 184*(2), 110–117.

England, A., Freeman, T.P., Murray, R.M. & McGuire, P. (2017). Can we make cannabis safer? *The Lancet Psychiatry, 4*(8), 643–648.

Green, B., Kavanagh, D. & Young, R.M. (2004). Reasons for cannabis use in men with and without psychosis. *Drug and Alcohol Review, 23*(4), 445–453.

Gregg, L., Haddock, G. & Barrowclough, C. (2009). Self-reported reasons for substance use in schizophrenia: A Q methodological investigation. *Mental Health and Substance Use: Dual diagnosis, 2*(1), 24–39.

Large, M., Sharma, S., Compton, M.T., Slade, T. & Nielssen, O. (2011). Cannabis use and earlier onset of psychosis: A systematic meta-analysis. *Archives of General Psychiatry, 68*(6), 555–561.

Leweke, F.M., Piomelli, D., Pahlisch, F., Muhl, D., Gerth, C.W., Hoyer, C., Klosterkötter, J., Hellmich, M. & Koethe, D. (2012). Cannabidiol enhances anandamide signaling and alleviates psychotic symptoms of schizophrenia. *Translational Psychiatry, 2*(3), e94.

Marconi, A., Di Forti, M., Lewis, C.M., Murray, R.M. & Vassos, E. (2016). Meta-analysis of the association between the level of cannabis use and risk of psychosis. *Schizophrenia Bulletin, 42*(5), 1262–1269.

Potter, D.J., Clark, P. & Brown, M.B. (2008). Potency of delta 9-THC and other cannabinoids in cannabis in England in 2005: Implications for psychoactivity and pharmacology. *Journal of Forensic Sciences, 53*(1), 90–94.

Schubart, C.D., Sommer, I.E., Van Gastel, W.A., Goetgebuer, R.L., Kahn, R.S. & Bok, M.P. (2011). Cannabis with high cannabidiol content is associated with fewer psychotic experiences. *Schizophrenia Research, 130*(1–3), 216–221.

Sevy, S., Robinson, D.G., Napolitano, B., Patel, R.C., Gunduz-Bruce, H., Miller, R., McCormack, J., Lorell, B.S. & Kane, J. (2010). Are cannabis use disorders associated with an earlier age at onset of psychosis? A study in first episode schizophrenia. *Schizophrenia Research, 120*(1-3), 101–107.

Spencer, C., Castle, D., & Michie, P.T. (2002). Motivations that maintain substance use among individuals with psychotic disorders. *Schizophrenia Bulletin, 28*(2), 233–247.

Wade, D. (2005). Cannabis use and schizophrenia. *American Journal of Psychiatry, 162*(2), 401.

12 Black voices and the deafness of whiteness
Colin King

This chapter explores the pain, fear and cultural forms of bereavement faced by black, Asian and minority ethnic mental health service users when they share their voice-hearing experiences as personal, spiritual and authentic truths and these then come to be understood as 'symptoms' of their diagnosis. It reflects on my own conversion from a black mental health survivor to a social work practitioner. It explores the clinical and cultural meanings of whiteness that are contained in the voices that I hear and the changes that are needed to empower a new co-production to understand the voices of people that try to diagnose me. The challenge is to ensure that voice hearing has an important and not automatically pathological status in the assessment, diagnosis and support planning for and with members of black, Asian and minority ethnic communities. I examine how mental health professionals may helpfully engage voice hearers from black, Asian and minority ethnic backgrounds to draw on their experiences to enable greater equality in understanding the experience of hearing voices in the mental health assessment framework.

Whiteness as the radio of my disorder

> This young man was admitted from Ashford Remand Centre on 24th November 1977. He was on remand for several charges. While in the remand centre he was seen by Dr X and admitted there. It seems that his present illness started at the beginning of the previous year following a series of unpleasant events – his father stabbed him with a chisel in the face and forearm. He was also stabbed in the chest by a friend of his sister and treated at Guy's Hospital. When he was admitted, he said that he had been troubled by hearing voices that were linked to his death and the death of his mother. We found that, although he went to bed early, he was unable to get up in the morning and often slept late because of the voices. He also tended to be weepy and very irritable. His appetite was diminished and he was constipated. After admission, there were several episodes during which

he lost his temper and became physically aggressive towards other patients. Because of his high arousal state, he was treated with phenothiazine as well as an antidepressant, and he was diagnosed as suffering from schizophrenia and manic symptoms. His depression seemed to improve; his thoughts about death receded and he became much livelier.

This quote represents the clinical voice of a white female consultant who wrote this report about me in 1977. I heard this voice on my admission and during my stay and it said that I was a 'schizophrenic and a manic depressive'. The voice pounded in my head and it reinforced my fears. After a now total of four mental health assessments and four admissions, I continue to hear the same voices from the same professionals who discuss how my cultural heritage and my personality have become medicalised. My life has been a combination of white noises and voices. These sounds have been present in my home, in my school and inside both the prison and the mental hospital where I was placed. I kept hearing the voices of white philosophers, white teachers, white prison officers and white clinical practitioners – sometimes internally and sometimes externally, and sometimes these voices seemed to merge into a form of voice hearing that has traditionally been considered a sign of pathology, like schizophrenia.

I have continued to hear these voices, but also started to listen to them more carefully. In this way, I have come to understand them as voices from my past, and in doing so I have made sense of my life. In this process of sense making, I was inspired by Foucault's (1967/2001) book on madness and civilisation. It helped me to understand the idea of hearing voices as an expression of how other people have seen, treated and spoken about me negatively, and how I do actually hear voices saying similar or the same things inside my head, too. What is interesting is how I feel that the voices that I do hear (which others associate with a diagnosis of schizophrenia in me) are essentially also reflecting the contents of the voices expressed by other people. These do, for example, seem to have their origin in a philosophical age that constructed me as biologically and socially inferior, deviant or politically different. These are the voices that emerged through the period between the 15th and 18th centuries at a time when black men were perceived as uncivilised, brutish and incapable of emotions. Hearing these kinds of voices haunted me and drove me from living at home and attending school to being kept against my will in a psychiatric hospital when I was 17 years of age.

Learning point 1

- How can voices like those I heard help us understand why white professionals fail to understand black people's voices?
- Can we challenge psychiatric services that are routinely dominated by white thinking and white professionals to really hear black people's voices when they are assessing black people?

Again, I want to make a distinction between voices heard as telling me I have no worth that are external, and the voices of white theorists, such as Foucault (1967/2001), that I hear outwardly but that have also become internalised. This helps me to understand how these white voices are attributed with the knowledge and power to observe and classify me as mad. I do, however, also hear the voices of other theorists inside my head who offer me the opportunity to listen to my own voice when I explore the complexity of race and diagnosis as a lived experience. What I hear at night, when I am distressed, is the terror of the white voices, with their power to discriminate and damage black people. This power and discrimination have contributed to the deaths in the psychiatric system of many people, like David Bennett (died 1998) and Sean Riggs (died 2008), to name well-known cases, who died after the use of physical restraint by mental health staff and the police, respectively. These voices have followed me throughout my life: to a cell in a mental hospital, and now in my practice as a social worker. These voices operate like a radio station. In another radio station, they also represent distressing voices. That is, I hear my family speaking to me, again as external voices. These are voices that I have listened to, as they represent my despair. They represent my sense of fear and separation and remind me how I feel inferior due to the colour of my skin. They are distinct from actual classic voice hearing, as they are there as voices I cannot locate. They are heard in moments of trauma, of sitting on the sofa, shaking, not able to locate who owns the voice.

White voices permeated my perception of my family, my heritage and my identity as being different. I heard these voices when my father took his last breath at the age of 49. Even when I witnessed my father's heart stop and I knew that this physical frame that had abused me and terrified me for 22 years had died, I was still not free of the voices that saw me as mad. A white doctor pronounced my father dead in an uncaring way. I left the building and started to walk towards school. It was at that point that I heard a voice that I associated with the negativity of the black family, which I thought came from the same radio, but a different station. I found that these voices of negativity sounded like those of a school system.

> *Learning point 2*
> - Do you hear voices talk about you in relation to your family?
> - Could you create a tape of what your family members say about you in relation to your family?
> - Could you create an edited tape of what professionals have said about you and your family?
> - After listening to these tapes, identify the voices that you hear about yourself.

Within the school setting, Coard (1971) suggests that Eurocentric voices have contributed to 'how the West Indian child is made educationally subnormal'. In this new radio station, I was hearing the voices of Burt (1955), Jensen (1980) and Eysenck (Eysenck & Eysenck, 1969), who were demonising my intellect, as expressed by the teachers, when I was a black child. My voice hearing developed into a sixth sense and the whiteness continued to shape the voices that I heard. The voices told me that I was stupid and slow and that I lacked the ability to learn. These voices in the white world of schooling contributed towards my ongoing sense of feeling inferior. I vividly heard the voice of Galton (1869), which was racist and told me that I was incapable of being civilised. I was entering the first part of a classification system of mental disorders in which I heard my psyche telling me that I was inferior. These voices told me about the European norms of family life and the norms of a European educational system. My voice hearing, like a radio station, could now detect how I was being constructed within frameworks that measured me as being unintelligent. I was now aware that, when I went to school, these haunting voices were waiting for me. For example, one voice said to me, 'You are black, and you are not intelligent enough to be educated. This is where black men end up' (as in, not amounting to anything). It was a message that I have remembered throughout my life.

At secondary school, the voice reinforced my experience with teachers and classmates and told me that I was ugly, feared and less than human. The voice sounded like that of a new presenter who had recently joined the educational radio station. I also heard white colonialist teachers who thought that black men were monkeys who couldn't be taught and could only be caned. When I was 16 years of age, I failed all my exams. I had heard internal voices of dislike and a voice that told me to kill myself. My anguish and disappointment built up in my organs and I felt an intense sense of internal hatred. My ego died, cremated inside the furnace of wanting to look like a white man and behave in a white way. The voices then moved to a new place, which was the mental health ward. My voices of self-hatred followed me to the mental health setting of youth custody, where I was to become a mental disorder.

Learning point 3

- In what ways does voice hearing transfer from one setting to another, especially in terms of you/the voice hearer being stigmatised as being different?
- What types of things do your voices say? What is the tone and pitch of the voices? What different people do you hear speaking to you?
- Can you identify whether the voices make stereotypical comments about your race, gender or other cultural issues?

Now I heard the voices of practitioners inside the mental health zones of the prison and the ward setting. Powerful voices told me about models of mental illness and diagnostic frameworks. These voices constrained me to a psychiatric bed and I heard myself being diagnosed by white voices. I listened to these voices and they made me angry. I wanted to die. I heard the voice of a professional white female who offered me a cell as an appreciation of my madness, as I had answered the doctor's questions and said that I was 'hearing voices at night'. They were the historical voices of my own cultural oppression. However, this personal relevance had not seemed of any interest to the assessing doctor. In the assessment of the professionals, I could hear how they were making use of Freud's (1949) thinking, asking me if I had thoughts interfering with my cultural and racial worlds. I could also hear in their language and treatment of me how they were agreeing with Herrnstein and Murray (1994), who said that I was a living example of a 'dysfunction'. Through my own internal voice, I was attempting to run away from their stereotypical pathologising. The volume and intensity of these white assessing voices meant that I struggled to see my supposed mental disorder for what it actually was: my attempt as a black man to escape from my own internal fears.

In the mental health ward, I heard the prison officer's voice and the psychiatrist's voice. These voices reminded me that I was mad. In both the prison and the ward, the displays of black despair often end up with the person being restrained or locked in a room. Black people are subjected to medication, incarceration and control. Black voices are not heard standing up to the powerful voice of whiteness that labels a black male as mad when he resists the idea of being seen and treated as mad.

Consequently, at night, I heard voices that verbalised my suicidal thoughts. I heard voices telling me to self-harm. I had developed my own internal radio stations of despair that I would tune in to at times. I became my own radio presenter with my own voice that repeated to me what was written in the diagnostic manuals used by psychiatrists. I was encouraged to see my experiences as 'symptoms' that fitted with white mental health professionals' lists of symptoms of 'mental disorders'. This experience represented a cultural bereavement, as I had lost my sense of worth as a black man and I became just another person in a system that did not see hearing and listening to my voice as being important. This had negative consequences for my practice as a mental health practitioner later on.

Learning point 4

- Have you heard voices that make you think that you are suffering from a diagnosis of mental illness that was given to you because of your race?
- Can you think of others who have gone through similar experiences?
- Are your voices saying what other people say about your mental health?
- Can you think of ways that you can deal with these voices?

Last night a DJ saved my life

During my transition to becoming a mental health professional, I undertook a personal inquiry into how the voices of whiteness that I had heard, as a survivor of white psychiatry, as an expression and form of discrimination and trauma, had contributed to the devastation in the lives of black men in the statutory location of the hospitals where I worked. I explored how my white voices that I heard when I was a black social worker activated racism, as many of these voices drew on the European theories (Kant, 1788/2004; Hobbes, 1651/1985) that had previously been used to assess, classify and imprison black young men like me. In the process of being discharged from the ward through to becoming an approved social worker (which, in the UK, allows me to be the deciding professional to section people to be held in a mental health hospital against their will), I was empowered to use white voices to section other innocent black men in the same cultural spaces of hospitals. It was a form of entrapment, and it contributed towards my third admission. After sectioning a black man, I walked into my office and the voice told me to jump out of the window in order to end this personal saga of the injustice that had contributed to many black men being sectioned when I could see no reason for them being detained against their will.

I wanted to die in order to stop hearing these voices. The voices represented the psychosis inside whiteness that was unconscious, unsaid and undisclosed. I worried about colluding with practices that had been used to devastate the lives of black men – for example, through violation, restraint, control, through being sectioned and through being overly medicated and violently restrained. I wanted to disempower the voices of these theories by showing that black men's mental health issues could be understood in a different way, where there was less emphasis on diagnosis and treatment. I realised that I was misrepresenting black men when I undertook mental health assessments in the community and transported a black person to the ward of a hospital. I was representing a statutory organisation that has no respect for black men like me. I was engaged in a form of cultural bereavement where I felt a sense of loss in relation to the positive voices of the lived black experiences. These are voices that are never heard by white practitioners who adopt European diagnoses that stop them being sensitive to their impact on the black experience. They tune into their stations in which their DJs' voices discuss the pathologies of black men unchallenged. These voices are rarely exposed. As a survivor and practitioner, I still hear voices of my own despair that tell me that I am mentally disordered. As a practitioner, I hear external voices that say I am inferior in my attempts to challenge their impact on black men where I am committed to making black voices creditable. These voices of black empowerment offer the potential to change how I understand my world, the external voices I hear that cause my inferiority, and the actual voices I hear as being based in a reality that causes distress.

Learning point 5

- There has been very little literature on black people hearing voices. Can you think of any books that cover these issues?
- Could these books contribute to better healthcare for black people who hear voices?
- Can we trust mental health services to understand these voices of black people?

Conclusion

It can be difficult to differentiate between voices that psychiatry traditionally labels as signs of illness and those that represent a culturally dominant white paradigm in psychiatry and in the legal and educational systems. It may not be important to distinguish the two, but learn to listen to the truth of trauma and discrimination expressed in these experiences. Learning to listen to all of these voices and taking them seriously necessarily demands a personal revolution in approach and practice.

References

Burt, C.L. (1955). The evidence for the concept of intelligence. *British Journal of Educational Psychology, 25*(3), 158–177.

Coard, B. (1971). *How the West Indian child is made educationally subnormal in the British school system: The scandal of the black child in schools in Britain*. New Beacon Books.

Eysenck, H.J. & Eysenck, S.B.G. (1969). *Personality structure and measurement*. Routledge & Kegan Paul.

Foucault, M. (1967/2001). *Madness and civilisation*. Routledge.

Freud, S. (1949). *An outline of psycho-analysis*. W.W. Norton & Co.

Galton, F. (1869). *Hereditary genius*. Macmillan & Co.

Herrnstein, R.J. & Murray, C. (1994). *The bell curve: Intelligence and class structure in American life*. The Free Press.

Hobbes, T. (1651/1985). *Leviathan* (C.B. Macpherson (Ed.)). Penguin Classics

Jensen, A. (1980). *Bias in mental testing*. The Free Press.

Kant, I. (1788/2004). *Critique of practical reason (Kritik der praktischen Vernunft)*. Dover Philosophical Classics.

Part two

Emerging social and therapeutic approaches to working with voices

13 Voices, values and values-based practice: engaging with what matters in voice hearing

David Crepaz-Keay and Bill (K.W.M.) Fulford

This chapter explores, through the experiences of three voice hearers (Natalie, Liam and Susan[1]), the role of values-based practice in the context of voice hearing.

The chapter is divided into a number of short sections. We start with Natalie's story and the values challenges presented by the tragic outcomes of the way people responded to her voice hearing. This is followed by a brief overview of values-based practice as a skills-based approach to working with values challenges in healthcare. We then return to Natalie's story to illustrate how values-based practice might have made a difference to the way she was treated. We end with Liam and Susan's stories for further illustrations of the role of values-based practice in working with people who hear voices.

A note on how to read the chapter

As a skills-based approach (see below), values-based practice is better understood by 'doing than saying'. Hence, as you read this chapter, think about the values and other issues that come up for you, rather than just accepting what we say. If you read the chapter in this way – actively engaging with the text rather than just passively reading it through – you will develop your own skills for working with the complex and sometimes conflicting values associated with voice hearing.

Section 1: Natalie's story and the values arising

In this section we tell Natalie's story and then look at the values arising. As indicated above you may want to think about the values in Natalie's story for yourself before looking at what we have to say.

---

[1]. All three stories are based on the experiences of real people, with their names and other biographical details changed to protect confidentiality. Natalie's story has been published in her own name (Crepaz-Keay & Binns, 1997).

Natalie's story

Natalie was accompanied by angels. They used to sing to her and she to them. Natalie would often dance with her angels and, although she caused no problems, she was regularly taken to hospital and prescribed antipsychotic medication. Natalie refused to take the medication because she believed that it killed her angels. In her mid-20s she was detained and put on depot medication. Natalie took her own life and left a note saying she couldn't face living without her angels.

The values arising in Natalie's story

In healthcare contexts there is a tendency to equate values with ethical values. However, as the term is used in values-based practice, values includes but is not confined to ethical values. It covers anything that is important or matters to those concerned.

Identifying the values in Natalie's story involves thinking about what is important or matters to Natalie and also to other people involved. Both sets of values, as we describe later, are important for values-based practice.

One way to identify the relevant values is to go through the story highlighting Natalie's values in one colour and other people's values in another colour (we have used italic and bold in the example in Box 13.1). You may be surprised at just how many values you can pick out by 'close reading' the text in this way.

Think imaginatively about what mattered or was important both to Natalie and to others concerned (relatives perhaps, or friends and staff). What might have driven them to take the actions they did? Their values may be implicit rather than explicit in the text. But use your imagination to 'hunt the values'. We will see later in the chapter that thinking imaginatively about implicit values is really important for values-based practice.

Now think about your own experience of voice hearing (or that of someone you know). Is this experience similarly rich in values?

Box 13.1: Finding the values in Natalie's story

> Natalie was accompanied by *angels*. They used to *sing to her and she to them*. Natalie would often *dance* with her angels and though she **caused no problems** she was regularly **taken to hospital** and **prescribed antipsychotic medication**. Natalie *refused* to take medication because she believed that it *killed* her angels. In her mid-20s, she was **detained** and **put on depot medication**. Natalie *took her own life* and left a note saying *she couldn't face living without her angels*.
>
> Key: italics = Natalie's values; bold = other people's values

We have given our own highlighted version of Natalie's story in Box 13.1. Again, values are far wider than just ethical values. As Box 13.1 illustrates, values include *anything that matters or is important* to those concerned. Values in this inclusive sense (Natalie's values and the values of other people) are written all over Natalie's story.

Natalie's own values (what mattered or was important to her) are largely explicit in this story. Thus, looking at the *italic* highlighted text, we see the importance to

Natalie of her voices: they were the voices of *angels* – that is to say, they were the voices of benevolent supernatural beings – and they mattered so much to her that she *took her own life* because she *couldn't face living* without them.

Other italic text picks out Natalie's values implicitly. Thus, Natalie *refused* medication because she believed it *killed* her angels. Implicit here is the importance to Natalie of her voices (corresponding with the explicit expression of this value as just outlined). Other passages point to some of Natalie's other values. *Singing* and *dancing* are among these. Unlike the terms 'angel' and 'problem' (above), 'singing' and 'dancing' are not explicitly evaluative. But, in the context of Natalie's story, it is clear that they *mattered a good deal to her*. There are many other ways of interacting with angels. What mattered to Natalie was to be able to sing and dance with them.

The values of other people in Natalie's story (highlighted in **bold** text) are more implicit than explicit. This is why we have to 'hunt the values'. We have to use our imaginations to think what might have been important or mattered to those concerned and so might explain the actions they took.

The phrase **caused no problems**, for example, indicates that Natalie's voices, and her reactions to them (singing and dancing) had no untoward consequences for other people. But this begs the question, who triggered Natalie being taken to hospital, and why? Clearly, someone's values (something that mattered or was important to someone other than Natalie) must have been in play here. So we have to use our imaginations to think through the range of possibilities.

Given the tragic outcome of Natalie's story, it is perhaps natural to attribute ill intentions to those concerned. After all, if Natalie's singing and dancing with her angels really 'caused no problems', was it ethical (or even legal) to subject her to involuntary treatment? Did other people (relatives, for example) find Natalie's singing and dancing embarrassing? Were staff being pressured by relatives to 'do something about it'? Were there management targets for 'throughput of cases' to be met? Any or all of such negative values may have been in play.

Yet staff may also have been well intentioned in the actions they took. Most people entering the caring professions do so because they want to help people. In professions like medicine and nursing, this generally means treating symptoms and curing diseases. In mental health contexts, voice hearing is widely assumed to be a symptom of a disease (a psychosis of some kind). Such 'diseases' are linked with an increased risk of suicide. Evidence-based guidelines furthermore suggest that antipsychotic medication is effective in treating psychoses (National Collaborating Centre for Mental Health, 2009). In contemporary mental health practice, suicide prevention is a major value for (it matters a great deal to) everyone concerned. That is to say, suicide prevention is a value that is shared not only by service users and staff but also by managers, policymakers and the general public. Understood in this way, therefore, staff may have felt they had a positive obligation – perhaps even a legal duty – to ensure Natalie took her medication.

So what went wrong? How did potentially well-intentioned actions aimed at preventing suicide end up apparently provoking it? And how might Natalie's story have come out differently? This is where values-based practice has a potential role to play. First, though, just what is values-based practice?

Section 2: Values-based practice

Everything in values-based practice starts from two main messages:

- People's values, what matters or is important to them, vary widely.
- We have to find out what matters or is important to someone from the person themself.

Values-based practice builds on 10 key process elements that together support balanced decision-making within frameworks of shared values (Table 13.1).

Table 13.1: The elements of values-based practice

Values-based practice	Brief definition
PREMISE	
Mutual respect	Mutual respect for differences of values
TEN PROCESS ELEMENTS	
Four clinical skills:	
1) **Awareness**	Awareness of values and of differences of values
2) **Knowledge**	Knowledge retrieval and its limitations
3) **Reasoning**	Used to explore the values in play rather than to close down on 'right answers'
4) **Communication**	Especially for eliciting values and of conflict resolution
Two aspects of clinical relationships:	
5) **Person-values-centred care**	Care centred on the actual rather than assumed values of the patient
6) **The extended multidisciplinary team**	MDT role extended to include values as well as knowledge and skills
Three principles linking values-based practice and evidence-based practice:	
7) **Two feet principle**	All decisions are based on the two feet of values and evidence
8) **Squeaky wheel principle**	We notice values when they cause difficulties (like the squeaky wheel) but (like the wheel that doesn't squeak) they are always there and operative

9) Science-driven principle	Advances in medical science drive the need for values-based practice (as well as evidence-based practice) because they open up choices and with choices go values
Partnership in decision-making:	
10) Partnership based on dissensus	Partnership in decision-making based on the values of those concerned remain in play to be balanced sometimes one way and sometimes in other ways according to the circumstances of a given case

The first and foundational skill for values-based practice is raised awareness of values and the surprising diversity of individual values. Get raised awareness and, as we illustrate further below, you will also get the need to use the other skills (reasoning, knowledge and communication) to find out what values are in play. Get raised awareness and you will get the importance of a service model that is person-*values*-centred (focusing on what is important to the person concerned rather than to services) and delivered through an extended multidisciplinary team (more on this below). Get raised awareness and you will also get that values-based practice is a partner to, not a substitute for, still less an opponent of, evidence-based practice (we also say more about this below). Get raised awareness, finally, and you will also get the importance of the outputs of values-based practice in balanced decisions made within frameworks of shared values.

Section 3: Values-based practice and Natalie's story

So what would a values-based understanding of Natalie's story look like? And how might values-based practice have delivered a different and more positive outcome?

Table 13.2 sets out the elements that we think are of particular relevance to understanding and responding to Natalie's story. Our comments have, of course, to be caveated with the fact that we lack first-hand understanding of the situation. That said, it does seem clear that there was little awareness of Natalie's values among those responsible for repeatedly prescribing antipsychotics (and, ultimately, forcing her to have depot medication).

Table 13.2: Elements of values-based practice highlighted by Natalie's story

Values-based practice	✓ main areas highlighted
PREMISE	
Mutual respect	No respect for what mattered to her
TEN PROCESS ELEMENTS	
Four clinical skills:	

1) Awareness	Positively evaluated voices – mattered above all to her; values of clinicians to 'treat' voices
2) Knowledge	The evidence is there
3) Reasoning	
4) Communication	No one asked her
Two aspects of clinical relationships:	
5) Person-values-centred care	Her treatment was not person-values-centred
6) The extended multidisciplinary team	
Three principles linking values-based practice and evidence-based practice:	
7) Two-feet principle	Applies – values in how her 'problem' was understood
8) Squeaky wheel principle	Applies – evidence (treating voices) seems obvious so 'think values'
9) Science-driven principle	
Partnership in decision-making:	
10) Partnership based on dissensus	No evidence of – far from shared she had no agency – pure Montgomery (see page 121)

Awareness of values is, as noted above, fundamental. Had anyone listened to Natalie (an essential component of the communication skills for values-based practice), they would have been left in no doubt just how important her voices were to her. Knowledge too could have been important. There is extensive literature indicating the very different and often positive ways in which people may value their voices.

Building on this awareness, further elements of values-based practice come into play. Mutual respect, for example, the premise of values-based practice, is essential if Natalie's values are to be taken seriously. This is so even where services are committed to a person-centred approach. If staff 'write off' Natalie's values (attributing them, for example, to 'lack of insight'), they may still impose treatment in what they take to be her best interests.

This is why person-values-centred care is important to values-based practice. As we noted in Section 1, staff may well have taken this approach guided by a 'medical' model in which voice hearing is regarded as a symptom of a disease and thus assumed to be a bad thing, whatever the person hearing the voices thinks. This is why the two-feet principle of values-based practice (all decisions 'stand' on the two 'feet' of values and evidence) (see Table 13.1) is important in Natalie's story. As Table 13.1 indicates, the two-feet principle reminds us that values as well as evidence are important in all aspects of healthcare decision-making, including, as in Natalie's story, diagnostic assessment.

What this means in practice is that, even if a medical model were an appropriate way of understanding Natalie's story, what was important to her about her 'symptoms' would still be vital to any decision about how to 'treat' them. This is true in values-based surgical care, for example – an area at the very heart of the medical model (Handa et al., 2016). So why should it not be true in values-based psychiatric care (to the extent that this is guided by the same medical model as surgery)?

Finally, then, what would values-based practice have to say about what should be done? As Table 13.1 indicates, values-based practice supports balanced decision-making within frameworks of shared values. There is, as we noted earlier, at least one shared value here: the importance attached by everyone concerned to preventing suicide. In many situations there may be a difficult balance to be struck with countervailing values such as that of the patient's freedom of choice. Positive risk management, as it is called, raises challenging values issues. But, in Natalie's story at least, it seems clear that, since her voices were 'causing no problems', and given their overwhelming importance to her, the balance of risk comes out unequivocally on the side of respecting her freedom of choice.

Section 4: Values-based practice and Liam and Susan's stories

In this section we consider Liam's and then Susan's stories along essentially the same lines as Natalie's story. As in Natalie's story, there is a sense in which values-based practice as a whole is relevant to both. Both, however, as we will see, highlight elements of values-based practice not covered in our account of Natalie's story.

Liam's story: saved by the phone

Liam was in his late 20s and had been hearing voices for more than 10 years. His voices would tell him he was useless and ugly and that everyone hated him and was staring at him. For many years, he refused to leave his flat because he thought people would hurt him. He then found he was able to manage his voices by swearing loudly at them. Although this improved his day-to-day life, it caused significant problems when he started going out. His swearing meant that people did start staring at him, avoiding him or even getting into altercations with him. After joining a hearing voices support group, he was able to negotiate with his voices while he was out, using phrases like, 'I can't deal with this now, I'll speak to you later'. This significantly improved his day-to-day life but still made him stand out when he was in public spaces. (Note: This was before mobile phones were invented. Now Liam holds one of these to his ear when he is negotiating with his voices, and no one gives him a second look.)

As with Natalie's story, Liam's values are evident from the start. Where, however, Natalie valued her voices positively, Liam valued them negatively. Many of the elements of values-based practice noted in connection with Natalie's story are thus relevant with Liam's: the importance of the values of others, of a person-values-centred approach, of balanced decision-making, and so forth.

However, Liam's story highlights two further elements of values-based practice. First, it shows the importance of the *extended* multidisciplinary team. In values-based practice, different team members bring to clinical care not only a range of knowledge and skills but also a range of values. This range of values is important as a resource for meeting the corresponding range of values presented by clients and patients. This in turn contributes to more balanced decision-making on person-values-centred care (Colombo et al., 2003).

The 'team' in question is not limited to health and social care professionals, but may extend to other agencies (housing, the police, education). Crucially in Liam's story, it included the members of a peer support group. Such a group brings precisely that combination of knowledge, experience and values that meets the needs of an individual voice hearer.

The second element of values-based practice highlighted by Liam's story is the importance of scientific and technological developments. There is a tendency to mistrust science and technology. This is fuelled by all-too-common misuses of evidence-based guidelines to override rather than complement an individual's values. This is why the science-driven principle of values-based practice spells out that science and technology actually drive the need for evidence-based practice and values-based practice to be used as partners. Why? Because scientific advances open up choices in healthcare, and with choices go values (Fulford et al., 2012; see also Box 13.2). The operative advances do not, however, have to be in medical science. In Liam's story, his choices, as the final note tells us, were opened up by the invention of the mobile phone.

Susan's story: it's the law!

Susan is in her 40s and her voice is her companion. She is well known in her small town and can often be seen on buses or in her favourite café, chatting away to her 'companion'. She gets angry if people interrupt her conversations but is otherwise polite and friendly. She has had a number of jobs but they never last and she currently lives reasonably well in her own small bedsit. She has only occasionally been harassed, but this is rare and, after the police cautioned someone for disability hate crime, people mostly leave her to her own devices.

Once again, then, values are all over Susan's story. Like Natalie, she values her voice positively. It is her companion. Like Liam (at least later in his story), there is no conflict with other people's values. Living as she does in a small town, it seems that Susan has established what amounts to a relationship of 'live and let live' with her community, consistent with the values-based premise of mutual respect.

Susan has, nonetheless, experienced occasional harassment. In values-based terms, then, there are at least some people in her community who are outside the circle of mutual respect. And, being outwith the premise of values-based practice, it was dealt with in Susan's story using another tool from the values toolkit of healthcare – the law (anti-discrimination legislation). Susan's story thus highlights the importance, when working with values, of being ready to draw appropriately on the full set of tools available from the healthcare values toolkit.

Conclusion

Although we have focused throughout on values-based practice, it is important to emphasise that values-based practice is very much a partner to evidence-based practice. This point is emphasised in Box 13.2. It is not that we need one or the other; we need both.

Box 13.2: Values and evidence

Values-based practice is, from theory (Fulford, 1989) to practical applications (Fulford et al., 2012), a partner to evidence-based practice.
The two feet principle (see Table 13.1) is about never losing sight of the values, particularly (as in our three stories) in diagnostic assessment. The '3 Keys' programme offers a values-based approach to mental health assessment (NIMHE/CSIP, 2008; Fulford et al., 2015).
The squeaky wheel principle is about never losing sight of the evidence. That people's voices are often (as with Susan) benign or even (as with Natalie) positive is widely ignored, even though the evidence has been available for many years (Johns & van Os, 2001).
The science-driven principle takes 'evidence *and* values' as a pair. Liam's use of his mobile phone is emblematic of the many contemporary technological advances promising improved self-management, not only in bodily health (for example, in diabetes) but in mental health too (see for example, Bikson et al., 2008).
Small wonder, then, that the 'values *and* evidence' partnership underpinning values-based practice is increasingly also underpinning medical law (Montgomery v Lanarkshire Health Board, 2015; Herring et al., 2017) and regulation (GMC, 2008), and the best of evidence-based practice too (Sackett et al., 2000[2]).

Shared decision-making, based on evidence and values working together in partnership, may seem a long way from the day-to-day experience of many voice hearers. However, there is increasing pressure on services, at least in the UK, to work in this way, following a 2015 Supreme Court decision called the Montgomery judgement (Montgomery v Lanarkshire Health Board, 2015). This ruling makes shared decision-making based on evidence and values the legal basis of consent to treatment in all areas of health and social care. Had Natalie had the benefit of this Supreme Court decision, perhaps she and her angel voices would be alive today.

---

2. See also the preface to all the NICE guidelines – for example, www.nice.org.uk/guidance/ng12 – and scroll down to the section 'Your Responsibility'. This includes the phrase: '... When exercising their judgement, professionals and practitioners are expected to take this guideline fully into account, alongside the individual needs, preferences and values of their patients or the people using their service.'

References

Bikson, M., Bulow, P., Stiller, J.W., Datta, A., Battaglia, F., Karnup, S.V. & Postolache, T.T. (2008). Transcranial direct current stimulation for major depression: A general system for quantifying transcranial electrotherapy dosage, *Current Treatment Options in Neurology, 10*(5), 377–385.

Colombo, A., Bendelow, G., Fulford, K.W.M. & Williams, S. (2003). Evaluating the influence of implicit models of mental disorder on processes of shared decision making within community-based multi-disciplinary teams. *Social Science & Medicine, 5,* 1557–1570.

Crepaz-Keay, D. & Binns, C. (1997). *Dancing with angels: Involving survivors in mental health training.* CCETSW.

Fulford, K.W.M. (1989). *Moral theory and medical practice.* Cambridge University Press.

Fulford, K.W.M., Dewey, S. & King, M. (2015). Values-based involuntary seclusion and treatment: Value pluralism and the UK's Mental Health Act 2007. In J.Z. Sadler, W. van Staden & K.W.M. Fulford (Eds.), *The Oxford handbook of psychiatric ethics* (Chapter 60). Oxford University Press.

Fulford, K.W.M., Peile, E. & Carroll, H. (2012). *Essential values-based practice: Clinical stories linking science with people.* Cambridge University Press.

General Medical Council (2008). *Consent: Patients and doctors making decisions together.* General Medical Council.

Handa, I.A., Fulford-Smith, L., Barber, Z.E., Dobbs, T.D., Fulford, K.W.M. & Peile, E. (2016). The importance of seeing things from someone else's point of view. *British Medical Journal, 354,* i1652.

Herring, J., Fulford, K.W.M., Dunn, D. & Handa, A. (2017). Elbow room for best practice? Montgomery, patients' values, and balanced decision-making in person-centred care. *Medical Law Review, 25*(4): 582–603

Johns, L.C. & van Os, J. (2001). The continuity of psychotic experiences in the general population. *Clinical Psychology Review, 21*(8), 1125–1141.

Montgomery v Lanarkshire Health Board (2015). Case details. The Supreme Court. www.supremecourt.uk/cases/uksc-2013-0136.html

National Collaborating Centre for Mental Health (2009). *Schizophrenia: Core interventions in the treatment and management of schizophrenia in adults in primary and secondary care.* National clinical guideline number 82. British Psychological Society/Royal College of Psychiatrists.

NIMHE (National Institute for Mental Health in England) & CSIP (Care Services Improvement Partnership) (2008). *3 keys to a shared approach in mental health assessment.* Department of Health.

Sackett, D.L., Straus, S.E., Scott Richardson, W., Rosenberg, W. & Haynes, R.B. (2000). *Evidence-based medicine: How to practise and teach EBM* (2nd ed.). Churchill Livingstone.

Further information

For more information on all aspects of values-based practice including a reading guide and free downloadable materials, please go to the website for the Collaborating Centre for Values-based Practice in Health and Social Care, St Catherine's College, Oxford at: https://valuesbasedpractice.org/more-about-vbp

For information on a voice-hearers network hosted by the Centre and convened by David Crepaz-Keay, please go to: https://valuesbasedpractice.org/what-do-we-do/networks/

14 An invitation to dialogue: what we can all learn from Open Dialogue and Hearing Voices Networks

Olga Runciman and Iseult Twamley

In this chapter, psychologists, Open Dialogue (OD) practitioners and Hearing Voices Network (HVN) members Olga Runciman and Iseult Twamley, one a voice hearer and one a family member, will share experiences of being in and working with networks in crisis, families and people with unshared realities. In particular, we wish to explore the contribution of the values and practices of dialogue that are common to OD and HVNs and that we have found profoundly helpful when working with voices.

Hearing Voices Networks are part of the Hearing Voices Movement (HVM). Both OD and HVNs offer alternatives to a biomedically based approach to hearing voices. For many voice hearers, their social network and professionals, the biomedical approach to hearing voices can privilege the expertise of the mental health professional, pay insufficient and reductionist attention to the context and life experience of the voice hearer (that is, not enough interest in really understanding the context within which these experiences occur), and rely heavily on psychotropic medication and hospitalisation as forms of treatment. The dominance of such a biomedical approach may result in some very questionable views on how seriously people with certain diagnoses should be taken, as is highlighted by the following quote by the former chair of the Danish psychiatric foundation:

> It is open to question whether schizophrenic patients, with their lack of insight into their illness and their cognitive deficiencies, are able to assess their own situation and to evaluate and describe their psychic state and the positive/negative effects of the medication given to them. (Larsen & Gerlach, 1996).

However, notwithstanding such ongoing attitudes in the arenas of mental health practice and research, there is now also a paradigm shift occurring in the field of mental health practice and research, driven by the hopes and pressures from services users, family members and practitioners to have more rights-based mental health services, with less emphasis on medication and hospitalisation (Johnstone & Boyle, 2018; United Nations Office of the High Commissioner, 2019). Some mental health services in various Western countries are consequently starting to shift towards a more inclusive and collaborative practice across disciplines, in which service users, family members and the wider communities are more actively involved.

The awareness that there is an identified need for a human rights-based approach to mental health that privileges the voice and understandings of the voice hearer and allows each person to find their own understandings and supports as is right for them, is growing and increasingly supported by formal and informal mental health bodies and organisations (CMHNN, 2015; United Nations Office of the High Commissioner, 2019). We hope to speak in this chapter about the respective contributions of both the OD and HVN approaches and what they can offer voice hearers, families and professionals in finding a new way to talk to and support each other. Specifically, we will be looking at:

- the **similarities and differences** between the OD and the HVN approaches using the seven principles of OD
- the challenge of **'being with'** each other when distressing voices are present
- presenting principles and values from OD, and how they may help us all to listen to **hear all of the voices** in the room and within people
- **power and uncertainty** – how lived experience can offer a pathway for connection to 'the other' and what can be learnt from that wisdom, drawing on the dialogical experience of HVN meetings.

We hope that the chapter will offer hope and guidance for all who live with distressing voices, and those who love them or hope to connect with them.

Open Dialogue and Hearing Voices Networks

As internationally active OD trainers, we are quite aware of the increasing interest shown in recent years by various mainstream mental health organisations and social care services in a variety of Western countries in being trained and helped to implement the valuable contribution that OD 'dialogic' approaches can make to their services. OD is a values- and principles-led approach to the delivery of care that involves network involvement and shared decision-making. It has already found some improved outcomes over the usual offer of services (Seikkula et al., 2011; see also Chapter 27 by Mark Hopfenbeck in this book).

Similarly, HVNs take a two-pronged approach in which voice hearers work together in shared activism for better understandings and support. Among the key foundations are the community self-help groups where people gather to share their unusual or unshared experiences and together try to create meaning and understandings (Intervoice, n.d.).

Rather than using particular strategies or interventions, the collaborative and dialogical practice that characterises both OD and HVNs demonstrates a philosophical and ethical stance in the way that therapeutic conversations are conducted (Anderson 1997, 2001). They thus express a postmodernist approach that maintains that human reality is created through social construction and dialogue.

Within this way of dialogic working, we meet each other from a not-knowing stance, or the position of a curious and respectful learner. The voice hearer is the expert on their concerns, struggles, goals, and preferred outcomes. In an OD practice setting, this may take the form of the practitioner(s) engaging with the client and their social and relational network (those people that they feel are important in their lives), to understand and resolve the current crisis. Within HVNs, as they are peer led and community based, voice hearers engage with each other, in group dialogues, to explore shared and unique meanings and understandings.

Few have contemplated drawing on the knowledge of HVNs and OD and combining this knowledge where possible. Yet, when we look at the seven principles from OD in the chart below, we can see some remarkable parallels between the HVN and OD approach, albeit from very different positions of power, acceptance and structure. Both approaches are quite explicit in putting similar ethical values and principles at their heart and both appear to have the potential to address at least some of the changes hoped for and demanded by many service users and some professionals, as highlighted above. As there has been a lot of collaboration and mutual endorsement, as well as some critiquing in practice, between the two approaches in recent years, it seems only right to be considering the respective differences, similarities and contributions in more detail, which is what this chapter will do.

The origins of HVNs and OD

HVNs and OD emerged separately around the same time in the late 1980s and came into being in response to voice hearers' needs not being met by the established mental health systems. Both introduced the then novel idea of valuing and honouring the voice and expertise of the person suffering the distress. Both approaches respectively developed skills, theories and ways of helping through learning and cooperating together, where transparency in the process was paramount for all. 'Nothing about me without me' was a value that drove the development of both methodologies.

One significant difference is that, right from the start, the HVNs valued professionals playing a role in the wider movement, even though the HVNs themselves were driven by people with lived voice-hearing experience. In contrast, OD, which was originally developed by professionals (such as psychiatrists and psychologists), did not invite those it is intended to help to play an active 'helper' role. This only really changed in any significant way when Open Dialogue UK started the first ever Finnish-model, three-year OD practitioner training in the UK in 2015. Some people who were active within the HVM felt that OD could offer a good complementary alternative and formal structure for the implementation of many of the values that were already considered important and being lived out within the HVM. The OD approach seemed to offer a vehicle within which at least some important values could be integrated better into mainstream service provision. As a consequence, some very active members of the HVM and HVNs, along with Open Dialogue UK, initiated a dialogue with the OD trainers and pointed out the need for greater 'expert-by-experience' involvement, and so the first five people with lived experience were trained as full OD practitioners (Olga being one of them).[1]

Comparing OD and HVNs

Using the seven principles of OD as a basis on which to compare the differences and similarities between this approach and the HVN approach, it is possible to see just how much their values and ideas seem to overlap.

Table 14.1: Similarities and *differences**

	'Bottom up' HVN A space for multiple truths/*Power imbalance less prevalent here*	'Top down' OD A space for multiple truths
1	Immediate help	Immediate help
2	Network/*The group of voice hearers is the network; all are in 'the same boat'*	Network/*Person in crisis gathers a network of their choice working with therapists/OD practitioners*
3	Flexibility/mobility	Flexibility/mobility
4	Responsibility/*Group and voice hearer are jointly responsible*	Responsibility/*Professionals and network are responsible*
5	Psychological continuity/*Groups continue, but people change in them.*	Psychological continuity/*Attempt to keep the same therapists/OD practitioners, or at least one of them, present over time*
6	Tolerance of uncertainty/*Very high, as there is no choice to lock someone up if what they say creates fear in others*	Tolerance of uncertainty/*Is an active choice and has to be learned – the most challenging concept for professionals*
7	Dialogical, listening, curiosity, acceptance, multiple truths, no dominant truth	Dialogical, listening, curiosity, acceptance, multiple truths, no dominant truth
8	Training/*No training – only experience needed before being able to offer support*	Training/*Fairly extensive therapeutic training needed as an OD practitioner before support can be offered*

* Please note, this is a very simple differential list and is meant to be an inspiration for further discussion rather than exhaustive.

---

1. http://opendialogueapproach.co.uk/training/full/

The most profound differences can be seen in the placement and power structures. For example, the OD approach is part of the established mental health system and operates *within* it, while the HVN approach is positioned largely *outside* of the mainstream provision of mental health services. Both have advantages and disadvantages. However, an awareness of these power structures and differentials often does not appear to be part of a differentiated mainstream mental health service discourse. Nevertheless, as highlighted above, the power disparities between psychiatric professionals and the psychiatric and related legal system and its patients are vast, leading to experiences of abuse for some. Based on our extensive international travelling as OD trainers, we are also aware of a deep wish for change among many mental health professionals and for humanity to have a far greater presence within psychiatry. We therefore believe that these two approaches, similar in values, but with different positioning within society, have something valuable to offer to anyone who is hearing voices or seeking to support people who hear voices.

> ### Learning point 1
>
> Before going any further, perhaps you would like to reflect on the following questions:
>
> - How do these values and ideas from OD and the HVN relate to your own ideas and practices?
> - What might it offer to you to draw on these two approaches with regards to hearing voices? What might be the challenges?
> - What might these values and ideas offer the person who is hearing distressing voices?

On being with vs about

In OD, we offer dialogue in crisis. Often when in crisis, we hope for certainty, so that we can know what is wrong and how to fix it. Traditional models of mental health services aim to meet this need for certainty. However, aspiring to certainty often creates the dynamic that dissent to a majority view is dismissed and voices go unheard.

When we hear/experience things that others do not, we are alone in an unshared reality. This can be the most damaging aspect of these experiences, for to be human is to be in a relationship with another person or other people. Typically, people who hear distressing voices and seek help have trauma in their lives (Varese et al., 2012), yet the consequences of this aspect of people's lives are often underestimated, or even ignored within traditional mental health service provision.

What we see, both in our Western societies and in biologically dominated mental health practice, is that unusual or challenging 'utterances' are not responded to, and are met by being ignored or a change of subject; or they are responded to with worry or a need to fix or diagnose. Family members may also feel unsure and scared in response to a loved one's unusual or unshared experiences.

In these situations, we regularly move from being with the other to othering and thinking 'about' them. This denial of someone's reality is quite literally mad making. As the psychologist, reformist and campaigner Lucy Johnstone writes, 'Re-defining someone's reality for them is the most insidious and the most devastating form of power we can use' (Johnstone, 2013). It is perhaps not accidental that this dynamic is also typical of abuse situations, where disclosing one's reality can have dangerous and isolating consequences for individuals caught in toxic situations.

Dialogue, in contrast, is not a direct route to certainty. Instead, it brings in new perspectives and understandings (which can initially feel less stable!). Dialogue also creates a richness that we will explore below. For now, we would like to acknowledge that talking and listening and feeling together can be extremely challenging in a crisis. It is helpful, however, when the emphasis is placed on creating a dialogue 'together'. If we don't reject or seek to change or define another's reality, we can instead bring a respectful and compassionate curiosity to a dialogue. If we remember that we can never truly know another, we can approach dialogue with an openness to learning something new about the person (and potentially ourselves).

The OD approach and the HVN approach both ask us to come out from behind the safety and distancing measures of diagnosis and treatment. Sadly, many mental health professionals' trainings either ignore or insufficiently address how to 'be with' such experiences, like hearing voices or other unshared realities, or be with strong and unpleasantly experienced emotions. Being with people in such a new way seems to be well described by psychologist and psychotherapist Tawio Afuape (2011), who writes: 'This way involves an opening of hearts with a willingness on the part of the therapist to have theirs broken.' In such dialogues, we have the opportunity and the challenge of being in a deeper relationship where capacity for change can come about both for oneself and the other, precisely because the emphasis is not primarily on changing an unpleasant feeling of reality; rather, it is on being with the uncertainty of that unpleasantness or distress.

In the OD approach, we take time to explore together what is happening and how it is understood and experienced by the various participants at an OD meeting. This means, for example, staying with words that are used and exploring what they mean for the speaker, while not assuming a shared understanding.

Ultimately, we hope to engage in a process of meaning-making where we are in dialogue with the people involved, so that we can create space for new understandings. This is a very different position to traditional models of 'giving' understanding (be this in the form of medical diagnoses or theory-bound formulations).

Family member perspective (Iseult): As a family member of someone who was receiving traditional mental health service provision, I was not included or invited into discussions of the voice hearer's care. Diagnoses, understandings and decisions happened outside of the network. There was no opportunity for shared meaning making – there was no opportunity to understand or hear about the voice hearer's experience – and in that, both the voice hearer and the family were left to manage as best as we could, separately and alone. OD could have offered us the opportunity to listen to each other and meet in the point of crisis.

Voice hearer perspective (Olga): As a voice hearer, I found becoming a patient led to isolation, fear and hopelessness, as decisions about my care were made for me, not with me. Meetings about me were held behind closed doors and I was left to try and explain this catastrophic crisis as best as I could to my bewildered family. Family meetings, when present, were informational in nature rather than dialogical. Although staff did their best, I believe that, had OD been an option, this crisis could have resulted in growth and healing rather than years of distress while being separated from each other.

Learning point 2

We invite you to reflect on the following questions:

- Dialogue asks of us, can we bring a compassionate curiosity to our own experience and to that of others? Are we willing to meet the other?
- Where in your life and practice have you experienced this?
- What supports might you need to create more space for 'being with' another person? What would that look like? Who might partner with you in this?

Many voices (polyphony)

Western mental health services tend to support adults separately from their contexts and their networks (Johnstone & Boyle, 2018). However, like all living beings, humans are also products of their environments. We believe that working with our communities provides the best opportunity for healing. Relationships with friends and family are also what people identify as being most important for their mental health recovery (Faulkner & Layzell, 2000).

Both in the OD approach and in the HVN approach, we bring the support of the collective to the situation, which may pinnacle in a famous catchphrase of OD: 'We never leave them alone.' This idea is core to both the HVN approach and to the OD approach. In OD, we encourage people to invite those who are closest to them to attend the meeting. HVNs, similarly, provide voice-hearing groups to share unshared realities and form a community for each other.

In these dialogical spaces we come together to create a shared language for the situation we find ourselves in. When welcoming all of the voices, including those heard only by the person who hears voices, it is important to create rich and real understandings. In this way of approaching distress, co-creating the story of our experience(s) is critical for ownership and agency over the way forward. In an article on 'Symptom or Experience: Does language matter?' (2013), Rai Waddingham, a well-known advocate, activist, consultant and trainer within the HVM, writes movingly of her experience of 'weaving her own story'

In our experience of holding OD meetings, hearing all the voices can be very challenging. Some voices can lead to a professional feeling anxious, so they move from a position of listening to interviewing and intervening. We have learnt instead to 'slow down… and move in'; that is, we give more space and time for these less heard (and sometimes less welcome) voices and become curious about these moments. This equally applies to us – it is important that we give attention and compassion to the voices within ourselves, and dialogical work actively invites us to be in dialogue with those voices as well.

When we consider *every* voice as expert, we aspire to listen without conditions and without aiming for a specific outcome. As Seikkula and Arnkil (2014) note when writing about the OD approach, this is a radical idea in both psychiatry and psychotherapy. It challenges all those who are present to be equally responsible for the 'answers' that may or may not emerge. It invites us to welcome different and dissenting perspectives, rather than aim for agreement. This is often a significant challenge for mental health professionals and systems, where there can be an assumption of primary truths that can be found through professional assessment (diagnosis being an obvious example), leading to 'appropriate' treatment. We even have a language that can pathologise disagreement: for example, when we talk of a 'lack of insight' or 'non-compliance'. When the service users' voices have equal weight, we need to be open to different understandings and solutions. We need to practise saying, 'I don't know', so that we foster a space where uncertainty can be valued. In our experience, this is ultimately more helpful in finding constructive ways forward, and more humane.

Multiple truths – that is, that there are many ways of seeing things that may be contradictory but all hold truth – are an important tenet of these approaches and we see this in full fruition in HVN groups. All who are present may share stories that are both separate from and also resonate with the stories of the others. Thus a sacred space connecting us to a reality that transcends our fears is co-created, where honouring the stories becomes the most healing aspect of all. The OD approach, offering common ground to create a joint language of understanding, can provide healing within the network and the person suffering distress. Thus, together, participants of OD network meetings and of HVN groups create a richness that exceeds what each could do separately.

Family member perspective: In traditional mental health services, voice hearers are often met alone, and their family (if met at all) are met separately. The information that is shared in such meetings is often short and un-nuanced – such as a label or diagnosis. Stories and truths held by the network about the voice hearer, the family and the life surrounding the current crisis are routinely not shared – stories that might shed important light on shared trauma or existing strengths. OD would offer an opportunity to hear from everyone that the voice hearer wished to invite; it would also offer the chance to hear different professional discussions and perspectives that are otherwise shared behind closed doors.

Voice hearer perspective: A system that has the power and the right to interpret a voice hearer's truths creates multiple moral and ethical dilemmas as well as the potential to harm: 'When we name you a "schizophrenic", we take away your speech and your ability to name yourself; we obliterate you.' The moral position that we must adopt [instead] is one in which we bear witness and resistance. To bear witness means accepting the reality of lives harmed and damaged by many things, including psychiatry.' (Bracken & Thomas, 2009). The HVN and the OD approaches allow these multiple truths to unfold and be present in equal value and can offer a chance for a more democratic health care system to evolve which is something most mental health staff long for.

> *Learning point 3*
>
> Things that may be of help to reflect over:
>
> - How willing am I not to know, as in: Am I willing to admit to not having the solution or the answer?
> - What happens to me, and to the dialogue, when I accept that I cannot fix the other person?
> - How can I invite the expertise of lived experience (including my own) into my work and into dialogues with others?
> - What voices do I find hard to hear? How can I create a space to hear all of the voices, even those that are challenging?

Tolerance of uncertainty

One of the principles of OD that is the most difficult to put into practice (particularly within the psychiatric context) is that of tolerating uncertainty. To be in the space of uncertainty can often cause distress, anxiety and a sense of a lack of control. When this is combined with mental health hierarchical systems that have already predefined who are the experts and who are not, uncertainty can become extremely challenging, and this may result in an instinctual desire to remove it. This can be particularly prevalent when risk situations occur and there is a perceived need to invoke legally sanctioned compulsory treatment.

The principle of tolerating uncertainty is also where the HVN and the OD approaches differ, and where we believe that the HVN approach can contribute in profound ways by providing skills to enable us to be present in a state of uncertainty.

Tolerating uncertainty is at the heart of OD. It means to give space to and value the importance of polyphony, thereby avoiding rapid conclusions and hasty decisions, while creating a sense of safety. We believe that the point of crisis is to have a place where new meanings and truths can be found. It can also be the place where we can feel most dangerously separate and unconnected. Therefore, it is the most important place to have dialogue. If we can't tolerate the uncertainty of what is happening, we resort to monologue, often resulting in attempts to take control and give primacy to professional or powerful voices and decisions.

Tolerating uncertainty is something to be learned by unlearning traditional psychiatric ways of thinking, while challenging power structures and the concept of control both systemically and personally. In this regard, positioning the OD approach within the mental health system opens the door to the ever-present risk of OD itself also exercising systemic power, such as in the use of force or coercion. On the other hand, a strength of working within the system is that this can lead to and inspire ways of humanising traditional mental health systems.

Tolerating uncertainty is the most important and most challenging principle of OD, and many of the other principles can be understood as ways of supporting us to stay with uncertainty. In our OD implementation in Ireland (Twamley, 2019), we grew to understand the importance of personal and structural supports within the system to allow us to develop our uncertainty muscles – for example, in reflective spaces, supervision and organisational policies.

HVN groups, on the other hand, work in constant uncertainty. There are no systemic power differentials other than those that are formed between people within the context of the relationships that are present. Therefore, when uncertainty is the norm, it paradoxically becomes less visible, fading into the tapestry of the stories that are being interwoven by the group. It strengthens the 'being with' that is necessary for co-creating a shared language when talking about that which has not yet found words.

Significantly, when the power to decide over another is not a possibility, it allows for conversations that often cause interventions elsewhere to be present. An example could be suicide. Rarely is it possible to find a space to discuss the wish to end one's own life and truly be listened to, with no interventions. Uncertainties in these situations must be borne and absorbed by the group – if we do not have the systemic power to stop or control it, dialogue *is* all that we have.

We would like to encourage you as professionals to invite these multiple voices in, be curious, embrace uncertainty and 'be with' the voices, so that it becomes possible to break through the barriers of fear and uncertainty, in order that your work with voice hearers becomes more compassionate and healing.

Family member perspective: As a family member, when a loved one starts to hear voices we do not hear, it can feel scary and wrong. We don't share the experience; we don't know what the voices are saying, or what the experience might mean. In particular, when distress is involved, we may feel helpless and unsure as to how to respond. In traditional mental health services, voice hearers may be taken away, through hospitalisation or private appointments, and families are no wiser as to how to 'be with' their loved one when they are discharged, or how to discuss these unusual experiences. OD takes the time to talk and understand together before making big decisions, and those decisions can be made with everyone important present. Equally, OD, in tolerating uncertainty, opens the possibility that voice hearing may be positive; may be understandable; may be lived with. These are all perspectives that family members might otherwise not have any knowledge of.

A voice hearer perspective: For many who begin to hear voices for the first time, it can be an uncertain and scary situation. If there is no possibility to explore and be in the space of 'not knowing' with others and instead you are subjected to treatment protocols to get rid of the voices, fear inevitably enters the picture. This fear becomes the dominating but often untalked-about underlying driving force on how families, staff and the voice hearer themselves interact. To be able to be curious about this unexplored unknown space opens the door to meaning making for all involved. I often wonder how many years of being in the mental health system could have been avoided if the HVN and/or OD perspective of tolerating uncertainty had been present, so meaning-making could have been a possibility.

Learning point 4

Perhaps you would like to reflect on the following questions:

- What does the feeling of uncertainty awaken in you?
- How does uncertainty affect dialogue in your experience? What about the interplay of power and dialogue? What personal or structural supports are available to you to support you in tolerating uncertainty? What other resources might be needed?

Conclusion

We hope that this brief introduction to the potential interplay between the HVN and OD approaches, as well as to the dialogical ideas that are so meaningful to us, has aroused a curiosity in you and a desire to learn more. OD, by being placed within psychiatry, has the potential to bridge and invite the multitude of voices that exist within the established system and, more importantly, the voices of those who are traditionally silenced: the voice hearers and their networks. HVNs add a whole new integral dimension to OD by being placed outside psychiatry, and by its rich knowledge and tradition for valuing the stories that people carry within them and its history of challenging systemic power structures. Together, they offer the possibility of implementing into practice a widely encountered deep wish among many mental health professionals for a paradigmatic change and for humanity to play a far greater role within psychiatry and thus become a reality. Approaching distress from a dialogical vantage point, as found in OD and HVN groups, can open doors to a whole new way of being.

For those of us who have walked that path have found our lives have become richer and more meaningful for it.

References

Afuape, T. (2011). *Power, resistance and liberation in therapy with survivors of trauma: To have our hearts broken*. Routledge.

Anderson, H. (1997). *Conversation, language, and possibilities: A postmodern approach to therapy*. Basic Books.

Anderson, H. (2001). Postmodern collaborative and person-centered therapies: What would Carl Rogers say? *Journal of Family Therapy, 4*(23), 339-360. doi: 10.1111/1467-6427.00189

Bracken, P. & Thomas, P. (2009). *Postpsychiatry: Mental health in a postmodern world*. Oxford University Press

Critical Mental Health Nurses Network (2015). *Best wishes from the CMHNN to the World Hearing Voices Congress*. [Blog]. https://criticalmhnursing.org/2015/11/04/best-wishes-from-the-cmhnn-to-the-7th-world-hearing-voices-congress/#more-376

Faulkner, A. & Layzell, S. (2000). *Strategies for living*. Mental Health Foundation.

Intervoice (n.d). *About Intervoice: Values and vision*. www.intervoiceonline.org/about-intervoice/values-vision

Johnstone, L. (2013, January 1).Time to abolish psychiatric diagnosis. *Mad in America*. www.madinamerica.com/2013/01/time-to-abolish-psychiatric-diagnosis

Johnstone, L., Boyle, M. with Cromby, J., Dillon, J., Harper, D., Kinderman, P., Longden, E., Pilgrim, D. & Read, J. (2018). *The Power Threat Meaning Framework: Towards the identification of patterns in emotional distress, unusual experiences and troubled or troubling behaviour, as an alternative to functional psychiatric diagnosis*. British Psychological Society.

Larsen, E.B. & Gerlach, J. (1996). Subjective experience of treatment, side-effects, mental state and quality of life in chronic schizophrenic out-patients treated with depot neuroleptics. *Acta Psychiatrica Scandinavica, 93*, 381–388.

Seikkula, J. & Arnkil, T. (2014). *Open dialogues and anticipations: Respecting the otherness in the present moment*. THL.

Seikkula, J., Alakare, B. & Aaltonen, J. (2011). The comprehensive open-dialogue approach in Western Lapland: II. Long-term stability of acute psychosis outcomes in advanced community care. *Psychosis, 3*(3), 192–204.

Twamley, I. (2019). Reluctant revolutionaries: Implementing Open Dialogue in a community mental health team. In H. Gijbels, L. Sapouna & G. Sidley (Eds.), *Inside out, outside in: Transforming mental health practices* (pp.93–115). PCCS Books.

United Nations Office of the High Commissioner (renewed 2019, October 7). *Special Rapporteur on the right to physical and mental health*. United Nations. www.ohchr.org/en/issues/health/pages/srrighthealthindex.aspx

Varese, F., Smeets, F. & Drukker, M. (2012). Childhood trauma increases the risk of psychosis: A meta analysis of patient-control, prospective and cross sectional cohort studies. *Schizophrenia Bulletin, 38*(4), 661–671.

Waddingham, R. (2013). Symptom or experience: Does language matter? *Mad in America*. www.madinamerica.com/2013/08/does-language-matter

15 Medication and voices: reflections from a relational perspective

Dirk Corstens and Joachim Schnackenberg

As workers in mental health organisations, we meet a lot of voice hearers who use psychoactive medications that are intended to silence voices, but do not do so. Others are suffering from unwanted effects of the medication. One could argue that the medication is not working. This we consider too simplistic. It is possible to live with voices without medication, but it doesn't mean that you can simply stop taking it. We promote choice. Tapering off medication is not always possible, but nor is it always impossible. In this chapter we want first to present evidence and then approach the prescription and taking of medication from a relational perspective, in order to promote choice.

While antipsychotic medication remains the main intervention offered to people who are distressed by their voice-hearing experience, it is important to emphasise that recent research findings have cast increasing doubt on their relative benefits over their unwanted effects.

In what follows, some key points of the current scientific discourse are considered in relation to medication. For a more detailed view, the second edition of Joanna Moncrieff's book, *A Straight Talking Introduction to Psychiatric Drugs* (2020), may also be useful.

Effectiveness of medication for voice-hearing related distress

Antipsychotic medication is primarily prescribed for people with diagnoses like schizophrenia or schizoaffective disorder. The assumption here is that it treats an underlying biological illness. However, there is no evidence to confirm that it does indeed treat such an underlying biological illness (Moncrieff, 2020), or that these diagnoses even have a firm biological causation that could be treated with medication (Johnstone & Boyle, 2018). Antipsychotics are in practice also often used to attempt to bring about symptomatic relief for people with other diagnoses, such as bipolar disorder or personality disorder.

It is also important to remember in this context that antipsychotic medication research has generally not specifically been designed to answer the question of whether the medication helps with voices-related distress specifically, but whether it helps in treating the assumed underlying illness. However, voice-related distress is one of the many experiences commonly called 'symptoms' that are considered in this type of research, and on several rating scales they are one of many experiences that are rated separately, alongside other experiences such as how clear the thinking is or whether someone's behaviour is considered to be normal. In this way one can see whether there is an impact on the voices-related distress too.

Meta-analytic studies (considered by most researchers to be the most reliable form of evidence available, as they summarise all relevant studies of a particular research question) have found that the newer antipsychotics are more effective than placebo for only 18% of people taking them over longer periods. Those 18% said to have benefitted also often did not meet the 20% threshold of symptomatic distress improvement that is normally considered to be a minimum clinical improvement (Leucht et al., 2009a). Looking at the 15 most widely used antipsychotics, the older-generation antipsychotics were just as effective as the newer ones (Leucht et al., 2013). When pooling all of the data in relation to antipsychotics' effects in acute episodes for people who take these medications over longer periods, only 9% were found to have at least a 50% improvement in symptom distress, which is considered to be a good response in research terms (Leucht et al., 2017).

These studies conclude that the medication's efficacy may have been overestimated and the placebo effect underestimated. They also pose the question whether improved methodology in recent years has led to smaller effects. At the same time, the authors are claiming that it shows that these medications are working similarly well to medication used in other areas of medicine (Leucht et al., 2009b). As is clear, some authors and practitioners consider this to be sufficient evidence for the importance that antipsychotic medication plays in the support of people who hear voices.

Others – as is normal in research and practice communities – question the methodology of the studies used to come to the conclusions of their effectiveness. For example, people in the placebo groups were often swapped over very quickly from taking antipsychotic medication to taking placebo medication, without an adequate tapering off process, which may have led to withdrawal symptoms that may have been confused for a relapse. There are many other factors that can be used to criticise the methodology employed, which, if taken into account, could indicate smaller positive effects of the medication (DGSP, 2018; Aderhold & Weinmann, 2020; Moncrieff, 2020).

There is also an increasing awareness of potential negative longer-term effects, such as increased mortality (Weinmann et al., 2009) and brain volume reductions (Huhtaniska, 2017). These are in addition to well-known side effects, such as tardive dyskinesia, sexual dysfunction and extra-pyramidal side effects (Moncrieff, 2020). It is also not clear if antipsychotic medication, if taken for longer than two years, does in fact help recovery (Sohler et al., 2015), and there is some indication that it may, in fact, hinder recovery processes in some people (Moncrieff, 2020; Harrow et al., 2021).

There are also some ongoing questions about exactly how these drugs work. While it is assumed that many of them work by decreasing dopamine activity in the brain, it remains unclear whether this is the main reason for the perceived benefits that some people consider these medications to have. Could it be that the reason for their perceived benefits is, for example, also down to their blunting effect on emotions or their restricting effects on thoughts and behaviour (Moncrieff, 2020)? It would seem to be a difficult ethical dilemma to justify prescribing medication against emotions, thoughts and behaviour – even if these can be perceived to be associated with some quite frightening or disturbing behaviour at times.

It is important to point out that this chapter is not trying to say that antipsychotic medication has no role to play. It clearly is one tool among many that are available. It seems important, though, to ensure proper informed consent has been given by the people who are taking the medications. This includes giving more information on the current knowledge on efficacy and unwanted effects (some of which we outlined above) and a greater emphasis on choice than appears often to be common practice at the moment.

Many of the above-mentioned problems with medication are increasingly widely recognised (Servonnet et al., 2021). This has, for example, also led to an increasing number of studies starting to look at the possibility of intermittent use of antipsychotic medication (DGPPN, 2019), and to research initiatives like the Antipsychotic-Induced Brain Changes (APIC) study, led by the University of Aachen and funded by the Federal Republic of Germany,[1,2] seeking answers to the question, 'Are antipsychotics neurotoxic or neuroprotective?'

The unwanted effects and, in the view of many, insufficient positive effects of medication have also led to the development of non-medication approaches to managing the distressing experiences, or 'symptoms', that are associated with diagnoses of schizophrenia or psychosis. Many of them are still in development, such as using MRI scans to help a person detect activity in their brains when they hear voices. Others, like some of the talking approaches introduced in this book, have been around for many years – even if only practised by some people so far.

In view of the many unwanted and limited positive effects, some people may feel they would like to stop or reduce their medication more significantly than their practitioners might feel happy with. It is important to remember that any reduction attempt should ideally be done in agreement with your supporting team and ideally in combination with working on alternative ways of coping with your experiences before, during and after the reduction process, such as an improved way of dealing with one's emotions (Hall, 2012; Schlimme et al., 2018).

---

1. www.rwth-aachen.de

2. www.rwth-aachen.de/go/id/feby?lidx=1

It is also important not to simply stop medication outright, but to do it gradually, since it is possible to experience potentially severe withdrawal symptoms. Such withdrawal symptoms may be made worse by, for example, the brain possibly having developed an increased number of dopamine neurotransmitters and also more dopamine receptors to balance out the suppression of dopamine and other activities through the medication (DGSP, 2015; Servonnet & Samaha, 2020). If one were to withdraw too quickly, then the brain would still be working overtime, so to speak, as if it was still working against the suppression through the medication. It is possible to become overwhelmed or psychotic simply by withdrawing too quickly before the brain has had time to adjust (this is sometimes referred to as rebound or super-sensitivity psychosis) (Moncrieff, 2020; Servonnet &, Samaha, 2020). This is why one needs to take time over it and be careful in the process.

For many years, reducing or stopping antipsychotic medication was not even considered to be possible or advisable and there are consequently still not enough studies on how to do this well. Many practitioners are not aware of, or do not have a lot of experience in, how to support people well in reducing antipsychotic medication. However, an increasing number of people have successfully come off antipsychotic medication or supported people professionally in coming off medication (DGSP, 2015; Schlimme et al., 2018). These experiences have now, for the first time, even been fed into a national guideline in Germany (DGPPN, 2019). It is good to consult these or other guidelines before embarking on a reduction of medication. Some key take-away points from these German national guidelines (DGPPN, 2019) include:

- There can be a number of physical, emotional and mental health-related symptoms associated with significant dose reduction or after a rapid stopping of antipsychotics. These symptoms can develop within days or weeks after reducing or stopping the medication, too, and often only improve after weeks. In practice, there can be a risk of confusing these withdrawal symptoms with a relapse.

- When reducing medication, this should be done in steps of roughly between 5% and 20% of the current dose, with a period of several weeks of stability on the reduced dose before reducing further. Based on experience, it is also clear that, before reducing down to a very small or zero dose, the last steps should be taken in very small reductions, with an openness to finishing the process on a low dose, if it is considered too difficult to stop completely.

There are also several good English-language sources of advice and information about how to come off psychiatric drugs (see, for example, Hall, 2012; Moncrieff, 2020, Chapter 9; Timimi, 2021, pp.102–107). The Mind website also offers helpful advice on the process.[3]

---

3. www.mind.org.uk/information-support/drugs-and-treatments/antipsychotics/coming-off-antipsychotics

For people who are considering taking, reducing or stopping their antipsychotic medication, British critical psychiatrist Joanna Moncrieff, who has published extensively on psychiatric drugs, advises that they ask their psychiatrist or support team some or all of the following questions (Moncrieff, 2020, p.169):

1. What sort of drug-induced state does the drug produce? What does it feel like to take it and how will it affect my mental abilities and my normal emotional reactions? How will it affect my body and what physical effects will I experience?
2. What happens if I use the drug continuously for weeks or months? Do the immediate effects persist or are they lost as the body adapts? Do other effects emerge? Do I need to keep increasing the dose to maintain the effect I initially wanted?
3. What is the evidence that the drug will help me with my particular problems? How large are the effects shown in research and will they make a meaningful difference to my life?
4. What are my chances of recovering or improving without taking drug treatment?
5. What alternative approaches could I try?
6. What is the shortest time I can take the drug for and get a worthwhile benefit?
7. What happens when I stop the drug? What withdrawal symptoms might occur? How severe are they, how long do they last and how can they be avoided?
8. What does research say about whether the drug causes long-lasting or permanent damage to some brain or body systems?
9. Will health services support me if I decide not to use drugs, or use them briefly and then stop them, even if this is not what is recommended?

According to Moncrieff (2020), mental health professionals do not yet have sufficient answers to all of these questions. However, it is important to ask them anyway and hope that the research community will increasingly pick up on the need to provide answers.

In what follows, Dirk Corstens will expand a little on what he has found helpful in his own practice as a psychiatrist.

What happens in mental health practice

'Can you help me to get rid of my voices'? A very understandable question, when you're tormented by voices. This is a request, though, that fits right into the medical model, the model most used by psychiatrists. This model perceives voices as a symptom of illness. Like bacteria have to be killed when they cause infection, voices have to be silenced, according to that approach. Medication is offered as a lifeline. The driving assumption is that voices *can* be silenced. Both practitioner and the voice hearer are afraid of the voices. They share the same aim. To get rid of them. As a practitioner, you do exactly what the patient asks. You think you help the patient to have a better life. And sometimes that seems to work. But often it doesn't. A missed chance, in my opinion.

'No, I don't hear voices at all'. As a practitioner, you have heard from people who are close to the patient – relatives, neighbours – that she (or he, of course, but I will use she here for convenience) is doing things that don't belong to her normal way of life. She is aggressive, she does dangerous things, threatens other people. This is not how she is, though. She speaks loudly when she is alone. Often, she screams. She makes other people feel afraid. There is a great pressure on you as a practitioner to do something in order to prevent her harming herself or others. Compulsory treatment is considered. Building up a relationship with someone who denies that they hear voices is difficult. If medication helps, it is often rejected when there is no compulsion to take it anymore. This can keep practitioner and voice hearer in a lifelong compulsory grasp.

There is no solid evidence that so-called antipsychotic medication helps *eliminate* voices, as we have outlined above. Most of the research literature on medication and voices is about schizophrenia, which is itself a highly disputable concept (Bentall, 2003, 2009), or about psychosis, which is different from hearing voices. Research has not been done on hearing voices as a single target for medication. Regarding psychosis, you need to treat six people who are getting antipsychotics over longer periods to have a response that is not even very strongly beyond the placebo effect *in only one person*. In research terms, this is known as numbers needed to treat (NNT) (McCarthy-Jones, 2017, p.216). This is not a very high success rate in my view! In our book, *Living with Voices* (Romme et al., 2009), which describes 50 recovery stories, most of the voice hearers ended up stopping their medication because it had not had a positive effect. In fact, it is shocking that medication is used so often by psychiatrists as the first-line treatment in psychosis and hearing voices. I would go further and say it is surprising that voice hearers are referred to psychiatrists and not to people who are *not* afraid of voices.

> *Learning point 1*
>
> I don't want to say that you should stop medication, or that you should taper down. What I do want is for you to start to think and talk about your medication in a considered way. Maybe your medication doesn't help for voices, but for other things. The following questions can perhaps help you to find out more about your individual reactions towards medication.
>
> - In what kind of situation did you start with your medication? How did you feel? What did the medication do then? In what way did it help you?
> - Can you write down what you think the effects of the medication – both positive and negative – are for you?

- Can you ask people around you, the people who know you well enough, what they think the effects are? And can you perhaps also list these effects?
- How is your relationship with the professional who prescribes this medication? Is this professional open to your own evaluation of the effects of the medication?

Below are three anonymised examples from my practice where medication is an issue, to illustrate how varied and complex the effects of antipsychotics are.

1. A 40-year-old woman approached me for help. She had been to a voices outpatient clinic six years previously and there she started the medication she still used (a high dose of aripiprazole, an antipsychotic). The medication was never reviewed, the dose was only increased. Now she was having a depot injection every three weeks. 'What are the effects of the medication?' I asked. She reported that the voices had not changed very much. She had gained weight. Her emotions were flat, the voices didn't cause so much fear anymore. But she still wasn't able to live on her own. From her point of view, she would have been happy for the medication to be stopped. No professional wanted – or dared? – to advise her to decrease the dose or stop the medication.

An alternative approach seemed very simple. 'When did your voices start?' I asked. 'When I was seven.' 'What happened then?' 'The sexual abuse by this man started then,' she answered. 'It continued for 10 years.' 'Do you hear *his* voice?' 'Yes, indeed.'

This is how we started our conversation, by relating her voices to what happened in her personal life. All the other voices she heard related to other, similarly significant or traumatising events. She started to learn to communicate with her voices. Writing about her voices helped her very much in coping with them. It is a struggle, though, to cope with difficult emotions related to sexual abuse. The medication, we both decided, could be tapered down gradually but not stopped at once. Now, after more than a year off the medication, she is still doing better than before.

2. A 60-year-old woman I have known for 20 or more years was hearing a lot of voices when I met her for the first time. Her voices made a great deal of sense in the context of her life story, but she didn't accept my framework for making sense of them. It didn't help her. The antipsychotic (risperidone) she already took helped to suppress her voices a little bit. The voices were more distant, yet they were always present and attacking her. Whenever she stopped her medication – which she did regularly because she (and her voices) hated to be dependent – she soon entered into a state of confusion and harmed herself and started to wander around. She had to be motivated by her peers to take her medication again, and eventually she got a depot that made her more 'emotionally stable'. But she developed severe tardive

dyskinesia (TD). My advice was to take clozapine, one of the few antipsychotics that don't cause severe TD. However, it does come with a lot of other unwanted effects, like weight gain. The weight gain was something her voices panicked about. She resisted. After a few years, though, an expert on moving disorders succeeded in talking her into taking clozapine. This had a dramatic effect on her voices. They completely disappeared with a dose of 100mg. She now only uses 25mg a day, a very low dose; we both think she is a different person, and she is free of voices. She still has tardive dyskinesia but it is less severe, and she is able to live her life and doesn't want to stop this very low dose of antipsychotics. She is glad that she got rid of her voices.

3. A young man, 19 years old, came to me with complaints (called symptoms in the medical model) that fitted into the category of schizophrenia. The young man asked me to give him medication to stop his voices. He was really afraid he might harm other people, which his voices urgently ordered him to do. I asked him if he was prepared to listen to my story of the findings of our research, and about my conversations with other voice hearers. I explained the idea that voices often make sense when you explore what actually happened when they emerged in your life. He agreed and we had a long conversation. In the next session, he told me how his voices were related to his personal history. This made his voices much calmer. We talked a lot about his voices, but also about his family and possibilities for work and education. The voices became his advisors after a while. That was 13 years ago, and he has never had to experience the effects of antipsychotics; he is able to cope with his voices and tell other people about this process. He is a peer worker now, supporting other voice hearers and teaching boxing. (An extended version of this story can be read in Knols & Corstens, 2011.)

These examples are stories that represent clinical practice and they tell me that:

1. The reason why people hear voices is often not addressed. The schizophrenia diagnosis is covering up the real story. This anachronistic diagnosis is almost never challenged in practice and this often results in people having to take medication for the rest of their lives (despite severe doubts from a research perspective about their limited positive and many negative effects, as stated in the first half of this chapter). This medication covers up emotions and sometimes ruins the body.

2. Choice should be the basis of prescribing medication. If you prescribe medication in a low dose, it sometimes really helps, but it can also cause severe side effects. Never give up looking for alternative solutions to low doses of medication and for ways to prevent or diminish side-effects.

3. Making sense of voices can prevent you from becoming a psychiatric patient. Stories from peers can be very influential in the recovery process for voice-hearers.

> *Learning point 2*
> - In what way does your medication help you to cope with your voices?
> - Do you talk about your voices with other people? Do you meet other voice hearers to exchange experiences? Do you make some effort yourself to meet other people who are able to listen to your story related to your voices?
> - There is a lot of information available about learning to live with voices. Have you looked for it?

I have heard stories from voice hearers who are very grateful to the psychiatrists who helped them with medication. But I have also heard many stories about people having bad relationships with psychiatrists – and not only when compulsory 'treatment' is at stake. In the relationship with a psychiatrist there are two parties: the voice hearer and the psychiatrist (who generally mainly prescribes medication). If you also count the voices, who have their own opinions, then there are three parties (or more). In the next section, I want to share what I think about how a voice hearer could approach a psychiatrist more successfully, and how a psychiatrist could be more patient centred in terms of how they prescribe medication, even it if it is in the context of compulsory 'treatment'.

It can help if you consider what you can do yourself in a relationship instead of blaming the other. It is often the case that voice hearers refer to 'the system' and psychiatrists use their powerful medical jargon (like 'schizophrenia' or 'psychosis').

How to deal with your psychiatrist

Psychiatrists are human beings. They have feelings, they want to help. Some you will experience as nice and some you will not. One psychiatrist will be liked by one patient and disliked by another. Because of the power they are given by society – the power to 'lock you up' in a psychiatric hospital and administer drugs against your will – there is a big power issue. But they must have good reasons to 'lock you up', reasons that in some countries have to follow strict legal processes. But they may use a language that is difficult to understand, the core of which is 'diagnosis'. I don't have the ability or the space to write a 'psychology of the psychiatrist', but I will share some thoughts.

First of all, I must confess that, as a psychiatrist, I do things wrong every day in my professional relationship with my patients. So what I write here is also addressed to myself.

At the first World Hearing Voices Congress in 2009, a lot of psychiatrist colleagues were attending. They were all surprised by the experience of the atmosphere of equality and connectedness in this two-day meeting with voice hearers, and they could honestly share that. But most of them were shocked by the recovery stories presented by three voice hearers at the start of each day. These stories suggested at best that psychiatry was of little support and at worst that their experience in the mental health system had been utterly traumatic. My colleagues experienced this as too harsh a critique of the mental health system; they couldn't believe that what they heard was true. Many psychiatrists don't appear to realise just how much power they exert. When they do become aware of it, it seems that most generally do not enjoy the fact that they have so much power.

In order to feel less powerless, it is therefore important for people who hear voices to find allies and use them. You can find allies in your peer group, your social network and through the Hearing Voices Network in your region or country. Share your experiences. Use an advocate in your contact with professionals if possible.

I have had the privilege of meeting hundreds of voice hearers who were not my patients. I became an ally and some of them became real friends. That doesn't mean I always do the right thing. Your psychiatrist often needs to be challenged. Personally, I like to be challenged; I feel at that point I am really working together with the person who wants my support.

There are, of course, committed and kind psychiatrists who can listen very well to their patients. You don't need much time to discover that. However, I would argue that 'kind' is not enough. Psychiatrists really need to work on the basis of equality. They try to challenge you and they should like to be challenged in return. But very few use the tools that were developed to help people make sense of voices (Longden et al., 2012). There are now more nurses, social workers and some psychologists, but also many voice hearers who are acquainted with the Hearing Voices Network approach. Ask for them, so that you can work with the psychiatrist. If need be, you can ask to work with a different psychiatrist, too. You do not need to ask for permission; you can simply tell them that this is what you need. That is your right!

Many psychiatrists use their power to prescribe their pills on the basis of selective reading of often outdated guidelines and ill-informed science (Whitaker, 2017). It can sometimes seem almost as though many do not read the critical literature to the end. It is not surprising that some people end up feeling that psychiatrists are easily offended by criticism. I found that many of my colleagues did not appear to be able to digest the critical anthologies by voice hearers about the circumstances in mental health care, because they considered it to be a *personal* criticism. And that's human! They think they are doing good, and they want to help voice hearers.

However, we must not be surprised if some voice hearers have therefore learned by experience to withhold personal information from the psychiatrist, if the main response is to be prescribed more medication. They have learned they need to be strategic in their conversations with psychiatrists.

The power and the pressure psychiatrists get from society and their employers are very hard for psychiatrists to deal with. You can see the effects of this pressure in statements like: 'I have no time to do an interview with a voice hearer, my caseload is too big', or 'I have to protect you from yourself and others from you', or 'I am not a psychotherapist'.

I hope it is clear, therefore, that you need alternative or additional information and to make your own choices. You don't *have* to trust the psychiatrist just because they are the doctor or the person in charge. You are in charge of your life and you can also think about what you find helpful for yourself. You should have a choice in this whole process. That is absolutely critical. So, do ask for options.

> *Learning point 3 (for the patient)*
>
> It's important to be critical of yourself and others regarding medication. Seek allies and information. You need people around you that you can trust. Make your own choices, based on proper information, not only on the opinions of one person.
>
> - Do you understand your own experiences? How are these experiences connected to your personal history?
> - Can you work with the people who prescribe your pills on an equal basis? How do they explain the effects of the medication? Do they listen to your experiences and take them seriously? Do they explain the positive and the negative effects (the 'side effects')?
> - Do you get well-informed choice? Do you get alternatives?
> - Can you avoid a power struggle? How?

My advice to my fellow psychiatrists

When a voice hearer has never had medication and seeks help or is sectioned

The first step when considering medication should be *wait and listen*. A good and often fruitful guideline from Open Dialogue practice is to wait at least three sessions before you start medication. In Open Dialogue, the social network around the person is also asked to come up with ideas about what could be done. You're not alone! Antipsychotic medication should be a choice, not the first-line treatment (Morrison et al., 2012, 2014). Some of the talking or other approaches in this book may be as effective or more effective than medication, and less harmful. They can also help with people who do not want to take pills.

So, first try to make sense of the voices, with the help of the person's social network or individually, and only start medication when the patient's anxiety is too overwhelming. Even at that point, it may be helpful to consider the use of an anti-anxiety medication first (e.g. a benzodiazepine like diazepam or lorazepam), rather than going in with an antipsychotic medication straight away, as it may be just as effective and it may be possible to use it over a shorter period (Moncrieff, 2020).

When a voice hearer has a long history in mental health services

I must confess that I am biased because I have met so many voice hearers who have been in psychiatric services for a long time without positive results. Many are disappointed because they didn't get any choice – only medication. Many voice hearers in mental health services have never been informed that there are alternative ways of going about things. This may be because many mental health professionals also do not know about alternatives or are not confident in applying alternatives, like the ones introduced in this book. They may therefore also not know that there are different ways of going about living with voices or understanding them or that something like recovery is indeed possible. The question, 'What happened to you in your life that things have turned out as they have?' (Johnstone & Boyle, 2018) may never have been put to them because they have been given a diagnosis like schizophrenia, which has long been considered primarily biologically caused (although this view is slowly changing in research and even more slowly in practice). However, asking such questions could be absolutely crucial and pivotal to creating new openings. It offers a chance for the person's story to be revealed, which can really make a difference for them and for how they are treated by others. Recovery begins with owning your own story and learning to share it. Often medication is not the solution here.

Hearing voices is not a symptom of psychosis. Hearing voices, in our understanding, is a human response to life. If a person does not learn how to deal constructively with voices, they might come across as experiencing psychosis (as the voices might become overwhelming and lead to behaviour and feelings that they and others do not understand straight away). However, in this way, we would also say that psychosis is a human reaction to circumstances and life's challenges, too (Razzaque, 2014; Romme & Escher, 2013). Try to understand this relationship. Perhaps, as a therapist – and as a psychiatrist you're a therapist too, whether you like it or not – you're responsible for the treatment, but the goal is recovery. It is teamwork, and the patient must find his or her own journey. You could work with a psychologist or nurse, or – even better – an experienced voice hearer who has the time to build up a relationship with the patient hearing voices so that together they can work to make sense of their voices. There are several approaches introduced in this book that can also be helpful. It is also helpful to support self-help groups for voice-hearers. There is so much more to do than prescribing pills. And if you prescribe pills, then I would recommend that this should be done for a short time at a low dose while other self-work and community work is also supported. Often, simply changing circumstances can contribute tremendously to recovery. In this process it is really helpful, therefore, to also build connections with the primary person in their life who really believes in the voice hearer.

> *Learning point 4 (for the psychiatrist)*
>
> As a psychiatrist, can you be patient when it comes to the process of prescribing pills? Can you postpone it and first listen to the person concerned and to his or her social and support network?
>
> - What are the benefits in the short and long term for prescribing medication?

- What are the disadvantages?
- If the person concerned were your child, what would you do?
- Do you help to organise support from others for your patients?
- Do you help the patient to feel safer?

My advice to the patient's support network

Your unconditional support is of greatest importance. Read the chapters in this book and the recommended reading. Find your own way to support the voice hearer. Try to listen, understand, and ask what is needed. Accompany the voice hearer in mental health settings (if that is where they are getting some support) and challenge the options that are offered if you feel they are insufficient.

Which medication?

Personally, I support the 'drug-centred' model proposed by Joanna Moncrieff (a professor of critical psychiatry and practising psychiatrist in London). The drug-centred model focuses our attention on the impact that drugs have on the body and the brain (as opposed to the disease-centred model, which is the more usual approach, and believes psychiatric drugs work by correcting a hypothetical underlying brain abnormality), and on all the possible consequences that drug-induced alterations can have on how people think, feel and behave (Moncrieff, 2013a; 2013b; 2020).

Benzodiazepines

Voice hearers often prefer benzodiazepines over antipsychotics to diminish anxiety. But they can also be a trap since people can develop tolerance and dependence quickly. Sedation is a common side effect. Use them only for a short time.

Antipsychotics

Sometimes antipsychotics are helpful when people experience a high level of anxiety. At this point, everything in their environment may take on a personal and often frightening meaning (which is called 'psychosis'). It is in a therapeutic context, such as in an Open Dialogue meeting, a self-help group, conducting the Maastricht Hearing Voices Interview, or a cognitive-behavioural session, that the patient is encouraged to make sense of their voices. In these settings, it may be rational and productive for the psychiatrist to hold back on prescribing antipsychotics. I would also advise low doses if and when antipsychotics are prescribed.

Sometimes people take antipsychotics for a longer period and report that they have been helpful (according to them or their network members). However, it is important to remember that, as indicated at the beginning of this chapter, in the long run, and after an initial period on medication, there is some evidence that people may do better with little, reduced or no medication. However, more research is needed (Harrow et al., 2014; Moncrieff, 2020). We do not yet have a good insight into who recovers better with or without antipsychotics from the start. It should therefore ideally be an individual decision whether to take antipsychotics, not take them, or taper them off. Even though this is supported by legislation in many countries (in Germany it is even in the practice guidelines, as reported above), the experience in practice is often different for users of mental health services.

Emotional work

I would like to give a brief additional example of how important emotional work can be. I was once working with a voice hearer who slept 16 hours a day and had difficulty in speaking because they were taking high doses of antipsychotics. After we had worked out that his voices represented bereavement and a depressive reaction, I suggested gradually stopping the antipsychotics and prescribed him an antidepressant instead, as he preferred to continue to take some medication. His voice disappeared and he could be discharged from hospital. This is not to say the voice disappeared as a result of the antidepressant. It seemed clear that the work with him on his bereavement had also helped.

In conclusion

As we explained at the beginning of this chapter, there is no research evidence of proper quality that has singled out a specific effect of medication on hearing voices (Moncrieff, 2020). Much research therefore doesn't justify any generalisation whatsoever about the treatment of hearing voices (Corstens et al., 2013). It is 'bad science', in other words. Many scientific articles can end up being advertisements for the pharmaceutical industry (DGSP, 2018). We have therefore tried to set an agenda for research that could benefit voice hearers from *their* perspective (Corstens et al., 2014). Almost all mainstream research is based on the eradication of the voices, which contrasts with our starting point, based on our practice and research findings, which is that voices have meaning and can be or become supportive. The question is, 'How do we measure successful support or accompaniment or treatment?' We argue that the relationship between the voices and the voice hearer should be the primary target in scientific research, as opposed to the eradication of the voices, as it is only when the relationship with the voices is not as constructive as it could be that voices can become overwhelming and make everyday life difficult.

My conclusion is that it is important to listen to and talk with voice hearers, try to understand the personal reasons for hearing voices and work through the problems that are related to that. Medication – in a low dose – can be of support temporarily, but should never be the first or even the main line of treatment, as is often still commonplace and in many guidelines worldwide.

References

Aderhold, V. & Weinmann, S. (2020, July 27). *Neue leitlinien schizophrenie: Bitte auch weitersenden. (New guidelines on schizophrenia: Please forward).* (Email circular containing guideline DGPPN (2019) S3-Schizophrenia critique). (Personal communication, available from second editor).

Bentall, R. (2003). *Madness explained: Psychosis and human nature.* Penguin Books.

Bentall, R. (2009). *Doctoring the mind: Is our current treatment of mental illness really any good?* NYU Press.

Corstens, D., Longden, E., McCarthy-Jones, S., Waddingham, R. & Thomas, N. (2014). Emerging perspectives from the Hearing Voices Movement: Implications for research and practice. *Schizophrenia Bulletin, 40*(4), s285–s294.

Corstens, D., Longden, E., Rydinger, B., Bentall, R. & van Os, J. (2013). Treatment of hallucinations: A comment. *Psychosis: Psychological, social and integrative approaches, 5*(1), 98–102.

Deutsche Gesellschaft für Psychiatrie und Psychotherapie, Psychosomatik und Nervenheilkunde e.V. (DGPPN) [German Association for Psychiatry, Psychotherapy and Psychosomatics]. (2019). *S3-Leitlinie Schizophrenie [S3-Guideline schizophrenia].* DGPPN. www.awmf.org/uploads/tx_szleitlinien/038-009l_S3_Schizophrenie_2019-03.pdf

Deutsche Gesellschaft für Soziale Psychiatrie (DGSP) [German Society for Social Psychiatry]. (2015). *Neuroleptika reduzieren und absetzen. Eine Broschüre für Psychose-Erfahrene, Angehörige und Professionelle aller Berufsgruppen. [Reducing and stopping neuroleptics: A brochure for experiencers of psychosis, families and professionals of all groups of professionals].* Deutsche Gesellschaft für Soziale Psychiatrie.

Deutsche Gesellschaft für Soziale Psychiatrie (DGSP) (*German Society for Social Psychiatry*) (2018). *Memorandum der Deutschen Gesellschaft für Soziale Psychiatrie zur Anwendung von Neuroleptika (3. Auflage) [Memorandum of the German Society for Social Psychiatry on the Use of Neuroleptics (3rd Ed.).* DGSP. www.dgsp-ev.de/fileadmin/user_files/dgsp/pdfs/Publikationen/DGSP_Memorandum_zur_Anwendung_von_Neuroleptika_2018.pdf

Hall, W. (2012). *The harm reduction guide to coming off psychiatric drugs.* Icarus Project. https://willhall.net/comingoffmeds/

Harrow, M., Jobe, T. & Faull, R. (2014). Does treatment of schizophrenia with antipsychotic medications eliminate or reduce psychosis? A 20-year multi-follow-up study *Psychological Medicine, 4,* 3007–3016.

Harrow, M., Jobe, T. & Tong, L. (2021). Twenty-year effects of antipsychotics in schizophrenia and affective psychotic disorders. First view. *Psychological Medicine,* 1–11. https://doi.org/10.1017/S0033291720004778

Huhtaniska, S. (2017). Long-term antipsychotic use and brain changes in schizophrenia – a systematic review and meta-analysis. *Human Psychopharmacology, 32*(2). doi: 10.1002/hup.2574

Johnstone, L., Boyle, M. with Cromby, J., Dillon, J., Harper, D., Kinderman, P., Longden, E., Pilgrim, D. & Read, J. (2018). *The Power Threat Meaning Framework: Towards the identification of patterns in emotional distress, unusual experiences and troubled or troubling behaviour, as an alternative to functional psychiatric diagnosis.* British Psychological Society.

Knols, M. & Corstens, D. (2011). Tuning in: A story by a patient and a therapist about making sense of voices. *Mental Health Today,* Nov-Dec, 28–32.

Leucht, S., Arbter, D., Engel, R.R., Kissling, W. & Davis, J.M. (2009a). How effective are second-generation antipsychotic drugs? A meta-analysis of placebo-controlled trials. *Molecular Psychiatry, 14,* 429–447.

Leucht, S., Cipriani, A., Spineli, L., Mavridis, D., Orey, D., Richter, F., Samara, M., Barbui, C., Engel, R.R., Geddes, J.R., Kissling, W., Stapf, M.P., Lässig, B., Salanti, G. & Davis, J.M. (2013). Comparative efficacy and tolerability of 15 antipsychotic drugs in schizophrenia: A multiple-treatments meta-analysis. *The Lancet, 382,* 951–962.

Leucht, S., Hierl, S., Kissling, W., Dold, M. & Davis, J.M. (2009b). Putting the efficacy of psychiatric and general medicine into perspective: Review of meta-analyses. *The British Journal of Psychiatry, 200*(2), 97–106.

Leucht, S., Leucht, C., Huhn, M., Chaimani, A., Mavridis, D., Helfer, B., Samara, M., Rabaioli, M., Bächer, S., Cipriani, A., Geddes, J.R., Salanti, G. & Davis, J.M. (2017). Sixty years of placebo-controlled antipsychotic drug trials in acute schizophrenia: Systematic review, Bayesian meta-analysis, and meta-regression of efficacy predictors. *American Journal of Psychiatry, 174*(10), 927–942.

Longden, E., Corstens, D., Escher, A. & Romme, M. (2012). Hearing voices in biographical context: A framework to give meaning to voice-hearing experiences. *Psychosis: Psychological, social and integrative approaches, 4*(3), 224–234.

McCarthy-Jones, S. (2017). *Can't you hear them? The science and significance of hearing voices.* Jessica Kingsley Publishers.

Moncrieff, J. (2013a). Models of drugs action. [Online.] https://joannamoncrieff.com/2013/11/21/models-of-drug-action/

Moncrieff, J. (2013b). T*he bitterest pills: The troubling story of antipsychotics*. Palgrave Macmillan.

Moncrieff, J. (2020). *A straight talking introduction to psychiatric drugs* (2nd ed.). PCCS Books.

Morrison, A., Hutton, P., Shiers, D. & Turkington, D. (2012). Antipsychotics: Is it time to introduce patient choice? *The British Journal of Psychiatry, 201*, 83–84.

Morrison, A., Turkington, D., Pyle, M., Spencer, H., Brabban, A., Dunn, G., Christodoulides, T., Dudley, R., Chapman, N., Callcott, P., Grace, T., Lumley, V., Drage, L., Tully, S., Irving, K, Cummings, A., Byrne, R., Davies, L.M. & Hutton, P. (2014). Cognitive therapy for people with schizophrenia spectrum disorders not taking antipsychotic drugs: A single-blind randomised controlled trial. *The Lancet, 383*(9926), 1395–1403.

Razzaque, R. (2014). *Breaking down is waking up.* Watkins Publishing.

Romme, M. & Escher, A. (Eds.) (2013). *Psychosis as a personal crisis: An experience-based approach.* Routledge.

Romme, M., Escher, S., Dillon, J., Corstens, D. & Morris, M. (2009). *Living with voices: 50 stories of recovery.* PCCS Books.

Schlimme, J.E., Scholz, T. & Seroka, R. (2018). *Medikamentenreduktion und Genesung von Psychosen.* Psychiatrieverlag.

Servonnet, A., & Samaha, A.-N. (2020). Antipsychotic-evoked dopamine supersensitivity. *Neuropharmacology, 163.* doi: 10.1016/j.neuropharm.2019.05.007

Servonnet, A., Uchida, H. & Samaha, A.-N. (2021). Continuous versus extended antipsychotic dosing in schizophrenia: Less is more. *Behavioural Brain Research, 5*(401). doi: 10.1016/j.bbr.2020.113076

Sohler, N., Adams, B.G., Barnes, D.M., Cohen, G.H., Prins, S.J. & Schwartz, S. (2015). Weighing the evidence of harm from long-term treatment with antipsychotic medications: A systematic review. *American Journal of Orthopsychiatry, 86*(5), 477–485.

Timimi, S. (2021). *A straight talking introduction to children's mental health* (2nd ed.). PCCS Books.

Weinmann, S., Read, J. & Aderhold, V. (2009). Influence of antipsychotics on mortality in schizophrenia: Systematic review. *Schizophrenia Research, 113,* 1–11.

Whitaker, R. (2017, May 21). Psychiatry defends its antipsychotics: A case study of institutional corruption. *Mad in America.* www.madinamerica.com/2017/05/psychiatry-defends-its-antipsychoticscase-study-of-institutional-corruption/

16 Voice hearers at work
Caroline Moughton

The life and work experiences of people who hear voices span a wide range, from those who have not yet experienced sufficient opportunities to be able to work to those who feel able to pursue successful professional careers. This chapter explores some practical tips that may be helpful for voice hearers who have found their life, hearing voices and potential support experiences quite difficult when seeking and holding down jobs. At the same time, as with most other things in life, it is important to remember that everyone follows their own path in this – there is no one golden route.

Starting small to build up your confidence is good advice for anyone, but many voice hearers actually also have had to negotiate and survive some very traumatic, difficult and distressing realities, both in relation to their voices but also other experiences, such as being the victims of abuse and bullying in their personal lives and sometimes also in mental health services. They have therefore had to be much stronger people than they, or others, often perceive them to be. If this applies to you, too, it may be helpful to view yourself not just as a victim of a difficult life (that definitely, as well), but also as a very strong person. You will likely already have had to show much more strength in dealing with the experiences in your life than a lot of other people. In this way, finding and retaining work could be seen as yet another battle that you can both survive and win, even if it does not always feel straightforward along the way.

A note of information: some might find this chapter too cautious, too pessimistic about the world of employment and its likely response to knowing you hear voices. I think it is important to be realistic and tell it like many people experience it. Yes, there are laws against discrimination on grounds of mental disorder or disability, but there are numerous subtle ways of discriminating that are very hard to prove. My aim here is to ensure you feel you have some sense of control over your employment situation and conditions and over what you disclose and keep to yourself.

Applying for work

Do you reveal your voice hearing?

A key issue to consider is whether to share the sensitive information that you hear voices. Many people choose to hide this from a potential employer, as they fear it will make them appear less attractive in a competitive job market. Voice hearing continues to be widely seen as a sign of craziness, dangerousness and of being out of control, and people may be reluctant to work alongside known voice hearers.

You may, of course, be successful in your career, while keeping your voice hearing secret from your colleagues and your employer. Later in this chapter, we look at ways to manage your voices without telling your employer.

However, you may feel that you could benefit from getting more help with getting into the workplace, especially if you have few or no qualifications and little or no formal work experience so far (perhaps because you have been overwhelmed by your voice hearing and related traumatic experiences in the past). In this case, you may want to consider being more open about your voice-hearing experience or find another way of talking about this period of not being in work so that it does not go against you so much. In the UK, voluntary sector organisations such as The Shaw Trust and Remploy can provide extra help for people with a history of having received psychiatric support, such as:

- help with identifying skills, interests and preferences and suggestions of different kinds of jobs
- basic skills training (such as computer skills and so forth), if you haven't had a chance to develop these yet
- getting experience – volunteering can be an opportunity to learn skills and develop social skills that your experiences so far have prevented you from learning
- arranging work experience via established links with employers
- support with completing job applications
- interview preparation
- a job coach to help you learn how to do a new job
- support in telling an employer about your voice hearing (if that is what you have decided to do, after discussing the pros and cons). If the voluntary or similar organisation does not have a particular expertise in employment and voice hearing, you could, for example, contact a local Hearing Voices Network for extra support in thinking this through.

In practice, many people choose not to reveal their voice hearing when applying for jobs, for a variety of reasons, including those mentioned above. There may be further opportunities to share this information later in the job-seeking process, but it may not ever be necessary. It is illegal in the UK for an employer to discriminate against a potential employee on the grounds of a disability or a mental health condition, but (as mentioned above) discrimination can be difficult to prove, and an employer may give another pretext for turning down your application.

In contrast to this, lived experience of hearing voices can be considered an asset in some jobs, such as being a peer support worker in a mental health setting. In such a case, you may want to show how your own experience will help you to support others.

Sasha's experience

I've been hearing voices since childhood and I've found lots of ways to manage this over the years. Being in a workplace and having to manage the voices felt quite daunting at first, as I didn't want to look weird or do things that would bring too much attention to myself. When I began working in a busy, noisy office environment with a new team of people, I felt my voices worsen. In hindsight, I probably could have anticipated this, as being surrounded by lots of people speaking and new people are both triggers for me.

Each workplace I have been in has brought new learning about how I can manage my voices. This has included developing strategies, such as feeling able to tell a few trusted people in my team that I hear voices and feeling I can confide in them, and using a workplace WRAP (Wellness Recovery Action Plan) that I share with my supervisor. I also put on headphones to listen to music if the environment feels overwhelming. It also helps to be able to get up and go for a five-minute walk when I know a change of environment will help.

I have discovered from colleagues' feedback that when I think I'm acting strangely or reacting to voices at work, they can't really tell. Being able to have this kind of conversation has made me feel much less self-conscious and more confident. This leads to me feeling more comfortable, and my voice hearing becomes manageable, even reducing in the workplace.

Writing a job application

A good job application is your chance to give specific evidence of how you meet the employer's person specification for the job. Voice hearers who have little previous employment experience may be able to demonstrate the requisite skills and experience from outside a work situation, such as through volunteering: for example, 'My good interpersonal skills were used when I intervened and defused an angry confrontation between two volunteers.'

It is useful to give a positive explanation of any gaps in your employment history: for example, 'I took time out to pursue my creative interests' (when you were unwell and used art to help manage your voices). Some employers may even find it impressive (which, of course, it is) to hear that you have worked through any pre-existing mental health difficulties. However, you need to be quite confident that a potential employer does feel that way before considering disclosing this information.

Make the most of your achievements. If you experience your voices as critical of your job application process, it may be hard to do yourself justice in the process. Ask a friend or family member to look over your application to make sure you are not underselling yourself. Alternatively, you may already have found a way of using that criticism to your own advantage, by asking the voices about their original intentions in criticising you – which may be very protective (e.g. they may be flagging up that this may not be the right job for you). If you do not want to, or feel unable to engage with the voices by dialoguing with them in this way, you could take it as a challenge to 'show them', so to speak – which, in turn, may even be one of the reasons why they are being so critical in the first place, as they may actually be intending to spur you on to do your best.

Preparing for an interview

Think in advance how you are going to answer possible questions. If you have had a previous job, you may be asked why you left. Some voice hearers decide not to name what happened and to speak generally about it: 'I had a breakdown, but I have recovered and feel I am now able to look after myself better.' You can simply say that you don't want to go into details.

Think about how you will deal with your voices during the interview. You are likely to be feeling anxious, like most people in an interview, which might increase your voices. You could try negotiating with your voices that you will listen to them later, which will only work if you have previously practised this and the voices have learned that you really do keep your side of the bargain and really do listen when you say this to them. If you are distracted by your voices, you can ask the interviewer to repeat the question. You may also want to consider saying something like: 'I am sorry, I was still thinking about our previous point, so I did not quite catch everything you were saying.'

Before the interview, an employer may ask you whether you want to disclose any disability or long-term health condition so that they can make any necessary reasonable adjustments for you, so you are not disadvantaged at interview. Most voice hearers would probably not be willing to tell the employer about voice hearing at this stage. Some may not consider their voices to be a sign of disability or a mental health condition. If someone does decide to disclose that they hear voices and may find this difficult at times, they could request help at interview, such as being accompanied by a support worker to reduce anxiety. However, to be honest, unless you are applying for a job where these kind of special adjustments are commonplace, experiences such as yours are particularly and expressly welcomed and you know that the employer would deal well with such a disclosure and not discriminate against you, you would be wise not to mention the voices at this point.

If you haven't had much experience of doing job interviews, you might find it useful to practise beforehand. You should definitely research how to get to the location, and allow extra time so that you are not agitated if you encounter delays that might make you late.

You should be told in advance if the selection process includes any practical tests, presentations or auditions, to give you a chance to prepare. If you are giving a presentation, make clear notes to take with you. If you are distracted by voices while giving the presentation, be open about it: calmly admit that you have lost focus and pick up where you left off. For example, you might say, 'Sorry, I lost the thread there. The main point I'm making is that …' or, 'Sorry, I am a bit nervous. What I was trying to say, is…'

Finally, a gentle reminder that it is never a good idea to use alcohol or street drugs before an interview.

Don't be discouraged if you don't get the first job you apply for. Most people apply for several jobs before they are successful. And remember too, the job may not be right for you: the interview is where you get to meet your employer and can decide for yourself if this is an environment and a group of people who you think you can work with.

How to manage at work as a voice hearer

Congratulations if you've been offered a job. Now you need to think about how you will manage being in the workplace. Everyone has their own particular needs and challenges when they enter a new employment. Yours happen to include voices. Jobs and workplaces are all very different, but here are some general tips.

Dealing with your voices

Use normal social breaks during the day if you need time out to talk and/or listen to your voices – for example, during toilet, smoking or lunch breaks. If you can, negotiate with your voices that you will listen to them in breaks but not during work time. If you find your voices less intrusive when you are with other people, you might want to eat lunch with colleagues. Alternatively, you may prefer to use lunch breaks for some quiet time. If colleagues ask why you don't join them, tell them the truth: 'I need a bit of quiet time to myself at lunch.' There is nothing abnormal or unusual about that.

If your voices tell you that you are useless, explain to them why: 'Yes, I'm feeling a bit insecure about starting a new job, but I am looking forward to the challenge.' So sometimes what they say may be worth considering. They may be trying to tell you something important about your work that you are trying to ignore. For example, they may say, 'You can't get this project finished,' which may be flagging up that you have a genuine problem with the project that you should raise with your manager and ask for additional input or resources.

Some people listen to their voices for a bit, then tell them to shut up. Most people find that if they ask their voices in a friendly way to be quiet and the voices know that you will give them time after work or during breaks, this is more likely to work (see Chapter 18 on experience focused counselling for more input on the similarities between relating well to voices and to people).

David's experience

Hearing voices is for me often an indicator of other issues that I may need to address. Being in an environment in which I can articulate my experience of hearing voices without being judged in a diagnostic fashion gives me an opportunity to start to address things that may be causing my voices to surface. Working in environments that allow me to pace my own work so that I can complete tasks when I'm feeling at my best and focus on my voices when I need to significantly helps reduce the negative impact of the voices on both my work and my mental well-being.

I do my best to make sure that I get enough sleep. I also need to have plenty of fresh air and exercise. At work, I find that it helps to be treated as a human being, rather than as a collection of symptoms. My job allows me to have autonomy and agency over the workload. Fortunately, I have a supportive manager, who both focuses on what I am able to do and helps with any aspects of my work that may need to be changed or delegated. I like working in a small office that has minimal distractions. This is a much better environment for me than a noisy, open-plan office. I can choose to work from home, apart from when travel is absolutely necessary. I will often choose to go into the office to do face-to-face meetings, as I find virtual meetings difficult if I am having difficulty with my voices.

John's experience

When I have worked as a nurse, managing my anxiety levels has helped me to live with voices. At one point I found it helpful to have my caseload reduced (although this was not done on account of my voices), as this meant that I was under less pressure and was less anxious. As a mental health nurse, I have been able to work largely semi-autonomously and build in my own 'reasonable adjustments', which include breaks, when I might go to another space like a quiet café or a library, or go for a swim at lunchtime. Where possible, I take short walks (instead of using public transport), so that I can have physical exercise.

Sometimes I would dialogue with the voices in my head during my breaks, which was like talking to a friend inside my head (instead of out loud). My voices stop me from feeling lonely and help me feel better about myself, which has a positive impact on my work. I have also found it helpful to attend peer support groups for voice hearers, and on occasion to see a psychotherapist on a one-to-one basis, because this has enabled me to reframe some of my experiences of my life at the time in a positive way, enabling me to integrate more of myself. I also find maintaining a regular sleep pattern critical in helping maintain my overall mental health and sense of wellbeing. A good sleep pattern helps me to keep my anxieties at a lower level, which in turn reduces the frequency and intensity of the voices.

Sarah's experience

Working as a staff nurse, I had little understanding of where my voices had originated or why. The confusion was problematic for me, but I was able to adjust my shifts so I could avoid the crowded times on the ward. When the voices were unmanageable I would take sick leave.

On medical retirement, I had the opportunity to engage in intensive therapy (provided by a complex needs service), which helped me to understand my emotions and my relationship with my voices. It also gave me a multitude of coping strategies, which give me emotional stability and control of my voices.

Post-therapy, I work alongside other professionals and personnel facilitating post-therapy groups. I now deliver training, engage service users into services, and attend consultations at academic and government levels. All of these situations may cause emotional distress, yet we all have the opportunity for a debrief following every event. There is also a monthly supervision and, if required, a phone call to whomever I have been working alongside, for grounding and feedback. This gives me emotional support, thereby supporting my negative voice hearing. If my voices are not helping, then I know that my emotional wellbeing requires attention.

Learning point 1

Stigma and self-stigma can be major barriers to people who hear voices being able to obtain and hold down a job.

- What feelings and thoughts (e.g. fear, lack of understanding or knowledge, lack of confidence) might mean you hold on to a view of seeing someone (or yourself) primarily through the lens of their mental health difficulties?

Using ordinary language

There are ways of explaining your needs using everyday language, without having to mention the words 'hearing voices'. For example, 'I find it easier to concentrate in a quieter space'; 'I work more effectively if I can organise my own work'; 'I get anxious if things change at the last minute'. Your colleagues are likely to sympathise with these common concerns and be able to accommodate them, whereas there is still a lot of ignorant fear around mental health difficulty or hearing voices.

Express your preferences, rather than say what you don't like doing: for example, 'I prefer dealing with customers to working in the back room.' There is no need to say that this is because you find your voices less intrusive if you are interacting with other people. Alternatively, of course, you might say you prefer working in the back room (when you find client interface more difficult because of the voices).

You may find that you are able to talk about some of the effects of your voices, even though you don't talk about the voices themselves. For example:

- 'I sometimes find it hard to concentrate…'
- 'I find I work better if I sometimes take a break, then come back to a piece of work.'
- 'I like to do things as well as I can, so I like to re-check my work.'
- 'Meeting deadlines is not my biggest strength.'
- 'I like to have some time on my own when we have breaks.'

If you are finding it more difficult than usual to cope with the voices, you can explain why you are not well by talking about the impact without mentioning the voices: 'I'm not sleeping well at the moment'; 'I'm having relationship difficulties at the moment.'

If you can, identify a sympathetic work colleague who is willing to answer questions about your role, so you can check any queries easily. This may make it easier for you to cope with critical voices.

Talking with colleagues

Work is a social place and your colleagues will want to ask questions about your personal life. Plan how you will answer questions that are likely to come up. You don't need to share any personal information but you don't want to rebuff friendly overtures, so it's a good idea to plan and practise what you feel comfortable telling them. It is fine to give a brief response and then change the subject by asking them a question about themselves. Most people are very happy to chat about their lives and family.

It may be wise to wait until you know more about your new colleagues' attitudes to mental ill health before risking sharing personal information. You may not find it helpful to share this information with colleagues at all, and there is no need to.

Talking with your line manager

If your voices are critical of your work performance, you may find it useful to ask your line manager for regular feedback, so you have objective evidence to answer your voices. However, be careful not to overdo it; you don't want to come across as too low in confidence. Most line managers see the value in helping a new employee learn their job.

You may want to explain that you find certain situations or places more difficult. Again, this is not unusual among non-voice hearers. You don't need to go into the actual details.

Take up development opportunities that you would enjoy or be able to do more easily. Employers like people who want to develop their skills. Asking about opportunities demonstrates your enthusiasm, but also lets you shape your path. 'I'm really interested in doing a course on X, which would help me in my job' (when the alternative Y appears likely to be stressful because of your voices). Or volunteer to do particular tasks that you know you can manage, so you don't get allocated ones that you find difficult. This allows you to play to your strengths.

Try to check out your line manager's attitude to mental health issues before risking saying anything about your voices, and find out, if you can, whether they can be trusted to respect confidentiality.

If you have low self-esteem, you may habitually dismiss praise. Learn to ask for specifics about what you did well (so that you can do it again) and say thank you. If things have gone less well, again be specific: everybody gets things wrong sometimes, and we learn from our mistakes. Try to acknowledge that you could improve your performance: 'So if this happens again it would be better if I did X...'

Learning point 2

Can you think of examples in your life where you found good ways of dealing with a personal crisis so that it did not adversely affect your relationships and (if you have worked or volunteered) employment?

- What did you learn from that?

Using available flexibility for all staff

Options for flexibility vary depending on your role and work organisation. Just like everybody else, a person who hears voices can make choices that make it easier to function at work. Some people who are very successful in their roles have never told their employer that they hear voices. This is easier where people have autonomy to arrange their work lives.

What options are there for flexibility in working patterns? You may be able to choose a start and finish time. Some voice hearers prefer a later start, to avoid rush-hour travel. Some employers operate a flexitime scheme where you have to work core hours but have flexibility on start and finish times. This enables staff to 'bank' hours so that they can take time off if they are less well.

Part-time working may be a useful option, especially if a person has been unwell and does not feel able to work full-time yet. Working part-time also allows time for rest, exercise and attending medical appointments and support groups. Full-time employees may have an option to ask whether they can reduce their hours to part-time, either permanently or temporarily. If you receive social security benefits, this may affect the hours you can work, so take advice on this.

Some voice hearers find it stressful to use public transport or drive at busy times. Would it be easier to travel at quieter times? Are there possible routes that are less crowded, or that include a longer walk? Can you use flexitime to travel at less busy times? Are there options for working from home? Would this be helpful or not? It can be helpful to work one day a week at home, depending on the nature of your role.

Managing yourself in the workplace

Voices that can be experienced as critical can seem to demand your full attention (these voices might on occasion even seem to come from the colleagues around you). They can seem most disruptive of people's working lives, as they affect concentration, communication and task completion. For some people, voices can be neutral; for others, voices may be supportive in their work experience. Not surprisingly, meaningful experiences of work can diminish the negative impact of voice hearing (Craig et al., 2017). This may be comparable to the sense of self-worth that anybody – not just voice hearers – gets from working in a meaningful role. Again, as for anybody, so it is true for people who hear voices: to be successful at work one needs to develop effective strategies. Keeping a diary about your voices at work could enable you to reflect on and record the strategies that you have found helpful. Voices can respond inconsistently or unpredictably, so you need a variety of techniques.

Dealing with emotional ups and downs

Living with voices can be tiring, and leave you feeling emotionally fragile. In any job you can expect to work with people you like and dislike. Also, remember that everyone has bad days, so when a colleague seems grumpy or short with you, this may be about them, not you. Try to retain a polite, professional mask, regardless of how you feel inside.

Organisation

Develop excellent organisation skills to help overcome distractions from voice hearing. You might even develop a reputation for efficiency in the process. If the job and working conditions allow it:

- Plan your day, perhaps keeping an electronic diary or using your phone for meeting reminders.
- Keep your work area and any shared spaces such as kitchens tidy.
- Use reminder and organisational tools that work for you, such as notebooks, lists, post-its.
- At the end of the day, make a to-do list for the next day so you know what you have to do when you arrive the next morning.
- Depending on the nature of the job, you may want to develop your own reminder and orienting checklists, including photos (for example of particular equipment layouts).
- Set aside time for filing and archiving.

Time management

Time management may be more difficult if you are still finding it difficult to relate well to your voices. It may be a good idea to develop strategies. It is not a good idea to get a reputation for being late.

- Allow plenty of time for getting up and getting ready to leave for work.
- Allow sufficient time for travel to work by your preferred route.
- You may want to aim to arrive 10 minutes before your start time to allow a toilet break and to talk and listen to your voices before you have to start work.
- Where possible, arrange when you do what over the course of the day – for example, doing more complex, demanding tasks in the morning when you are less tired or at times when your voices are quieter.
- Avoid staying late at work; it is important to have enough down-time for yourself.
- Learn how long particular tasks take you so you deliver on time.
- Some people find it helpful to break bigger projects into very small, achievable chunks that they can tick off as they are completed. This gives a proof of progress to silence the critical voices. Don't take on too much overtime; it is important for you to rest.
- Take regular breaks, including lunch breaks.
- If a critical voice raises a difficulty, check if it is a valid concern. It may be something you should address.

Dealing with concentration difficulties

Where you find difficulties, suggest possible solutions for everyone. For example, if you sometimes lose track of what is being discussed in meetings because you are distracted by your voices, suggest that a summary of action points is circulated afterwards. This is likely to help other colleagues too.

If you can reduce additional distractions in your workspace, do so. If you are a desk worker, you may be able to move desks to a quieter area with fewer people passing by. Having difficulty concentrating in open-plan offices is commonplace.

If your voices are intrusive, can you listen to music or white noise through headphones? Some people find this helpful, but it won't be possible in many work environments.

Try to work out what you can do to make the most of your concentration. Is it better to concentrate hard for short periods? Does regularly changing activities keep you more alert? Would using colour to highlight documents increase the visual interest of your work?

If you find it hard to sit still for long periods, find reasons for regularly moving around, such as going to the photocopier or visiting another department.

Dealing with potential decision-making difficulties

Talk through decisions with colleagues and discuss their problems too: you will both gain from the additional perspective. Set out the advantages and disadvantages of alternative approaches and use this as the basis for a discussion with your line manager. Draft a response, but don't send it till the next day, in case you have further thoughts overnight.

If your voices are being critical, are they expressing valid issues that should be explored? Ask your voices for suggestions on how to proceed, but only implement these suggestions if you agree with their ideas.

Ask your manager or colleagues for feedback on a draft document, rather than struggling to produce a finished version. This may reduce critical voices. There is nothing unusual or wrong with being a perfectionist.

Managing your stress

Many voice hearers find that negative-seeming voices become stronger when they are stressed. At work, good organisation and time management will help you to make the best use of available time. Other tips include:

- Reflect on what has gone well/not so well. Make notes to discuss with your manager.
- Identify any problem areas and try to think of ways to improve – for example, if you are struggling with a task because you do it so rarely, could you do it with a colleague, so that you can remind each other of the process?
- Be prepared for disagreement. You have a choice as to whether to go with the other person's approach or challenge it.
- Some employers offer useful courses such as assertiveness skills or dealing with difficult customers.
- If under pressure, don't resort to alcohol.
- Ask for help if you are getting very stressed. Is your stress due to your voices, or are there other contributory factors such as a heavy workload, impossible deadlines or bullying? Workplace stress is increasing, and many organisations have a process for investigating and addressing it. However, this does not mean that it will automatically happen in a good way. Consider the pros and cons before initiating a formal process, which may itself be a source of stress.

Outside work

What you do outside work has an impact on you at work too. Tips include:

- Get enough relaxation and sleep.
- Use any tools you have developed for relating to your voices as constructively as possible. Seek additional learning opportunities – such as the various approaches introduced in this book.

- Try mindfulness, either through taking classes or via an app.
- If you are seeing a therapist, counsellor, GP or community psychiatric nurse, discuss with them any difficulties that arise in connection with work.
- If you are taking antipsychotic medication, take it regularly and go back to your doctor if the dose needs adjusting. Medication helps some people, but it can make others feel foggy and 'zombie-like' (for more guidance on this, see Chapter 15 on medication in this book).
- Keep attending hearing voices peer support groups if you have found them to be helpful.
- Ask a trusted friend or family member to tell you if they feel you are becoming overwhelmed and if this is likely to manifest in the workplace (your own experience may be quite different to how you are perceived by others).
- Block out regular holidays for rest and recovery.
- Use deep breathing and grounding exercises (if you find them helpful).

> *Learning point 3*
>
> Can you think of positive and inspiring examples of people – colleagues, peers, or in history – who have thrived in their working life and career because of their hearing-voices experience and what it brought to their work?
>
> - What can you learn from their stories?

Covid-19 and working implications

As I write this, we are still in the grip of the global coronavirus pandemic. This has had a massive impact on work. It has, in many cases, increased the difficulties for people in finding work, and thus also for voice hearers, as many jobs have been lost, changed or become insecure. Any related increased anxiety may, of course, also be reflected through the voices. Some voice hearers may have been cut off from their normal support networks, as social interaction with friends and family, social activities, exercise and access to talking therapies became severely restricted. For some people this may have meant taking additional medication to address issues such as insomnia.

Homeworking

During national lockdowns, homeworking has been an option for some people, but it has brought its own challenges. Some voice hearers have felt 'trapped' at home with their critical voices; they were isolated and missed the regular social contact with colleagues. For some, having to use the phone and online communication for meetings presented challenges, although others, who prefer to avoid face-to-face situations, found this advantageous.

Strategies for homeworking that anyone might find helpful include:

- Keep a regular routine of getting up, showering and dressing for work (even if you don't wear your formal work clothes).
- Make a detailed schedule for your work day, setting time periods to work on different tasks. Most people are more productive if they concentrate on a task for a limited period, then have a change. You could set alarms on your computer or phone.
- Make a task list, breaking work into smaller chunks. Tick them off as you complete them. This helps you to see that you are making progress, so that you can challenge your voices by evidencing that you completed these tasks today.
- It might be helpful for you to initiate regular reports to your manager, such as summaries of your progress, or highlighting any delays so they feel they are in touch with what you are doing. Essentially, you are making sure there is a chain of evidence about your work.
- It is okay to say, 'I'm finding it difficult to work from home.' Many colleagues may feel the same. Admitting that it is difficult may encourage people to share ideas about what can help.

Telling your employer you are a voice hearer

There may come a time when you decide to tell your employer that you hear voices, despite your initial reluctance. This may come about if you have been off sick and need further support or 'reasonable adjustments' on your return to work, perhaps to help you avoid becoming unwell again. Your return to work can be an opportunity to look at how you can be supported in the workplace and helped to remain well.

I just want to emphasise again, these are your rights under disability and employment legislation. Responsible employers encourage employees to disclose any disability or long-term health condition, including mental health conditions, so they can support them. This is because they have a legal responsibility to avoid discrimination and to make 'reasonable adjustments' where someone with a disability or long-term health condition is placed at a significant disadvantage because of that. Your line manager and human resources officers should seek guidance from an occupational health practitioner as to what are appropriate adjustments. You should be involved in the discussion too, especially since you should not assume that occupational health practitioners know about helpful adjustments for people who hear voices and may regard this as a matter for psychiatrists and medication, rather than practical changes.

With your employer's agreement, in the UK you can apply for support through the national Access to Work scheme.[1] The scheme provides a workplace needs

---

1. www.gov.uk/access-to-work

assessment, and may contribute to the costs of any support that is recommended. This can be useful if your employer doesn't know how to support you or is being unhelpful, because it involves an external assessor. Again, do not assume that these external assessors understand about mental health issues in the workplace. This book and the various Hearing Voices Networks might offer advice that you find more helpful. There are many things that your employer can do to support you, such as changes to your physical workspace, agreeing to flexitime arrangements, providing any helpful equipment, assistance with travel to work, and allowing you time off to attend medical appointments. You may also be able to access workplace coaching sessions.

An approach many have found helpful is the Wellness Action Plan (WAP), inspired by Mary Ellen Copeland's Wellness Recovery Action Plan (WRAP) (Copeland, 2005). This is a practical tool to help people identify what keeps them well at work, what causes them to become unwell, and what support they would like to receive from their manager to boost their wellbeing or speed their recovery. The *People Managers' Guide to Mental Health* provides further information for managers, and a template (CIPD/Mind, 2018).

Sickness absence

In the UK, if a worker is ill for less than seven days (including weekends), they do not have to give an explanation. Your employer may ask why and some voice hearers give another explanation, such as a chest infection, rather than the real reason, but you do not have to say. If you are ill for more than seven days, you will need to give your employer proof in the form of a 'fit note' from a GP, which would normally refer to your medical diagnosis.[2] A GP will normally give you a fit note for a limited period, and you will need to get another one at the end of that period if you are not better. Once you start to recover, the fit note may include recommendations on support you need in returning to work (such as a graduated return over several weeks). Your employer will usually continue to pay you while you are absent for short periods. This will be set out in your contract. For longer periods of absence, you may have to apply for Statutory Sick Pay.

This means that you will also need to think carefully about what you tell your GP. For many GPs, hearing voices is still an indication of a possible diagnosis of schizophrenia, and they think this means you cannot possibly cope with employment. Some voice hearers, understandably, prefer not to disclose that they hear voices and find alternative explanations. Many GPs are very happy to simply attribute time off due to stress. Remember: some people would say it is society's difficulty with treating voice hearers in a normal way that is the problem, and not the fact that they hear voices.

Your employer will normally want to remain in contact with you while you are absent, and will want to know when you are likely to be able to return to work. However, if you are very unwell you may not want or be able to communicate with

---

2. www.gov.uk/taking-sick-leave

your employer. In this case, you could ask a family member or friend to act as intermediary and to pass on messages.

Bullying and harassment

Sadly, some people experience bullying at work. This may arise for a variety of reasons – for example, simply because someone is seen as different. Although managers and human resources staff should prevent bullying, in practice they may themselves engage in bullying behaviours, and investigation of complaints may be flawed.

If you are unhappy in your current role because of bullying, you have various options. Your organisation may have a means of seeking support such as a harassment helpline, or an internal group of harassment advisers. If you are a member of a trade union, your local officers may be able to help you. If you are asked to attend any meetings to investigate a claim of alleged bullying (either as victim or perpetrator), you may have the option of taking a trade union officer or colleague with you. This will help to reduce your stress levels, and they can also make notes of the meeting for you. Everyone finds it difficult to concentrate in such a stressful situation, and you will have your voices also to contend with.

Some people who are unhappy in a particular work environment choose not to make a formal complaint but quietly look to see whether they can move to a different role within the same organisation. This can be presented as a move for career development, but also has the benefit of removing you from an unpleasant situation. Sometimes you may find the best thing for you is to simply hand in your notice. However, it is important that you take proper advice before you do this so that you know what this means in terms of any potential benefits payments you may or may not be entitled to.

It may feel risky to move on from a familiar job, but it is often rewarding to seek out new opportunities to develop further and flourish.

Conclusion

Many people find work rewarding and fulfilling, whether or not they are also living with hearing voices. We all have different needs and preferences and can contribute most successfully when our needs are met. People who live with hearing voices may need to be particularly thoughtful about what they would find helpful as they may have more variables to consider in their lives. Using ordinary language to frame their needs in a less stigmatising and pathologising way is a useful strategy and helps other people to understand. Careful consideration must be given to how open you are with your manager and colleagues about hearing voices. This is very dependent on the workplace culture. As the case studies in this chapter show, everyone does better at work when they can be honest and feel valued and supported.

References

CIPD/Mind. (2018). *People managers' guide to mental health*. [Online.] CIPD. www.cipd.co.uk/knowledge/culture/well-being/mental-health-support-report

Copeland, M.E. (2005). Wellness recovery action plan: A system for monitoring, reducing and eliminating uncomfortable or dangerous physical symptoms and emotional feelings. *Occupational Therapy in Mental Health, 17*(3–4), 127–150. https://doi.org/10.1300/J004v17n03_09

Craig, L., Cameron, J. & Longden, E. (2017). Work-related experiences of people who hear voices: An occupational perspective. *British Journal of Occupational Therapy, 80*(12). https://doi.org/10.1177/0308022617714749

17 Navigating university as a voice hearer
Deborah Altman

As a voice hearer, you can succeed at university. You may already be aware of this, as your experience of hearing voices may be positive or neutral, or you may already have found a way of living well with your voices, even if they are difficult at times. Alternatively, you may have heard or have already been advised by some mental health professionals or others that hearing voices may be a sign of a mental illness and that you are therefore likely to struggle at university. It may therefore be important to know that there are many people who feel they can live well with their voices, and some despite having used (or they are still using) mental health services for support because of their mental health experience.

It may also be important to know that not all mental health professionals and researchers agree that hearing voices is a sign of an illness or a disability. For example, the Hearing Voices Movement (a civil rights movement of voice hearers, professionals and laypeople), believes the experience to be a normal variation of human existence and not a sign of an illness, while understanding very well that these experiences can be overwhelming and make life difficult at times.[1] There are many people in this movement who have found a way of living well with their voice-hearing experience, despite having struggled with their voices in the past (Romme et al., 2009).

However, if you feel you are at a point in your life where you would like additional support in view of your voice-hearing experience, there is also plenty of support available at university if you know how to ask for it. This chapter aims to give you a few tools to help. We will also use the stories of two voice hearers, Mo and Emily (not their real names), who have successfully navigated student life.

It is well known that people may hear or begin hearing voices for a wide range of reasons, and for most their voices are not permanent or distressing (Understanding Voices, 2017).[2] There are sources of support available for young

---

1. See Intervoice – www.intervoiceonline.org
2. See also Hearing the Voice – https://hearingthevoice.org

people and adults who identify as voice hearers and who want to understand more about it.[3,4]

If you feel that your voices are beginning to affect your day-to-day activities, this could impact on your studies at university or your preparations and applications for a place at university. The website of Intervoice (an umbrella organisation for the international Hearing Voices Movement) has a support and recovery blog that gives some ideas of the different ways you may find your life being affected by the experience of voices.[5]

If you feel your voice-hearing experience is disrupting your studies, there will also be a range of student support services in your university. Most universities have a counselling service and mental health or wellbeing practitioners. These are usually centralised services that are available to all students, not connected with an individual department or school. In addition, most students have a personal tutor they can contact to discuss any wellbeing concerns that might affect their studies. Be sure you know who this person is and how to contact them.

If you are worried about your voices and fear they are having a negative impact on you and your ability to concentrate on your daily life, your studies or on your social relationships, you might also decide to discuss it with your GP. However, it is important to know in this context that many voice hearers would say that they have a painful history of engagement with medical and other mental health-related professions, as they felt they were being given little useful support and/or were only told about medication options and that their voices were a sign of illness. They were not offered any talking support, or other approaches described in this book. Some have found this support quite unhelpful or even damaging, and prefer to avoid involvement with these professionals, as they are not sure that what they offer will be helpful. At the same time, contacting your GP or another mental health professional could be useful as a means of accessing additional support. It is important to remember that different people find different things helpful.

Deciding about disclosure

It is important to remember that the decision whether to identify as a voice hearer is entirely your choice. If you are beginning to struggle with your studies, disclosure may unlock access to additional support systems within the university and externally. If you are thinking of disclosing to any individual or organisation, you may wish to check their data privacy arrangements. Counselling and medical services have strict protocols for client confidentiality, but other services generally share information within the university on a need-to-know basis, in the interests of meeting students' support needs.

It may also be important to be aware in this context that voice hearing is generally still considered to be a sign of a major mental illness by most mental

---

3. See Voice Collective – www.voicecollective.co.uk/
4. See Hearing Voices Network – https://hearingthevoice.org/looking-for-support/
5. See www.intervoiceonline.org

health and medical professionals. Hearing voices is widely regarded as a symptom of schizophrenia, a diagnosis that most mainstream mental health services still consider to be a chronic condition requiring long-term medication to manage. Many mainstream and associated mental health services, and even some university counselling services, are not yet familiar with some of the newer normalising and talking approaches to hearing voices introduced in this book.

> *Mo started his course at university and did not define himself as a student with a disability. He had experiences of voice hearing and sometimes felt anxiety around this, especially when he couldn't focus on anything but the voices. He was worried about how this might affect his studies. At other times, he found his voice hearing to be a positive and helpful experience. He was hesitant about whether he identified as a 'student with a disability' and whether he could therefore access university support services.*

Mo could, in fact, access help from the university support services, even if he did not regard himself as having a disability. Neil Alexander-Passe (2018) offers an interesting discussion in a journal article on the question of mental health, disability and difference.

You may decide not to disclose that you hear voices for a number of reasons, for example:

- You may have good control over your voice-hearing experience and do not feel you have a need for additional support.
- You may have adequate support from external people or services, and do not realise that the university can offer individualised, academic-related support.
- You may fear that information about you will be shared widely across the university, including with other students, and that you may experience discrimination as a result.
- You may worry that this information will be passed on to prospective employers.

The following points may be helpful with your decision about whether or not to disclose that you hear voices:

- Your voices may change without warning or at stressful points in the year, such as examination or assessment periods.
- You could be offered additional support if you registered with the university disability or wellbeing support service.
- Universities and colleges have policies to protect your sensitive personal data and deal with issues of discrimination, harassment and bullying. This may help to reassure you. You will be able to view these on the university's website.

> *Learning point 1 – whether to disclose*
>
> Deciding how and where to disclose that you hear voices can determine the level of support available to you at university.
>
> - Deciding about disclosure:
>   - Disclosure is a many-staged process, involving thinking about people around you and what they will do with the information. They might include friends, family, colleagues, teachers or supervisors. You do not have to disclose to all of them right away; you don't need to disclose at all if you are not comfortable with it.
>   - Make a list of people who might need to know that you hear voices. Think about disclosing this to them and next to each one write 'Now', 'Later' or 'Never'.
> - Support for your transition to university:
>   - Like any person first attending university, it is important that you have some personal support in place to help you make sense of university systems and procedures. Who could you ask to fulfil this role? It could be a friend, a member of your family, or someone you know from a support group. It is helpful if they have also been to university.

University disability support services

If you have decided to access the university's disability service, you may already have tried to access support from the university's centralised services, and you may have reached a point where you feel you need additional support from your department or tutors to enable you to achieve in your studies.

University disability services can help you in seeking further support, on the basis that your voice-hearing experience is affecting your day-to-day life and can therefore be described as a disability. This does not mean that you need to identify yourself as disabled just because you are hearing voices. As we said at the beginning, there are many people, including mental health professionals and researchers, who would say for good reasons that voice hearing does not need to be, or even should not be, considered a sign of an illness or a disability, despite some people finding the experience very difficult to live easily with. It ultimately remains your choice how you self-identify, which of course is true both in the context of voice hearing but also more generally in life: we do not need to believe the labels other people choose to give us.

Universities work with the legal definition of disability, as stated in the Equality Act 2010 (HM Government, 2011):

> A person has a disability for the purposes of the Act if he or she has a physical or mental impairment and the impairment has a substantial and long-term adverse effect on his or her ability to carry out normal day-to-day activities.

The role of university disability services is to simplify arranging disability-related support for all aspects of your studies. Universities have a legal responsibility to make 'reasonable adjustments' to learning and teaching activities to enable access for disabled students and the disability service advises them in carrying out this duty.

Universities vary in terms of the name they give to their disability support services. Some are called disability and mental health support; some support voice hearers through their counselling and mental health service; some use more generic titles such as 'wellbeing', 'support for students', or 'inclusive support'. Universities welcome contact from disabled students in advance of starting their course, to ask questions or arrange an informal visit. Once you have applied, making contact with the disability service and your department can help you familiarise yourself with university services and facilities and prepare you for starting your studies.

> *Mo attended a confidential meeting with the university disability and mental health adviser to discuss his anxiety about his voices and decide what to do next. He didn't feel comfortable declaring too much information to his lecturers but was reassured to hear that he could still receive adjustments for his course based on the information he was happy to share. He was also comforted that his medical evidence would be stored confidentially by the disability and mental health advisers and would not be shared with his lecturers.*

What to be aware of before contacting the university's disability service

Some form of medical confirmation will be required by the university's disability service, such as a letter from your GP or other medical practitioner. This would confirm an ongoing mental health disability and state how this affects your day-to-day activities or studies. Remember that you can choose how you describe your need for additional support to your GP or other medical practitioner. Some people, especially if they are unsure whether they will get a helpful response, may choose to find a language that is more generally accepted and not considered to be indicative of major mental illness. So, they may not talk about hearing voices and will use other words to describe their mental health, such as general stress, difficult thoughts, relationship difficulties and so on. We are not encouraging you to lie but just to be mindful of how you want to present yourself and how you want to be perceived.

The university disability service has a responsibility to share information with others at the university who need to know. However, they must not circulate it more widely than necessary and may only store it and use it in order to carry out their role. In particular, sensitive personal data will never be shared with other students. Again – as stated above – you can double-check with the service what information would be passed to whom before you make any detailed disclosure.

If you choose to disclose your voice hearing to the disability support service, the adviser may have local knowledge of hearing voices support groups, such as service-user groups or student-led groups. This could be particularly useful for students coming to study from elsewhere in the country or from overseas.

> *Learning point 2 – do you identify as having a disability?*
>
> These questions may be helpful when deciding whether you could be considered to have a disability.
>
> - What does the term disability mean to you?
> - Would you describe yourself as a person with a disability?
> - Looking at the legal definition in the Equality Act 2010, could you be described as a person with a disability?
> - Is this a term you would want to self-identify with or not? What would be the pros and cons for you?

Support from other students

It is important to remember that you are not the only student who hears voices. Other students who hear voices have successfully completed their studies before you, and you may be able to learn from their experience.

Some students who self-identify as having a disability belong to support networks that meet either in person or via social media. These groups offer valuable support, helping you to meet people who understand your experience and to learn that you are not alone. Student-led groups can also make an effective contribution in raising awareness and informing university policy about acknowledging and accommodating groups such as voice hearers who feel in need of additional support.

You may find there is already a support group for students who hear voices in your university or in the local area. There are now many national, regional and local hearing- voices networks offering self-help, training and support for people who hear voices or who have other unshared sensory or reality experiences (for example, the UK Hearing Voices Network[6]).

Emily's story

During her PhD, Emily helped to set up an unusual experiences peer support group in Oxford for people who live with voices, and/or other unusual experiences. Sharing experiences – at your own pace – in a safe, confidential

---

6. See Hearing Voices Network – https://hearingthevoice.org

space, with others who understand, can help. This group changed to meeting online when the Covid pandemic broke out.

Being a student, and a voice hearer, Emily wanted to learn strategies from others that would help her to study. In her memoir, Emily's Voices (Knoll, 2018), she tells her therapist, 'I'm in a power struggle with the voices. It's them against me, and I have to win.' Mostly the voices gave broken commentaries, picking on things that had happened; just a phrase here and there. Emily found it helpful to ignore what the voices said for an hour. Then she would try talking back to the male voice in her head for a minute or two. She sometimes told the voice to 'Shut up and go away!'

Emily had a mentor (for her academic work), and he encouraged her to plan her workload so that she felt less anxious. She used highlighters and post-it notes when she read books or journal articles, as this helped her to absorb new information. A student (who was studying for a PhD on a similar topic) read the chapters that Emily had written for her thesis, and offered feedback, tracking their changes to her work. Emily also gave the other students feedback on their thesis chapters. Emily found that this process encouraged her to keep going with writing her thesis.

Support from within the university

When you contact your university disability service, they will probably invite you to a meeting with a disability adviser. This is your opportunity to talk about the impact of your voices on your day-to-day activities, and to disclose any other difficulties or disabilities, such as a chronic health condition or dyslexia. Your disability adviser will remind you about the likely demands of university life and your studies. Together, you can then produce a learning support plan.

This learning support plan is a report shared between the disability service and key contacts in your department, such as departmental administrators and course and module leaders. Each university or college has their own name for this report: for example, individual student support record (ISSR), individual learner support record (ILSR), student support recommendations (SSR), disability support notification (DSN) and so on. Your disability adviser will be familiar with the university's systems and procedures, so will be able to advise on the type of support requests likely to be agreed by the university. They will then write these into your learner support record.

The reasonable adjustments recommended by your disability adviser might include increased access to tutors, practical classes taken in a smaller room, a separate room for examinations, extensions to coursework deadlines, and so forth. The recommendations are personalised, to help you manage your voices at times of increased stress. For example, if your voices are less intrusive in a smaller, quieter environment, this can be arranged for examinations. Having extended time to complete coursework may help to reduce the feeling of pressure, allowing you more space to engage in dialogue with your voices (which a lot of people find helpful when it is done in a constructive way), or extra time for relaxation activities. Postgraduate students may benefit from recording their meetings with their supervisors, if their voices stop them from paying full attention during the meeting, thus giving them a record of the meeting they can replay later.

Mo found it particularly helpful to have tailored support for the times when he found his voice hearing distressing. This included having a smaller exam room and being seated close to an exit in case he needed a rest break; extra time for all of his exams; access to extensions for assignments if needed and use of a quiet workspace in the library.

> *Learning point 3 – Before you apply to a university*
>
> If you are thinking of using the university's disability support service, you could try the following to learn more about what it offers:
>
> - Choose three universities you might consider applying to.
> - Go to their websites and find out the name of their disability support service.
> - Remember, the service may be located in a counselling and/or mental health service.
> - Find out what support they offer for students with mental health support needs.

If you are seriously considering applying to a university, write an email to the disability service asking them what support they offer people who feel they need additional support with their voice-hearing experience.

Inclusive practice

Most universities are working towards a model of inclusive practice. They are developing teaching and learning activities that aim to include students from wide variety of cultural and social backgrounds, thus reducing the need for individual disability-related adjustments.

One inclusive practice used in many universities is the centralised recording of lectures. You may find this a helpful resource if your voices interfere with your concentration or stop you paying attention during lectures. Lectures are recorded automatically, then made available via the university's intranet, usually within 24 hours. This means you can access the recordings after the lectures to help you complete your notes or use them for revision for exams. Universities vary in how widely they use centralised recording. Some lecturers may choose not to record their sessions, for personal or professional reasons.

Most universities post additional course materials on the university's intranet, such as module outlines, assignment briefs, lecture slides and reading lists. As for any other university student, it is recommended that you make good use of university online systems, to help you stay informed and up to speed with the requirements of your studies.

University online systems can also be of great benefit if you feel anxious about social contact. Most universities have an online library that, depending on the subject being studied, may contain a good proportion of the reading material for your course. Your university user name and password give you secure access, so the virtual library and course materials can be accessed from anywhere.

Finally, as for any other university student, most lecturers are available for you to ask questions if you have missed a class or need further explanation of a topic. Formal lectures are often quite large and there may not be opportunities to ask questions. Some lecturers prefer to be contacted by email to arrange a meeting; others publicise a time (sometimes known as 'office hours') when they are available to see students.

The development of online learning in response to Covid-19

In 2020–21, in response to the Covid-19 pandemic, universities had to adapt to provide online learning experiences. This has led to an expansion of inclusive learning and teaching practices in many universities. Many more learning resources are available online and students can access these at any time, not just in scheduled lecture sessions. This has benefitted some students, including some voice hearers, who may prefer to work alone or at certain times of day or night. It has also helped students who have some anxiety around social interactions. It is hoped that these practices will continue even when social distancing requirements are no longer in force.

External funded support

If you decide to obtain medical evidence that confirms a disabling condition, UK students may be eligible to apply for the Disabled Students' Allowance (DSA). This is a government fund that subsidises additional costs you may incur for any disability-related reason. It is not a cash benefit; it is provided to eligible students in the form of equipment, software or human support required to enable you to participate and achieve in your studies.[7]

You can apply for DSA if you are normally resident in the UK. You apply to your funding body (for example, Student Finance England) and will be assessed by them to discuss your study-related needs. If you have another disability, such as dyslexia or a mobility impairment, you can submit additional medical evidence to confirm this and the study needs assessment will take it into account at the same time.

Your university disability adviser can explain the process and help you with your application for DSA. The benefits from DSA can make the difference between staying on and dropping out of your course, or between scraping through and

---

7. See www.gov.uk/disabled-students-allowance-dsa

getting a good degree. As a voice hearer, you might qualify for funding for meetings with a specialist mentor, which could help you develop strategies for managing your experience of voices and coping with the varied demands of your studies. If you also have a disability or specific learning difficulty, you may find that symptoms of that condition, such as chronic pain or the challenges of academic reading, may increase the impact of your voices. Of course, relating well to voices can also be influenced by a myriad other experiences, such as relationship difficulties, having too much to do, and so forth.

DSA is separate from any support you may be receiving from local service providers, as it relates specifically to your studies. DSA is not means tested and does not need to be repaid. Furthermore, it is provided in confidence so other students or lecturers need know nothing about it.

If you decide to disclose a disability and apply for DSA, you can do so up to six months in advance of starting your course. This means you could have the support in place from day one, which would help to smooth your transition into higher education.

Mo had access to specialist mental health mentoring through the Disabled Students' Allowance. He arranged ongoing meetings with the mental health advisor when he felt that he needed further support or liaison with his course team.

At the time of writing, DSAs are available to undergraduate and postgraduate students who are UK residents, and to postgraduates on research-funded studentships. However, please note that the regulations are frequently reviewed and you should check for the latest update with your funding body or disability adviser.

> *Learning point 4 – Have the previous sections helped you to determine what support you might need?*
> - What would be your concerns about studying at university?
> - Review the above points about reasonable adjustments for disabilities, external funded support and inclusive practice at universities. How could these help to address your concerns?
> - What other support might you need for studying at university?

Final points

1. The disability adviser is one part of the support services available to students at university.
2. The level and nature of support offered depends on your decision about what you are disclosing as a voice hearer, and on obtaining medical evidence.

3. If you choose to disclose that you are at times struggling with voices, you may be entitled to disability support through the university as well as to funded support through Disabled Students' Allowance.
4. If you do not disclose that you find your voice-hearing experience difficult at times, you may still benefit from inclusive learning and teaching practices at the university, and from student-led support groups.

Like many students, Mo had some ups and downs throughout his degree, but he loved his course, enjoyed meeting new people and found that support services enriched his experience.

Acknowledgement

This chapter was written with generous support from Emily Knoll, Megan Barker and Hannah Griffin.

References

Alexander-Passe, N. (2018). Should 'developmental dyslexia' be understood as a disability or a difference? *Asia Pacific Journal of Developmental Differences, 5*(2), 247–281.

HM Government. (2011). *Equality Act 2010: Guidance.* Office for Disability Issues. HM Government.

Knoll, E. (2018). *Emily's voices: A memoir.* Knoll Publications.

Romme, M., Escher, S., Dillon, J., Corstens, D. & Morris, M. (2009). *Living with voices: 50 stories of recovery.* PCCS Books.

Understanding Voices. (2017). *What is hearing voices?* [Online]. https://understandingvoices.com/wp-content/uploads/2019/09/wihv_FINAL-1.pdf

18 Experience focused counselling (Making Sense of Voices)

Joachim K. Schnackenberg, Oana-Mihaela Iusco and Senait Debesay

Since its beginning in 1987, the Hearing Voices Movement (HVM) has been very influential in the de-pathologisation and normalisation of hearing voices, arguing instead that they might be an understandable reaction to life events. Voices can thus be used positively for a person's recovery journey. This chapter will give an overview of experience focused counselling (EFC), also known as Making Sense of Voices.

Background

Traditional assumptions about hearing voices as representing a key symptom of an assumed, biologically based diagnosis of 'schizophrenia'[1] are increasingly coming under challenge in the literature and in research (McCarthy-Jones, 2012; Murray, 2016; Harrison et al., 2018).

Instead, hearing voices and similar experiences are now recognised as being experienced by a significant minority (about 7.2%) of the general population, and will continue over the longer term for about 20% of them. However, only about 7.4% will attract a diagnosis of psychotic disorder (Linscott & van Os, 2013). In other words, for a significant number of people, hearing voices is not experienced as frightening, distressing, pathological or unusual enough to seek mental health support. Environmental factors, such as trauma and social inequalities – rather than brain disease or dysfunction – now appear to be evidenced much more convincingly as key precipitating or perpetuating factors in hearing voices (Bailey

---

1. 'Schizophrenia' and related 'symptoms' are put in inverted commas to clarify that this concept (as well as several other diagnoses in psychiatry) lacks sufficient scientific reliability and validity (Murray, 2016; Johnstone & Boyle, 2018). The science and debates around the validity of psychiatric diagnosis and medication should accordingly be openly discussed with clients, so that they can make properly informed choices about any support that might be offered (Schnackenberg & Burr, 2017).

et al., 2018; van Os, 2018). As antipsychotics have now also been shown to be more limited in their effectiveness (Leucht et al., 2017; Moncrieff, 2020) and possibly more damaging (decreased brain volume, increased risk of death and other major life-changing consequences) than has long been thought (Murray et al., 2016; Moncrieff, 2020), there is a growing recognition of a significant need for a real paradigm shift in theory and practice towards alternatives. Some of these alternatives include non-diagnostic, non-medical approaches to supporting or accompanying voice hearers (Murray, 2016; Johnstone & Boyle, 2018).

These insights are not new to the Hearing Voices Movement (HVM, see Box 18.1). The HVM would also contend that it is not the hearing of voices itself that can lead to far-reaching, negative personal and social consequences for the voice hearer; rather, the voice hearer may not yet have found a constructive way of understanding and relating to their voices (Romme et al., 2009).

Box 18.1: The Hearing Voices Movement (HVM)

> The HVM originates in research, insights and social action initiatives by psychiatrist Marius Romme and science journalist Sandra Escher, based in Maastricht, in the Netherlands, and voice hearers with and without psychiatric experience. It has now become a social emancipatory civil rights movement (Hearing Voices Cymru, 2018) within which voice hearers, professionals and interested allies are committed to an approach to voice hearing that is de-pathologising, normalising and strengths orientated. It emphasises the potential of voices to be understandable reactions in the context of a person's traumatic life experiences. It also seeks to address power imbalances within relationships, psychiatry and society. The organisation of social networks, self-help groups and alternative approaches are an essential part of this worldwide network (see www.intervoiceonline.org; Romme et al., 2009).

The HVM proposes that a learnable, more constructive way of dealing with voices can reduce the negative consequences and even has the potential to enrich the life of the voice hearer (Romme et al., 2009). By taking an interest in the everyday life of voice hearers within a genuinely trusting and dependable relationship, people – be they mental health professionals, counsellors, peers, family or other supportive individuals – can take on a key role in accompanying voice hearers on their recovery journey (Schnackenberg & Burr, 2017). These are the 'accompanying persons' we refer to in this chapter.

This focus by the HVM on recovery contrasts with the classic mainstream understanding of 'schizophrenia' as a chronic, primarily biologically based disorder, within which the potential meaning and intention of the voices and what they say in a person's life context are not considered relevant (Romme & Escher, 2000). In addition, both experience from practice (Schnackenberg & Burr, 2017) and recent developments in the scientific discourse point to the fact that hearing voices is found in a number of psychiatric 'diagnoses' and that differences in the voices cannot be attributed to any specific diagnosis to any meaningful extent (Aleman & Laroi, 2008; Waters & Fernyhough, 2017).

Experience focused counselling

Experience focused counselling (EFC), also known as Making Sense of Voices, the Maastricht Approach or Working with Voices, is a non-pathologising, non-diagnostic approach based on the HVM principles, which can be learned and partly or completely applied – depending on the role and situation – by anyone who is accompanying a person who hears voices. This includes any of the mental health-associated professions and also paid and unpaid peers. Even family or people close to the person hearing voices may benefit from the insights of this approach (Romme & Escher, 2000; Schnackenberg & Burr, 2017).

EFC focuses on making sense of a person's voices within their life context and accompanying the voice hearer if they want to work on reducing any related distress. Practice-based experience and evidence from research also suggest a central role for voices in understanding other psychiatric 'symptoms', such as 'delusions' and 'formal thought disorder', as well as life conflicts that might need to be worked through (Schnackenberg & Burr, 2017; Schnackenberg et al., 2018a). A 'delusion', 'formal thought disorder' or 'social withdrawal' may, for example, turn out to be, respectively, an attempt to explain the origins of voices (e.g. aliens), a reaction to voices interrupting the flow of thought or a reaction to disruptive, threatening voices. Similarly, a voice encouraging the person to hurt themselves may turn out to be a prompt to spur them on to seek to regain control in an emotionally overwhelming situation that may itself be associated with unresolved traumatic experiences.

This principle can be extended to other experiences categorised as 'symptoms' of 'mental disorder' too. Thus, voices are transformed from supposedly representing a key symptom of schizophrenia – and thus ultimately incomprehensible and meaningless in the person's life context – to representing not just a key to understanding past and current distress (Schnackenberg et al., 2018a; 2018b) but also to being an understandable key in the recovery process. In this way, using EFC can also help to turn what was formerly deemed psychotic (that is, not understandable in the person's life context) into understandable and therefore non-pathological reactions.

EFC can be used with any 'diagnosis' and none. The main criterion should be whether a person is distressed by their experience of voices, visions or other non-shared realities, not whether a particular diagnosis has been given (Schnackenberg & Burr, 2017; Schnackenberg et al., 2018b). The voices may be variously (and not exclusively) experienced as spirits, God, the devil, gods, coming from plants or animals, forms of telepathy, messages from the radio and so forth, and it is more helpful to use the terminology used by the voice hearer, rather than insisting on one's own (like 'voices' or 'hallucinations') (Romme & Escher, 2000). EFC can also be applied to working with visions, smells, feelings, tastes or other similar sensations that may not be understood straight away. It may then be helpful to ask what the vision, taste and so forth is saying or seems to be saying if it could speak. In that way one can make these experiences similarly accessible as voices.

> **Learning point 1**
>
> The current scientific and practice discourse demands a complete paradigm shift of attitude and behaviour in professionals and laypersons alike, not simply the use of different language or techniques. Putting the above described new insights into practice will not work if we insist that people who hear voices and/or have similar experiences are unwell or somehow different and should therefore be treated differently.
>
> - What fears and positive possibilities does the notion that the voice-hearing experience is a potential key to understanding a person's distress within their life context bring up for you? Are you fearful, disbelieving, curious, enthusiastic…?
> - What are you learning about yourself when you reflect on your reactions, whether they be fearful or curious?
> - How can you become more accepting and wanting to understand voice hearers and their voice-hearing experience as a non-pathological experience?

The rest of this chapter will provide a brief overview of EFC theory and practice.

Experience focused counselling

Based on the authors' many years of practice experience and involvement with the HVM, there are a number of insights that have turned out to be important when applying EFC in practice. Some of the basic principles of EFC (adapted from Schnackenberg & Burr, 2017, p.137–140) can be described as follows. The process should always:

- be voluntary
- not be guided by fear, although it is acknowledged that fear has a valid protective function
- attempt to create a sense of safety
- seek regular feedback from the voice hearer and the voices about what is helpful and what is not and then adapt the approach as necessary
- be subjective – it is led by the views and beliefs of the voice hearer.

The EFC practitioner:

- is able to sit with uncertainty
- respects the voice hearer's limits (e.g. via regular reminders that the person must/may watch his/her boundaries and need only speak about what they want and at their speed)

- conducts conversations on equal terms
- offers their own views but never imposes them
- takes a positive attitude
- imparts confidence and hope.

The EFC practitioner believes or knows that:

- acceptance, compassion and recognition count
- voices have meaning
- all behaviour is meaningful in a person's life context
- voices often express emotions and thoughts that are unwanted or rejected by the voice hearer
- avoidance may worsen levels of distress
- life is a teacher
- mistakes are okay
- the key to understanding the voices can be found in a person's history.

In EFC practice, it is important to remember that many voice hearers who are in receipt of psychiatric services may bring very difficult or traumatic unresolved conflicts. It is therefore important – wherever possible – for the professional to avoid the use of force or exploiting the inequalities in power between them and the voice hearer. At the same time, it is also important to note that it is possible to process, or find a good way of dealing with, difficult and traumatic experiences that might be connected with the voices, both with, but also without, the use of explicit trauma therapy. What is most important is that it happens at the pace of the person and in the way they want (Read et al., 2007).

The EFC approach also suggests the use of normalising, de-pathologising language, such as talking about 'hearing voices' instead of 'auditory hallucinations', and 'non-shared realities/views/beliefs' instead of 'delusional thinking'. It includes tools such as the *Working with Voices* workbook (Coleman & Smith, 2003) and the Maastricht Interview, Maastricht Report and Maastricht Construct (see below), as well as supporting the voice hearer to speak, indirectly or directly, to the voices to try to understand them, their intention and their significance in the person's life (Romme & Escher, 2000; Corstens et al., 2012; see Chapter 19 in this book for more detail). The whole process should be collaborative and led by the voice hearer. Its aims may include, for example, to work out the meaning and function of the voices in a person's life and enable them to establish a better relationship – one of mutual understanding rather than fear, for example – with the voices.

Voices are seen as having important messages for the recovery process. For example, they may become more aggressive when the voice hearer does not hold their boundaries. As the voice hearer improves their boundary setting, the voices may reduce or even fall silent. Other experiences (aka 'symptoms') might also reduce at the same time. For instance, an explanation that the secret service produces the voices might fall away when the voice hearer understands the voices to be an expression of their own conflicts. Even 'formal thought disorder', social withdrawal and other such 'symptoms' often associated with psychosis may reduce (Schnackenberg & Burr, 2017). It is not surprising to learn that an EFC process can thus also support a careful reduction of antipsychotic medication (Romme et al., 2009).

For some people, the EFC process can be anxiety provoking, as they and the persons accompanying them may be reluctant to engage acceptingly and/or positively with the voices. This is not surprising when we are reminded that the voices may be connected with hitherto unresolved difficult or traumatic life circumstances (Schnackenberg et al., 2018a; Varese et al., 2012), even if this is not automatically obvious to the voice hearer or the professional early on in the EFC process. The reluctance may, of course, derive from an understandable fear of not being taken seriously, of being locked up or of having their medication increased. A hesitant, avoidant or careful response from the voice hearer may have a protective intent and can be validated as such. The EFC practitioner may therefore want to clarify that they will not send the person to hospital or increase their medication (only if they can guarantee this, of course). Finding a constructive and validating way of dealing with the fears of people accompanying the voice hearer (particularly if they are mental health professionals) and voice hearers can take time (Schnackenberg & Burr, 2017), but it is time well spent.

The EFC approach can be used in hospital and community settings; even a time-limited, partial application of EFC can have a beneficial impact (Schnackenberg & Burr, 2017; Schnackenberg et al., 2017). Usually, the process starts with the EFC practitioner seeking to establish a trusting rapport with the voice hearer, followed by the (formal or informal), voice hearer-led application of the Maastricht Interview, and then the Maastricht Report and the Maastricht Construct. The Maastricht Report is a structured and ordered summary of the interview. The Maastricht Construct aims to identify the purpose or function of the voices in the person's life context. Voice dialoguing, or talking with the voices, whether directly or indirectly, may help clarify their intentions and motivations, and the voice hearer's understanding and acceptance of the voices.

Following this process of 'decoding' the intended purpose of the voices beyond the often metaphorical, symbolic or exaggerated language used by them and understanding the life circumstances of the voice hearer, the voice hearer may choose to work on areas that they would like to change in their life. For example, if a function of the voice turns out to be a reminder to the person to stand up for themselves, set boundaries and express their needs more assertively, then the voice hearer may decide to work on improving these areas. The voices will often, in fact, have good ideas as to how to do this. The whole process can be supported by helpful attitudes towards the voices and the voice hearer (see basic principles of EFC above) and by improving on the voice hearer's coping strategies for voices and emotions (as indicated below).

The Maastricht Interview

The semi-structured Maastricht Interview is often used as the main tool to facilitate relating in a normalising, conversational, genuinely interested way with the voice hearer and their voices. As voices can be experienced as overwhelming and chaotic, its structure and clarity can help both the voice hearer and the person accompanying them to engage with the voices and the EFC process with less fear. It consists of the following components:

1. The nature of the experience – what is it like and how does the voice hearer perceive the voices?
2. Characteristics of the voices.
3. Personal history – when did the voices start?
4. Triggers of the voices.
5. Contents – what do the voices say?
6. Explanations – how does the voice hearer explain the voices?
7. Impact of the voices on daily life.
8. Balance of relationship of the voice hearer with the voices.
9. Coping strategies of the voice hearer for the voices.
10. Childhood experiences – both difficult and positive experiences.
11. Treatment history – what has been tried?
12. Social network – who knows about the voices and how do they react?
13. Questions – any questions about the process.

(See Romme & Escher, 2000; Schnackenberg & Burr, 2017 for more detail.)

Helpful coping strategies

As a basic principle, it seems that strategies that work well or not well in non-voice-hearing relationships with people (that is, from person to person) also work well or not well in relationships with voices. We also know that dealing with problems is generally more helpful than trying to pretend they are not there. When applying this simple insight to the work with voices, it means that the more acceptingly we approach voices, related emotions, relationship questions or problems, the more likely it is that a good way of dealing with them can be found and related distress can be reduced significantly. Just as in person-to-person relationships, so it is in relationships with voices – what helps one person, does not necessarily help another person, or not at that time. Remembering that it is about relationships should hopefully encourage people to be able to engage – since we all have experience in what helps us and what does not in relationships and in conflicts. Also, just as in person-to-person relationships, it is never helpful to simply follow another person's opinion without checking first whether one thinks or believes this oneself. It is always important to find out what one wants to do oneself.

Some examples are (for more detail, see Romme & Escher, 2000; Schnackenberg & Burr, 2017):

- normalisation (giving examples of famous people who have heard voices, percentage of voice hearers in the general population, stories of coping and recovery, hearing about, learning from or meeting other voice hearers)
- talking about or with the voices
- writing down what the voices say
- thinking about what positions the voice hearer wants to take towards what the voices say and then expressing these positions
- listening and thinking about whether what the voices say is right or not
- not always taking the voices literally. Remembering that they also use metaphors, exaggerations and symbolic language – particularly initially, if they need to capture the attention of the voice hearer. A voice telling you to kill yourself or someone else could, for example, be a call for a necessary new start in life or for a dramatic change in a non-helpful relationship dynamic
- asking the voice to clarify what it means if you do not understand something or are initially hurt by something that the voice said
- assuming that the voice means well, or that you can turn it to your benefit. This can give the voice hearer confidence to ask questions differently right from the start, and so gives them a greater sense of control, even if it becomes clear that the voice hearer continues to only see the voices' intent as malign.

Helpful attitudes of the accompanying person

There are some attitudes that are felt to be helpful in the process of accompanying the voice hearer. In summary, the process ought to be strengths-focused (with a belief in the inherent ability of every person to recover), voluntary and trauma-sensitive in order to counter the experience of any trauma-related previous experiences or the invasion of personal boundaries, and with an understanding of how trauma and dissociation can be experienced (Herman, 1992). For example, the accompanying person might use invitational language, such as asking, 'What would you like to focus on?' or 'If you would like to talk about this, remember you only need to talk about what you want'. In this way, the accompanying person makes it clear that they feel able to hear about trauma and that they have dealt with any emotional resistance in themselves. The process should also be led by the voice hearer, and be collaborative and fear-free (i.e. not guided by fear), as much as possible. As with any support intervention offered in mental health services, a trusting relationship is the foundation stone.

Voices and emotions

Voices seem often to be connected to unexpressed and suppressed emotions and thoughts. The voices appear to express emotions that a person has thus far not been able to find an accepting way of dealing with (always for a good reason, such as not yet having had or been given the opportunity to talk about them or to process trauma-related emotions). It is therefore beneficial for the voice hearer to learn about helpful and accepting ways of dealing with emotions that are experienced as difficult. Such a process of increasing emotional acceptance can be greatly aided by the structured questioning of the Maastricht Interview, which can help the voice hearer to better understand and associate the voices in relation to specific emotions.

Speaking differently to and with voices

It may be helpful to remember that unexpressed emotions can often become exaggerated and that voices often use exaggerations or metaphors in order to get the voice hearer's attention, especially when they do not feel that the voice hearer is listening properly. In this way, there seems to be little difference from how human-to-human relationships can work in comparable situations. Within such an understanding, it may be beneficial to be inquisitive and as fear-free and friendly as possible, rather than confrontational with the voices. That is, if a voice says, for example: 'You are a parent murderer, you have committed crimes against your family,' it may be helpful for the voice hearer not to simply confront the voice by stating, 'How dare you?' and 'That is not true' and so forth. It may be more beneficial for the voice hearer to move on to say that this is hurtful for them to hear, and to ask with a truly open mind why the voice is saying that, and to continue to ask until a logical and (often) helpfully intended answer has been gained. The voice hearer may then, for example, discover that the voices are encouraging them to own their emotions, such as anger or sadness, which thus far they have perceived as difficult and have therefore rejected. If there are indeed unresolved and unspoken feelings about conflicts with others or themselves, the voices may then even move on to help the voice hearer find a way to reconcile themselves with those people or themselves, if that is what the voice hearer would like.

Acceptance of emotions

When emotions are increasingly accepted it is not unusual for the voices to become more positive or less frequent. They may even apologise or leave. Using language and expression that is less from the head and more from the gut may be more helpful in enabling a person to express themselves freely. This may possibly include physical expressions of emotions, for which they may find yoga helpful, or consciously used dramatic expression (such as hitting an object, while imagining it to be a previous assailant), or similar.

Within this process, accompanying persons can support the voice hearer by bearing witness to their current and past sufferings. Thus, an accepting way of dealing with emotions and voices can reduce the feeling of powerlessness and turn voices and emotions into helpful guides instead.

> *Learning point 2*
>
> Accompanying people who hear voices or have similar experiences towards greater acceptance of emotions they do not like or reject is a key skill for any person walking alongside them. It is helpful if the accompanying person is able to deal with their own emotions. It does not necessarily need specialist training in, for example, psychotherapy or similar. Sometimes there is fear that allowing certain emotions will lead to the person being stuck in this unpleasant emotion forever, and as a result they do not want to approach these emotions at all. However, based on our experience, people who allow themselves to feel unpleasant emotions within a boundaried process (that is, when they are going at their speed) also report that these emotions are self-limiting.
>
> - What kind of emotions would you rather not feel and how do you avoid emotions?
> - What is the result when you do not allow yourself to feel certain emotions? In your contact with people who hear voices, do you prefer them not to bring up related emotions?
> - What helps you to allow or express certain emotions that you consider to be difficult and would rather not feel when you are by yourself or with someone who hears voices?
> - Have you ever allowed yourself to feel emotions you consider to be unpleasant in a truly accepting and welcoming way? How long did the emotion last for and what was the result? Did you observe any change or improvement in your situation?

Practice example

This is an anonymised example of EFC in practice. Sandra is 30 years old and has been hearing voices for 25 years. She was diagnosed with anorexia as a teenager and with 'paranoid schizophrenia' at the age of 20. Sandra has now managed to achieve a balanced way of maintaining her weight; however, she continues to be really distressed by her voices. It is only about nine months ago that she first started talking about her six voices. It becomes clear during the Maastricht Interview that she assumes that they come telepathically from people both known and unknown to her. The voices are telling her that she should kill her mother and then herself. Sandra often gets very confused, finds it difficult to think clearly or express herself clearly and just does not know how to find a way through it all. Medication has sometimes offered some relief, in that she feels more dampened down. However, she cannot really tolerate the side effects. She has stopped her studies and has spent the last 14 years mostly at home with her mother, who looks after her. She is also in and out of hospital when the voices get too much for her.

Sandra was initially quite fearful about working with EFC and needed some ongoing validating and reassuring support from the EFC worker. Once she started EFC, she found the voices started to calm down. The more Sandra learned about how to relate to them and how to listen to them, using the Maastricht Interview and the Maastricht Construct, the more she understood they were not her enemies and she could increasingly relate to them as well-meaning friends. By asking the voices, she learned that they did not want her literally to kill herself or her mother but for her to become less dependent on her mother – which was, in fact, what she wanted. They were also encouraging her to take her life back into her own hands and not give up, as she seemed to be doing. Specifically, the voices were stating that she should face her fears – for example, that she should take action to process emotionally her experiences of sexual abuse and being bullied. They were suggesting specific ways of doing this by also seeking to motivate her to trust herself (again), to do more, set boundaries, express what she wanted, to go out by herself, mix with people and not to withdraw at home, as she had been doing. As Sandra began to manage to implement these encouraging prompts, the voices became less frequent, urgent, intense and negative. For the first time in about 17 years, Sandra began to feel she might be able to get her life back after all.

Differences between EFC and other talking approaches

Even though there are some similarities with other talking approaches, the openness towards talking directly or indirectly with and not against the voices and looking for a positive intention or use of the voices and in what they say within the person's life context, within a normalising and de-pathologising framework, may be a key difference to most other approaches. There are also early indications in research that it may be effective (Schnackenberg & Burr, 2017; Schnackenberg et al., 2017; Steel et al., 2019).

The use of EFC in practice and research

Increasingly, mental health practitioners, family members, voice hearers and mainstream mental health organisations (in countries including Denmark, Germany, Switzerland, Austria, the UK and elsewhere) have now started to use EFC, in acute, community and long-term rehabilitation settings. While the process of paradigmatic change requires a lot of patience and work by all parties involved, it has started and the feedback to the authors of this chapter (who work internationally as EFC trainers, supervisors and consultants) is that it is worth it, it is bringing positive results, and that it is often kindling a new enthusiasm for finding ways forward in the process of recovery for voice hearers and professionals alike.

Like other talking approaches, it is in the early days of developing a classic research evidence base, as its practitioners have preferred to use recovery stories as a way of moving forward instead.

> *Learning point 3*
>
> Many voice hearers describe the current standard mainstream psychiatric service response as being fear-driven, towards both them and their voices, often very limited in its helpfulness and potentially quite damaging in the short and long term. They describe the formal and informal use of force: for example, sections and the threat of sections and more medication; being pathologised; medication against their will and despite side effects; not being allowed to challenge professionals; not being seen in the context of their unique life history; not feeling that anyone takes a genuine interest in their experience and story; not being believed; being treated arrogantly, and being made to feel everything is their fault (for example, if they followed their medication regime properly, they'd be better). So this learning point is addressed to people working in mainstream services:
>
> - What has helped you not to be guided by fear but by trust? Can you apply this to your contacts with voice hearers?
> - Do you have times when you want to force your views on other people? What helps you not to do it?
> - What helps you in relationships with people you experience as bullying or otherwise unpleasant towards you when you can't just walk away from them? What do you do that you find helpful so that you do not end up losing your own sense of self-worth in such a situation?

Differences in the work with children and young people

Only a very few practitioners have extensive experience of using EFC with children and young people, and it is beyond the scope of this chapter to expand on it in any detail. You can find more about working with children in Chapter 20 in this book. It is worth pointing out, however, that when people respond to children's voices as though they are nothing extraordinary, the voices are more likely to be experienced positively, as they are often intended to be. Voices may also be representing important positive attachment figures for children and young people in otherwise overwhelming circumstances (Debesay, 2017).

Conclusion

In summary, we have learned from the voices and from voice hearers that voices can change from seemingly meaningless symptoms of distress or illness into helpful agents of recovery by both addressing unresolved, often trauma-related emotional conflicts and finding positive solutions for them. This process is helped by remembering that voices do not always need to be taken literally and that it is important to formulate one's own opinions and views and that it is never helpful to simply follow what a voice or another person says without understanding their intentions. Even then, it is important to remember that every one of us remains the author of our own lives and that we decide how much we listen or do not listen to the advice of others, including voices.

References

Aleman, A. & Laroi, F. (2008). *Hallucinations: The science of idiosyncratic perception.* American Psychological Association.

Bailey, T., Alvarez-Jimenez, M., Garcia-Sanchez, A.M., Hulbert, C., Barlow, E. & Bendall, S. (2018). Childhood trauma is associated with severity of hallucinations and delusions in psychotic disorders: A systematic review and meta-analysis. *Schizophrenia Bulletin, 44*(5), 1111–1122.

Coleman, R. & Smith, M. (2003). *Working with voices II: Victim to victor.* P&P Press.

Corstens, D., Longden, E. & May, R. (2012). Talking with voices: Exploring what is expressed by the voices people hear. *Psychosis: Psychological, social and integrative approaches, 4*(2), 95–104.

Debesay, S. (2017). Stimmenhören bei Kindern und Jugendlichen (Hearing voices in children and young people). In J. Schnackenberg & C. Burr (Eds.), with Furrer, M., Iusco, O.M. & Debesay, S., *Stimmenhören und Recovery: Erfahrungsfokussierte Beratung in der Praxis (Hearing Voices and Recovery: Experience focussed counselling in practice* (pp.127–68)). Psychiatrieverlag.

Harrison, P., Cowen, P., Burns, T. & Fazel, M. (2018). *Shorter Oxford textbook of psychiatry.* (7th ed.). Oxford University Press.

Hearing Voices Cymru (2018). *Thessalonika Hearing Voices declaration 2014.* https://hearingvoicescymru.org/about-2/thessalonika-hearing-voices-declaration-2014

Herman, J. (1992). *Trauma and recovery: The aftermath of violence – from domestic violence to political terror.* Basic Books.

Johnstone, L. & Boyle, M., with Cromby, J., Dillon, J., Harper, D., Kinderman, P., Longden, E., Pilgrim, D. & Read, J. (2018). *The Power Threat Meaning Framework: Towards the identification of patterns in emotional distress, unusual experiences and troubled or troubling behaviour, as an alternative to functional psychiatric diagnosis.* British Psychological Society.

Leucht, S., Leucht, C., Huhn, M., Chaimani, A., Mavridis, D., Helfer, B., Samara, M., Rabaioli, M., Bächer, S., Cipriani, A., Geddes, J.R., Salanti, G. & Davis, J.M. (2017). Sixty years of placebo-controlled antipsychotic drug trials in acute schizophrenia: Systematic review, Bayesian meta-analysis, and meta-regression of efficacy predictors. *American Journal of Psychiatry, 174*(10), 927–942.

Linscott, R.J. & van Os, J. (2013). An updated and conservative systematic review and meta-analysis of epidemiological evidence on psychotic experiences in children and adults: On the pathway from proneness to persistence to dimensional expression across mental disorders. *Psychological Medicine, 43*, 1133–1149.

McCarthy-Jones, S. (2012). *Hearing voices: The histories, causes and meanings of auditory verbal hallucinations.* Cambridge University Press.

Moncrieff, J. (2020). *A straight talking introduction to psychiatric drugs* (2nd ed.). PCCS Books.

Murray, R.M. (2016). Mistakes I have made in my research career. *Schizophrenia Bulletin 43*(6), 253–256.

Murray, R.M., Quattraone, D., Natesan, S., van Os, J., Nordentoft, M., Howes, O., di Forti, M. & Taylor, D. (2016). Should psychiatrists be more cautious about the long-term prophylactic use of antipsychotics? *British Journal of Psychiatry, 209*(5), 361–365.

Read, J., Hammersley, P. & Rudegeair, T. (2007). Why, when and how to ask about childhood abuse. *Advances in Psychiatric Treatment, 13*(2), 101–110.

Romme, M. & Escher, S. (2000). *Making sense of voices.* Mind Publications.

Romme, M., Escher, S., Dillon, J., Corstens, D. & Morris, M. (2009). *Living with voices: 50 stories of recovery.* PCCS Books.

Schnackenberg, J. & Burr, C. (Eds.), with Furrer, M., Iusco, O.M. & Debesay, S. (2017). *Stimmenhören und Recovery: Erfahrungsfokussierte Beratung in der Praxis (Hearing voices and recovery: Experience focussed counselling in practice).* Psychiatrieverlag.

Schnackenberg, J.K., Fleming, M. & Martin, C. (2017). A randomised controlled pilot study of experience focussed counselling with voice-hearers. *Psychosis, 9*(1), 12–24.

Schnackenberg, J., Fleming, M. & Martin, C.R. (2018a). Experience focussed counselling with voice-hearers as a trauma-sensitive approach: Results of a qualitative enquiry. *Community Mental Health Journal 54*(7), 997–1007.

Schnackenberg, J., Fleming, M., Walker, H. & Martin, C.R. (2018b). Experience focussed counselling with voice-hearers: Towards a trans-diagnostic key to understanding past and current distress – a thematic enquiry. *Community Mental Health Journal, 54*(7), 1071–1081.

Steel, C., Schnackenberg, J., Perry, H., Longden, E., Greenfield, E. & Corstens, D. (2019). Making sense of voices: A case series. *Psychosis, 11*(1), 3–15.

Van Os, J. (2018). *Environmental factors in schizophrenia.* Talk given at the conference, 'Schizophrenie im Dialog' ('Schizophrenia in Dialogue'), RWTH Aachen University, Germany, January 11.

Varese, F., Smeets, F., Drukker, M., Lieverse, R., Lataster, T., Viechtbauer, W., Read, J., van Os, J. & Bentall, R.P. (2012). Childhood adversities increase the risk of psychosis: A meta-analysis of patient-control, prospective- and cross-sectional cohort studies. *Schizophrenia Bulletin, 38*(4), 666–671.

Waters, F. & Fernyhough, C. (2017). Hallucinations: A systematic review of points of similarity and difference across diagnostic classes. *Schizophrenia Bulletin, 43*(1), 32–43.

19 Voice Dialogue

Ruth Lafferty and Rob Allison

This chapter aims to introduce the reader to 'Voice Dialogue', a form of communication that can be effective both for people who hear voices and for those who don't. We begin with a brief overview of Voice Dialogue before sharing our experiences of facilitating workshops aimed at enabling others to participate in it. One of us (RL) will then offer some personal insights into dialoguing with her voices and reflect on how these experiences have influenced her relationships with her voices and other people. Finally, we will offer suggestions for those wishing to learn more about this way of communicating with voices.

> *Learning point 1*
> What do you think is the purpose of communicating with voices?

Background

There isn't space here to describe in detail the historical and numerous accounts of voice hearing. But we will briefly set out a key assumption that we hold about it before discussing Voice Dialogue. In Western, industrialised societies, voice hearing is predominantly framed as a symptom of a biological illness. Biologically informed medical perspectives are predominant in psychiatric research and service provision, and these attribute voice-hearing experiences to one or more biological causes – for example, genetic, neurochemical and neurodevelopmental abnormalities – despite the lack of robust evidence to support the notion of a causal relationship (Schnackenberg & Martin, 2014).

Interestingly, however, findings from research increasingly associate voice hearing with previous trauma-related experiences. In fact, some researchers have found an index-related relationship, in which greater exposure to trauma leads to an increased likelihood of hearing voices at a later stage in life: the more trauma, the more the likelihood that the person will hear voices (McGrath et al., 2017; Cunningham et al., 2016; Read et al., 2005). We believe that anyone can hear voices and we remain open to different explanatory frameworks. However, in our experience, the voices can be traced back to the life stories of the voice hearer. The challenge is to understand how these stories connect with the voices.

Our assumption is rooted in our work with people who hear voices and our personal experiences, and is largely influenced by the seminal work of Marius Romme and Sandra Escher (Romme & Escher, 1989, 1993, 2012; Romme et al., 2006, 2009). Building on their research, the Hearing Voices Movement (HVM) began in the Netherlands in 1987 and became the inspiration for the Hearing Voices Network (HVN) and many other national, regional and local hearing voices groups and initiatives across the world. The HVM significantly differs from conventional psychiatry in that it accepts voice hearing as a real and normal human experience that can be understood. The approach in the HVM is to listen to a person's account of their voice hearing and help them to construct their own explanation. Romme and Escher argue that voice hearers' interactions with their voices reflect their relationships with their personal and social circumstances, which have regularly included very difficult encounters. According to Romme:

> … voices are the stories of threatening emotions; emotions of the person twisted by terrible experiences, hopelessness, feelings of guilt, aggression and anxiety. (Romme, 2009, p.9).

Voice hearing can be understood as having a protective function (Corstens et al., 2012). Construing voices in this way places importance on understanding and communicating with the voices, and this can be a turning point for many people who are distressed by their voices. This suggests that learning how to communicate with the voices and develop a better understanding of voices and the experiences of the voice hearer is a promising and exciting way forward.

We find the principles of Voice Dialogue very helpful for our understanding of voices. Developed by Stone and Stone (2011), it is primarily rooted in their personal experience and exploration of relationship difficulties. It is a means of exploring and communicating with voices in order to better understand them and what they are saying. Psychodynamic theories, such as Jungian psychotherapy, Gestalt and transactional analysis (and other therapy approaches) have similarities and may in part have been influential in its development. However, Voice Dialogue is very explicit in not being a therapy, although it may be experienced as therapeutic. It may best be described as a tool for personal growth.

Voice Dialogue should not be confused with approaches like relating therapy that emphasise assertiveness and setting boundaries in relation to communication with voices (e.g. Hayward, 2003; Hayward et al., 2017). Voice Dialogue is built on a relational framework and values assertiveness but starts from a benevolent attitude towards the voices and seeks to explore any emotions voices may describe and what the voices were originally and are currently hoping to achieve for the voice hearer. This, once decoded with the help of constructive communication (i.e. with Voice Dialogue principles), tends to be positive or can be used positively.

According to Stone and Stone (2011), we do not have a consistent single identity; instead, we consist of different 'Selves' or 'sub-personalities' or 'parts' or 'energies' – these terms are used interchangeably. The Selves help us to manage in our day-to-day social interactions. There are dominant Selves, which are the ones that are more noticeably present and are more apparent in their influence on how we manage social situations. Other Selves may be 'disowned', in that they may be less socially acceptable or have attributes we don't like. For example, we may have a dominant Self that we recognise as trying to please other people all the time, which we could refer to as a 'pleaser'. There may also be a Self that we recognise as being much more self-centred, where we only ever do things that are to our own benefit, which we could refer to as 'selfish'. The 'pleaser' may be endearing to others and help us to be accepted in social circles; the 'selfish' Self might be frowned on and rejected by others. If we want to be accepted by others, it would make sense to become a 'pleaser'. But constantly being a 'pleaser' can lead to us being more concerned about other people, at the cost of our own wellbeing. Of course, neither of these two Selves are helpful to our wellbeing if we promote one and exclude the other. The trick is to get a balance between our own self-interest and that of the community around us.

The theory of the Voice Dialogue approach has been found helpful to describe similar constructive communication processes with voices in the work of the HVM. Because members of the HVM have made some slight adaptations to the approach, and to differentiate it from working with 'parts', here it has come to be called 'Talking with Voices'. The principles of these two methods, such as learning to understand and communicate with different energies or voices, are closely aligned. What can be helpful when relating to the different Selves can also be helpful in relating to the voice hearer's different voices. This is not to say that we believe that voices and Selves are essentially the same – that is not important; however, the principles of relating to 'Selves' and voices do seem to be similar.

Stone and Stone (2011) point out that the disowning of 'Selves' that we don't want becomes problematic in the long term because each Self serves an important purpose. By pushing certain Selves away, we can end up not knowing what these Selves need and how they could actually be beneficial to us. They may also become unusually strong as a result and much energy must then be devoted to continue pushing them away. For example, a 'selfish' Self is only concerned with its own wellbeing, but to disown this would be, effectively, to disregard one's own wellbeing and not to understand that self-care might be the positive aspect of this 'selfish' Self. Similarly, to disregard a voice would be, effectively, to avoid trying to understand the meanings and potentially positive function related to it. Consequently, disowned Selves or voices leak back into our lives without our full awareness or understanding and in a way that can be unproductive or cause difficulty. For example, disowning a 'selfish' Self can lead one to become physically and emotionally exhausted both from pleasing others all the time and by trying to keep the selfish Self at bay. Likewise, disowning a voice can lead to one becoming fearful of the voice and its perceived intentions; keeping it away takes a lot of energy and the voice will likely become even more overwhelming.

> *Learning point 2*
>
> What do you think would be the potential benefits of and problems with communicating directly with voices?

Practising Voice Dialogue

We run Voice Dialogue workshops for people who hear voices and practitioners who work alongside them. We emphasise that participation in the workshop should be voluntary, for the professionals, the voice hearers and their voices. We start by focusing on voice hearers' life stories and identifying the characteristics of their voices before beginning to open up a conversation with the voices. We demonstrate how we would have a conversation with voices before asking whether other group members would like to ask questions or join a discussion with one of the voices. In this way, we begin a reflective cycle of learning through hearing about a person's history, examining whether there are clues in this history that might explain the voice profile (e.g. the name, age or gender of the voice, or how and what the voices communicate), and then sharing these insights in conversations with the voices in order to help understand who the voices are, why they have come into the person's life, and how to establish more helpful relationships between the voice hearers and their voices.

Key throughout this process is to be clear that the aim is not to get rid of the voices. Instead (as Stone and Stone also advocate), the aim is to increase understanding of voices and bring about greater harmony between the voices and the voice hearer. Just as it is unhelpful for our wellbeing if the 'pleaser' is always dominant or we are dominated by our 'selfish' side, so it is better to achieve a balance where we are considerate towards others and towards ourselves. In terms of voices, the aim is to help the voice hearer improve their relationship with their voices through learning about the voices and understanding the messages behind the words. In our experience, more gentle and courteous inquiry with the voices can help the development of more respectful relationships between the voice hearer and their voices and so reduce the distress associated with voices.

> *Learning point 3*
>
> How might someone facilitating a dialogue with a voice(s) help create a safe space for both the voice hearer and the voice(s)?

Experiencing Voice Dialogue

I (Ruth Lafferty) will now share some experiences of dialoguing with my voices. I have been hearing voices for 10 years. I heard one voice at first, and this increased to 15 voices over a two-year period. I was a psychotherapist when I started hearing voices. Transactional analysis, a form of psychotherapy, was one of the models core to my practice. Voice dialoguing was, therefore, perhaps easier for me to consider because of my familiarity with multiple chair work. I now use all of these voice experiences to inform my Voice Dialogue training practice.

I currently dialogue with my colleague and co-writer Rob Allison and with my partner. It is not common for voice hearers to dialogue as a training demonstration, but Rob and I regularly check whether this is still okay with my voices. It is meaningful for me to offer examples of my experience to other voice hearers and their workers. I am aware that people attending the training can feel that, because it works for me, it should work for any voice hearer. I am clear that I have found it transformational, but it's not for everyone and it's not the only way to develop a better relationship with voices. We are careful not to try to 'sell' voice dialoguing and become another coercive voice to voice hearers.

The felt experience of voice dialoguing is curious. I anticipated a spooky feeling, and a fear that my voices would run away with my mouth. It did indeed feel odd to allow a voice to use my mouth to speak from. However, it was part of my experience, and I assumed that my voices were desperate to speak, given how much I could hear them. It feels much less odd now and I am able to censor, to a degree, foul and abusive words. One of my fears is offending other people, especially those who are willing to talk with my voices. I also know that I can 'take back the mic', so to speak, and stop the voice from speaking. Equally, the voices can stop of their own accord and have sometimes left the chair before the formal ending of the conversation. A dialogue for me is typically only a few minutes long, as it can be tiring.

> *Learning point 4*
>
> What do you think might be useful for a voice hearer to know about Voice Dialogue when deciding whether to dialogue with one of their voices?

An important starting point in understanding voices, for me, is voice profiling. Profiling helped to bring some order and containment to what was a profound chaos of strong feelings, memories, abusive noise and new visual images. Profiling is an ongoing process, as the dialogue unfolds. My first experience was powerful. I soon had a sense of the hierarchy among the voices I had started hearing. Some communicated a greater sense of power and authority than others, and it was clear that the more dominant voices had more power than some of the younger and less authoritative voices. I found that voice profiling enabled me to identify more easily the different qualities and dynamics in the relationships between the voices.

One of the most dominant voices, who called himself Grande during my first Voice Dialogue, was the voice that pushed forward to speak to another during my initial Voice Dialogue training. I felt intuitively that he was the voice to dialogue with most regularly and to try to build a relationship with, as he felt like the most mature voice. I was scared of disobeying him in the early days. He would shout repeatedly if I did something 'wrong' in his eyes, such as go out of the house or talk to any male I didn't already know, and some that I did know if he considered them unsafe. He would also be critical if I made minor errors: for example, he'd shout 'Stupid idiot' if I dropped a spoon. I experienced him as highly critical and controlling of my every thought and action. He seemed to be in charge of all the other voices except one, called B, who he was in direct conflict with. They used to have regular powerful rows, with neither prepared to stand down.

B is the actual voice of someone who attacked me and the one that I am most intimidated by. He comes with a visual image of a man who is about 11 feet tall. Voice hearers often report that a voice has a visible aspect, either very clear or ghostly, and it may be important to discuss what this is like for them and if this changes during or after dialoguing.

Over time, I have experienced Grande as defending me from B, and in dialogue I sense his support for me and authority over this other voice. He now uses the kind of directive language and voice tone that he used to use toward me, instructing B to 'Shut the fuck up', 'Drop to the floor, you fucker', or 'Look at the floor', and saying, 'You are not wanted here', 'Fuck off and die' and so forth. These are harsh words, and the terms are absolute, with little room for negotiation.

B has now started to respond to this style of instruction from Grande and has generally become less vocal and moves away when Grande bears down on him. Grande no longer speaks to me in this way and, I believe, expresses something of the power that B used against me and that I would like to have had to use back to my attacker at the time. This new dynamic between them has changed the balance of power between all my voices and has been transformational in helping me feel safer in the world and increasing my confidence to disbelieve B's threats. However, I don't think this is the end of the transformational process as the content of the dialogue between Grande and B is still oppressive. I believe that, over time, we may achieve a negotiated neutrality between us all through Voice Dialogue. This might include involving another voice in negotiating between us, or negotiating directly with B, as I have with Grande.

I rarely dialogue with the other voices at the moment, except when I talk back to or with them when I am alone. Other voice hearers may want or need to dialogue with more than one voice when dialoguing. Grande holds a pivotal organising and safeguarding role, so it feels right at the moment to focus on developing my relationship with him. Being able to hear his side of what it's like living with me and hear him talk about the reasons for what he says and the way he says it helps me decode his real intentions, which are to protect me and keep me out of danger. This makes sense. In the past, I have been poor at identifying relational risk, and even when I have, I have been poorly equipped to respond assertively and protectively. Grande is my radar and I can now learn from him. And, as I improve my relationship with him, I have experienced shifts in my relationships with my other voices. They have become more organised and predictable, which reduces my threat responses.

> ### Learning point 5
> What do you think might be important in supporting a voice hearer to identify which voice to start voice dialoguing with?

Trust and safety

I have found it helps to let my voices get to know the people I dialogue with. They then experience them as a trusted other who doesn't judge me and, importantly, doesn't judge them. It is key that the dialoguing is respectful, with no ulterior motive to coerce the voice to another point of view or to challenge their way of being. A step forward in my relationship with Grande was hearing that he preferred to be called the leader, rather than the dominant. Just as we can all be sensitive to language, voices respond to being treated respectfully and having choices. When I am talking with Rob Allison, rather than dialoguing, I am always aware that Grande is listening and it matters that he and all my voices know they are regarded with respect. This ensures the process of dialoguing is grounded in a helpful trusting process.

Over time, I think Grande has experienced a growing relationship and has become more open to talking about his role and how he feels about life and living with me. Grande has become keener to dialogue and Rob has observed that his demeanour and the quality of his voice and phrasing has become less defensive. As a consequence, I am less anxious about what Grande might say and Grande can now negotiate with Rob, knowing that he will not be coerced. As I trust Grande more, Grande has started to trust me more.

My aim, from my early days of voice hearing, was to develop a better relationship with my voices and I try to live in a way that respects what they say, without being limited by them when their commands or accusations are destructive. I have found, however, that even their seemingly destructive commands can often be decoded and their underlying intention always seems to be protective. The paradox is the profoundly controlling and insulting way the voices come at me, and processing this can be lengthy and painful. Voice dialoguing can help cut through this kind of negative dialogue. Voice dialoguing makes it possible for the voices to have a conversation with a trusted other that is different to the kinds of conversation I can have with them alone.

When Rob dialogues with Grande, I can hear Grande talking with more directness and clarity about his protective role. I wonder why this is and believe it has something to do with the need for Grande and the other voices to be heard outside my internal community, as well as an observer effect: because someone outside of my Selves is witnessing what a voice is saying, perhaps they speak more plainly. It's not exactly 'best behaviour' but some kind of communication that is more direct. This is a hunch rather than absolute truth. Hearing about the tasks that Grande has set himself to try to keep me, himself and the other voices safe has allowed me to respect and understand why he feels he has to be so critical and coercive. His task is ultimately to keep me safe and he risk-manages my actions and interactions. For example, when meeting someone new, particularly male, he has in the past been very directive, shouting 'Walk away you fuckwit', 'No eye contact', 'Don't speak, shut the fuck up' and so forth. I understand that he didn't trust me to be able to see when I might be in danger of being exploited. I now understand why he is so critical and uses controlling and abusive language and I try to reassure him that I understand his concerns and will listen to him if he detects something that I have missed about someone or a situation.

I believe that, as a result of this cooperative stance and giving ground to Grande first, he is starting to trust me more and is less vocal. The key is decoding the language and the triggers for his elevated threat levels. I have learned to tolerate his approach and become curious rather than frightened, shut down or adversarial with him. The more I accept the way he comes at me, the more I can pick out the legitimate criticism. Processing after a dialogue is often the point when I make these connections and am able to resolve issues from the past. Over the past six years, the quality of the relationship has become more collaborative. Grande now speaks less, is less hostile, is quieter and gets less agitated and instructive in old and new situations.

> *Learning point 6*
>
> What can someone do to support a voice hearer to get closer to the voice in order to understand the reasons for the voice's manner toward the voice hearer?

Concluding thoughts

In our experience, Voice Dialogue is an intuitive method of communicating with voices. It has guided us through a creative process of making sense of the voices and developing a more helpful relationship with them. In turn, this has helped us to develop a more reflective approach to understanding how our relationships with people are somehow linked with how we relate to our voices. As such, the method can help redefine the voices and rebalance voice hearers' relationships with their voices.

Going forward, more research is needed to examine the effects of Voice Dialogue.

References

Corstens, D., May, R. & Longden, E. (2012). Talking with voices. In M. Romme & S. Escher (Eds.), *Psychosis as a personal crisis: An experience-based approach* (pp.166–178). Routledge.

Cunningham, T., Hoy, K. & Shannon, C. (2016). Does childhood bullying lead to the development of psychotic symptoms? A meta-analysis and review of prospective studies. *Psychosis, 8*, 48–59.

Hayward, M. (2003). Interpersonal relating and voice hearing: To what extent does relating to the voice reflect social relating? *Psychology and Psychotherapy: Theory, research and practice, 76*, 369–383.

Hayward, M., Jones, A.-M., Bogen-Johnston, L., Thomas, N. & Strauss, C. (2017). Relating therapy for distressing auditory hallucinations: A pilot randomized controlled trial. *Schizophrenia Research, 183*, 137–142.

McGrath, J.J., Saha, S., Lim, C.C., Aguilar-Gaxiola, S., Alonso, J., Andrade, L.H., Bromet, E.J., Bruffaerts, R., De Almeida, J.M.C., Cardoso, G., …WHO World Mental Health Survey collaborators. (2017). Trauma and psychotic experiences: Transnational data from the World Mental Health Survey. *British Journal of Psychiatry, 211*(6), 373–380.

Read, J., van Os, J., Morrison, A. & Ross, C.A. (2005). Childhood trauma, psychosis and schizophrenia: A literature review with theoretical and clinical implications. *Acta Psychiatrica Scandinavica, 112*, 330–350.

Romme, M. (2009). Important steps to recovery with voices. In: M. Romme, S. Escher, J. Dillon, D. Corstens & M. Morris (Eds.), *Living with voices: 50 stories of recovery* (pp.7–22). PCCS Books.

Romme, M.A. & Escher, A.D. (1989). Hearing voices. *Schizophrenia Bulletin, 15*(2), 209–216.

Romme, M. & Escher, S. (1993). *Accepting voices.* Mind Publications.

Romme, M. & Escher, S. (2012). *Psychosis as a personal crisis: An experience-based approach.* Routledge.

Romme, M., Escher, S., Dillon, J., Corstens, D. & Morris, M. (2009). *Living with voices: 50 stories of recovery.* PCCS Books.

Romme, M., Escher, S., Read, J., Van Engelen, S. & Corstens, D. (2006). Making sense of voices. *Acta Psychiatrica Scandinavica, 114*, 6–7.

Schnackenberg, J.K. & Martin, C.R. (2014). The need for Experience Focussed Counselling (EFC) with voice hearers in training and practice: A review of the literature. *Journal of Psychiatric and Mental Health Nursing, 21*, 391–402.

Stone, H. & Stone, S. (2011). *Embracing ourselves: The Voice Dialogue manual.* New World Library.

20 Experience focused counselling with children and young people who hear voices

Senait Debesay

Experience focused counselling (EFC) with children and young people is both similar and different to the work with adults, as developmental processes, for example, remain a focal point, just like in adult work, and a playful and creative approach to their experiential world also appears to be fitting. This is why knowledge about the pedagogy of play (such as Pohl, 2014), attachment theory (Bowlby, 1969), as applied to voices (Dillon et al., 2012), and emotional development (Dornes, 2000, 2006), trauma (Herman, 2015; van der Kolk, 2015) and the use of a de-pathologising story book (Subbiah, 2006) may also be helpful, as well as the work by Romme and Escher (2000) and Escher and Romme (2010), as applied in practice (Debesay, 2017). However, the basis of EFC with children and young people outlined in this chapter will be not so much the theoretical foundation but primarily my practice experience over the past 15 years, in a variety of settings, particularly as part of a community-based psychiatric service for children and young people. The structured approach of EFC does, however, help the practitioner to ask more targeted questions so as to better understand the experiential world of children and young people. All the practice examples in this chapter are anonymised.

Voices in young people are similar to those that adults hear, in that hearing voices might be seen as a natural resolution attempt, and should therefore not be ridiculed or seen as a problem in itself. However, this can unfortunately easily happen within the child's social environment. Failure to acknowledge and engage with the experience can undermine the natural processes of trust and expression. Instead, it is helpful to approach each child and each new situation like an island that is waiting to be explored by the accompanying person and the child, both full of curiosity, and not with an attitude filled with negative prejudices.

A fairly usual way of applying this approach in practice sees the building of rapport, followed by a formal or informal way of conducting the Maastricht Interview. It can be incorporated when the child is engaged in play or in normal conversation. A more formal use of the Maastricht Interview is potentially suitable for older children and young people. The interview process is followed by a report (if suitable) and a construct (see Chapters 1 and 18). Any related emotional or other life topics coming out of the construct can then be worked on.

How are hearing-voices experiences expressed?

Hearing voices can feature in various different diagnoses and non-diagnoses and can be apparent in various expressions and ways of behaving. It is, for example, not unusual to find voices disguised behind autistic, hyperactive or even selectively mute behaviour. EFC can thus also lead to a reduction of these kind of experiences.

It is also good to remember that the child's language development has not yet been completed and has been shaped by their social environment. Feelings may, therefore, not be expressed in a manner immediately understandable to adults. The child may also experience conflicts of loyalty towards their social environment. That is, a child may herself feel that something is not right – for example, when experiencing emotional or sexual abuse. In this context, it should not be surprising if the child were to try to keep something a secret while at the same time attempting to seek support. For accompanying persons, this means a need to engage with the child as creatively as possible, in order to both understand and speak their language and be able to relate to their experiential world. It is important to remember in this context that voices may express themselves in varied ways, such as like monsters (particularly if they are experienced as very powerful), or aliens, or even derive from animals.

Voices and emotions

As in adults, voices appear to express emotions and thoughts that the child or young person, for a variety of reasons, has not wanted or not been able to express. There may be religious, family, cultural or even personal reasons. Whatever the ultimate reason, essentially the child will not have felt safe enough to express certain emotions. Such a development is not really surprising when we remember that the expression of certain emotions, such as happiness, is acceptable in some societies and the expression of other emotions, such as anger, is not. The EFC process thus exposes the fact that voices represent – although often unconsciously – an attempt of the child or the young person to express precisely these kinds of emotions. This does not mean that emotions are always immediately identified as such through the voice-hearing experience. It is helpful, therefore, to use an open approach to the world of the child or young person, in order to better understand their language. Their use of metaphor may be very different in this context to that of adults, thus re-emphasising the importance of not being led by one's own ideas or prejudices towards the experience.

Voices can also serve as attempts to deal with a difficult situation in a more positive and life-affirming manner, even if a voice hearer does not agree that this is so. They will often use exaggerated expressions to express and point to a voice hearer's own underlying emotions, which thus far may not have been taken seriously enough. Rather than take the expressed emotion literally, a neutral approach may allow the voices' actual, originally positive, life-affirming intentions to become clear. A voice telling the voice hearer to end their life could, for example, turn out to be an attempt to prompt the child to make a necessary positive life change. However, it is not always clear to children and young people in this context that adults may react with fear and a desire to control the situation – for example, by admitting them to hospital. Such a reaction may in turn lead to a further undermining of trust in their own or other people's abilities to deal with a difficult situation.

> *Learning point 1*
>
> An eight-year-old child, who has been bullied at school for about six months, is saying in a convincing way that, based on what his voices are telling him, he is a ruler and a monster, and that he intends to kill a teacher and some of the other kids, too.
>
> - What kind of fears does this situation bring up in you and what would be important to you in terms of your own boundaries?
> - How can you manage to achieve/keep as neutral and positive a view as possible towards the voices and the voice hearer?
> - What might be a positive re-interpretation of his experience, within which the child could be supported to express emotions in a safe way that have thus far not been expressed?

> *Practice example 1*
>
> Anna is a six-year-old girl who is in contact with a (voice) dragon. As the accompanying person, I initially thought that the dragon appeared to be experienced as a negative and distressing figure. However, when I asked Anna, she explained that the dragon was always there for her and would protect her. She contrasted this with her father, who was regularly away on business trips, and her mother, who had difficulty in taking care of herself. This did not mean that Anna had already understood for herself what the meaning of the voice was. However, it was now clear to me just how important a sense of security and protection was to her.

EFC is therefore about creating a space within which all emotions may be seen, understood and accepted and a constructive way of dealing with feelings can be learned. Emotions will, of course, not normally come nicely packaged, categorised and neatly compartmentalised. Instead, they will inevitably relate to a mixture of relationship dynamics, thoughts and a range of interlinked issues. They may come across as somewhat chaotic in the child's overall presentation. I would therefore say that my role as an accompanier/supporter/counsellor in EFC work is to both allow for this chaos and be prepared to meet it with a structured approach. In this way, emotions can be better understood within their overall context, empathically related to and ultimately integrated, thus leading to more balanced mental wellbeing.

Voices and coping

When working with young voice hearers, it is very important to be guided by them, and not tell them which kind of coping strategies they should use. In practice, this means that, when a child comes to me and wants to draw, I encourage them and maybe ask what they are drawing and what the significance of the drawing is. At the same time, I would remember that they may simply have been socialised to say that they like drawing. I would therefore regularly ask the child what they would most like to do and then encourage them to do just that. It is through the stories that children tell when they are drawing or playing with toy blocks or other objects that I will increasingly get to know their experiential world. Children often have a rich fantasy life. This does not mean, however, that their stories and narratives are about topics that are not relevant to them. The stories may include a difficult situation at home, where the father regularly beats the mother, or a situation at school where the child is being bullied. An interesting observation from my experience in this context is that voices will often be representations of unexpressed anger.

> ### *Practice example 2*
>
> A 10-year-old boy, Ian, would regularly become physically and verbally aggressive at school. In conversation with me, he kept saying that he could not remember these aggressive outbursts. It became clear that he must have been dissociating. He said there was a monster that would essentially take charge of him in such situations. Ian did not like the idea of talking about the monster and he did not enjoy drawing either. But he happily took up my suggestion that he build this monster with toy blocks, as he did accept that something needed to change. As he recreated the monster, he gradually got to know it in conversations that I facilitated. In this way, he learned to deal with the monster in a better way. Ian had christened the monster Edward and understood that he would only turn up when Ian was not expressing his anger. The more he learned to express his anger in a safe and socially acceptable way, the less Edward appeared. This process was also helped by me supporting him to accept that it was okay to feel sad and angry about being bullied at school. In addition, I talked with his parents, as Ian had not yet learned that you do not always have to be happy. Eventually, the whole family transformed along with Ian, and found a new and accepting way of dealing with emotions.

Voices and identity

Voices can have a positive or negative impact on the identity of the child or young person. It very much depends on whether the voices are accepted by the child and those around them. When I am indicating that a particular way of reacting to the voices may be less helpful than others for the development and progress of the child, this does not mean I am assuming malintent on the part of those who are using that particular path. The various ways of dealing with the voices may all be well intended, but the particular chosen approach can have either a positive or negative impact.

It is also true that whether or not the child can learn to relate constructively to the voices or make positive use of them does, at least in part, also depend on whether the child finds herself in a socially difficult or a threatening situation. The more threatening to their existence the social situation is, the stronger the voices might be, and the harder it might be for the child to learn to relate well to the voices.

> *Practice example 3*
>
> Sixteen-year-old Faisal came to me for counselling support, accompanied by his mother. They had both been physically abused and threatened with their lives on several occasions by Faisal's father, the partner to his mother. Although the mother had separated from this man a few years ago, he continued to represent a threat, as he remained in regular contact with them. Faisal heard the voice of his father. At the beginning of our work, he was still very afraid of this voice and dissociated regularly. His biggest fear was that his father would return and physically harm him again. The EFC process thus revealed that Faisal continued to have a strong need for protection. As time went on, he also learned, however, how to assert himself better. He thus learned that he was not entirely powerless when faced with his father.

Of course, every child wants, in principle, to find a firm footing in life, in order to progress and take their future into their own hands. For this to happen, the child needs a safe foundation. Parents and others in their social network normally want to support the child in this process. It is also true, however, that the parents and their social network may be so busy with their own needs or aims in life that the child may not feel sufficiently seen.

The importance of play

The younger the children, the less able they are to express their feelings and fears verbally, even if we ask them. Using the medium of play helps me to understand the experiential world of the child in a much better way than the filling out of questionnaires. In play, a child may also keep a greater distance from their experiences, and from the accompanying professional, too. If I join in their play, the child can show me their world without having to fear potential conflicts of loyalty, feelings of guilt or negative consequences. They may feel more able to express that different voices represent the father, mother or other influential people or factors. Children are generally good at taking on different roles, too. I suggest to the child that I will offer them a space that they can use if they so choose. In this way, I leave the decision to the child as to whether and how much they want my support. I emphasise this explicitly in order that the child should have a sense of their ability to use their own compass to determine the direction of their ship. Being able to make their own choice in that way is particularly important, given that a child will often come to us for support as they have already experienced a loss of autonomy (e.g. via traumatisation).

In turn, this means being open to play or playing along with the ideas and the lead of the child. It is not unusual that I am used as this or that character, and that the child will also tell me when it is time to stop being that character.

An additional advantage of play is that children can break a taboo more easily in this context. Again, it is helpful that the very real conflicts of loyalty or guilt can thus be suspended. The world of play thus offers a protective space where the soul can express itself freely. The voices of the child can thus also show themselves without fear as they actually are.

Finally, we can use delving into their world of play to uncover some of the ways that the identity of the child has formed, too. To do this well and to understand the child, I will try to be as unbiased as I can. I might ask, for example: 'Who is Paul? Has he been hurt? How come he is in this or that situation?'

Thus, the use of play may even help us to integrate the voices better into everyday life.

Accompanying parents and the social surroundings

I normally wait for the right moment before I open up a supportive conversation with the parents or significant others in the child's social network. This may at times only be after an extended period of trust-building in the relationship. It is important that I phrase my observations and experiences in a language that fits with their experiential world. Parents often fear that their child is mentally disturbed. It is important to take these fears seriously and speak to them. It can be very helpful to give them a copy of the normalising and encouraging book *Children Hearing Voices* (Escher & Romme, 2010), and to talk about it if needed. If parents find it difficult to accept the voices of their child, it is important to accept where the parents and the children are at that point.

Working with parents thus often includes a lot of educational input, taking their fears seriously, not overwhelming them, but also trying not to be guided by their fears.

> *Learning point 2*
>
> A 16-year-old girl tells you about the voices telling her that she should kill both herself and her parents and threatening to kill her if she doesn't. She has been cutting herself to try to cope with the situation. The girl asks you how she can best deal with the situation. Your task is to deal with this situation in as fear-free and safe a way as possible.
>
> - What is your automatic first reaction?
> - How could you interpret such a situation in a positive way?
> - What does your reaction/intervention look like?
> - How would you counsel/accompany the parents?

Reflections

My work with children and young people hearing voices has shown me how resourceful children are and how well they can deal with situations that make a secure attachment difficult. My impression is that, in such circumstances, voices may represent the – mostly subconscious – attempt of the child to build up positive and life-affirming attachments.

Developing healthy attachments during childhood or adolescence is of great importance, as it is much more difficult during adulthood, even if it remains possible. In this way, it is possible to use the child´s attachment to their voices to enable positive attachment experiences if we take a non-pathologising and non-problematising approach to the phenomenon.

For professionals, this means that it is not actually important whether voices actually represent hallucinations or imaginary friends, but how we relate to these experiences. We should not judge the behaviour of children as problematic, but as an attempt to make the best out of the situation that they find themselves in. Even experiences like neglect and abuse can thus be overcome.

Finally, it may be important to emphasise again that EFC first and foremost represents an attitude and a motivation. For me, it is helpful to go to work every morning safe in the knowledge that I can say to the children: 'The sun is shining for you too and things can absolutely get better again, no matter which situation you are currently in.' Only then can I apply my knowledge of therapeutic methodology for the benefit of the children. In my experience, it is normally down to me if we are not moving on, not to the child. It may be that I have allowed myself to be guided too much by fear, or by my own methodology or experiences, and not by the creativity and the resources of the child.

References

Bowlby, J. (1969). *Attachment and loss (Vol. I): Attachment*. Basic Books.

Debesay, S. (2017). Stimmenhören bei Kindern und Jugendlichen (Hearing voices in children and young people). In: J. Schnackenberg & C. Burr C (Eds.) with Furrer, M, Iusco, O.M. & Debesay, S. *Stimmenhören und Recovery: Erfahrungsfokussierte Beratung in der Praxis (Hearing voices and recovery: Experience focussed counselling in practice* (pp.127–168). Psychiatrieverlag.

Dillon, J., Johnstone, L. & Longden, E. (2012). Trauma, dissociation, attachment and neuroscience: A new paradigm for understanding severe mental distress. *The Journal of Critical Psychology, Counselling and Psychotherapy*, *12*(3), 145–155.

Dornes, M. (2000). *Die emotionale welt des kindes*. Fischer Taschenbuch Verlag.

Dornes, M. (2006). *Die seele des kindes: Entstehung und entwicklung*. Fischer Taschenbuch Verlag.

Escher, S. & Romme, M. (2010). *Children hearing voices: What you need to know and what you can do*. PCCS Books.

Herman, J. (2015). *Trauma and recovery: The aftermath of violence – from domestic abuse to political terror*. Basic Books.

Pohl, G. (2014). *Kindheit – aufs spiel gesetzt. Vom wert des spielens für die entwicklung des kindes*. Springer.

Romme, M. & Escher, S. (2000). *Making sense of voices: A guide for mental health professionals working with voice hearers*. Mind Publications.

Subbiah, S. (2006). *Did you hear that? Help for children hearing voices*. WS Education.

Van der Kolk, B. (2015). *The body keeps the score: Brain, mind and body in the healing of trauma*. Penguin Books.

21 Understanding voices while living with dementia

David Storm and Ron Coleman

Many people who live with dementia experience hearing voices. These experiences are often seen as a symptom of the person's progressing dementia. The voices are rarely seen as potential messengers of the person's life history or disconnected memories or explored to consider their relevance to the person. It is essential, therefore, to look differently at the experiences that the person is finding distressing. This may open new avenues of understanding and acceptance of the voices, reducing distress as well as enabling alternative ways to be identified to help the person cope with any underlying reasons for their distress.

In Cumbria, following the work of Ron Coleman and Karen Taylor[1] (Coleman, 1999; 2011; Coleman & Smith, 1997; 2003), we have been exploring this approach with people living with dementia, often with dramatic successes. In the past they would often have been treated with antipsychotic medication (a widely used practice throughout the world, despite possible contraindications (All Party Parliamentary Group, 2008; Banerjee, 2009)). However, we have found that exploring the voice-hearing experience opens up alternative, non-medical pathways to reduce distress. The nature of the voices and their connection to the person may also help retain the person's identity. It has been extremely helpful to the person's carer/s if they find the voice-hearing experience of their loved one distressing.

---

1. Ron Coleman and Karen Taylor have been very influential trainers, consultants and mental health professionals within the Hearing Voices Movement and beyond in the past 25 years. They have been drawing on Ron's lived experience of hearing voices and recovery, as well as Karen's extensive experience as an innovative mental health nurse in the area of hearing voices, psychosis, trauma, self-harm and recovery in particular. Together they have innovated, pioneered, mentored and inspired voice hearers and mental health professionals and developed many now widely used approaches to constructive ways of approaching voice hearing, psychosis, trauma and recovery.

> *Learning point 1*
>
> Before you read any further, you may like to consider the following questions:
>
> - What do you think people's opinion of voice hearing in dementia might be?
> - When a person is living with dementia, what might the effects of hearing voices be for the person, and their carer(s)/family member(s)?
> - How might stigma affect people's perception of voice hearing in dementia?

The dangers of labelling

The labelling of 'symptoms' can also present difficulties for people living with dementia. The term 'behavioural disturbances' has been replaced by the term 'behavioural and psychological symptoms of dementia (BPSD)', defined as 'symptoms of disturbed perception, thought content, mood or behaviour that frequently occur in patients with dementia' (Finkel et al., 1996).

However, Macauley (2018) has suggested the need to examine the wording of BPSD as it stands. She writes:

> Many of these behaviours are human responses to unmet physical, emotional and/or psychosocial needs; responses that can easily be seen as normal in the light of feeling threatened or fearful. These responses may well be exacerbated by the medications being inappropriately used to treat them, as well.

This approach very much mirrors the greater understanding of the experience of voice hearing that has been developed over the past 25 years.

Ron Coleman has lived with hearing voices for 30-plus years, having been diagnosed with schizophrenia. Ron went on to be instrumental in the Hearing Voices Movement, recovering from the negative effects of mental health care and reclaiming his life and identity. Ron and his wife Karen developed their own, internationally acclaimed training and consultancy business, 'Working to Recovery'. A few years ago, Ron was diagnosed with Lewy body dementia, although this was not connected to his voice-hearing experience, which – as pointed out before – he had been having for many years prior to that diagnosis. Ron still hears voices, but they are part of Ron's lived experience and, clearly, his identity. It is vital for Ron that this element of his life is protected and not seen as a 'symptom'.

Ron's work has been the inspiration, the support and the driver for the discovery of an alternative approach to living with voices. This approach is core to the Hearing Voices Movement and the work of Marius Romme and colleagues in developing a greater understanding of voice hearing.

Below is Romme & Escher's (2000) core concept of making sense of voices:

- Hearing voices is in itself not a sign of mental illness.
- Hearing voices is experienced by many people without them becoming ill.
- Hearing voices is related to problems in the person's life history.
- To recover from the distress, the person has to learn to cope with their voices and the original problems that created them.

In addition, as Brooker (2007) observes:

> There is further evidence to suggest that behaviour that challenges may in fact be analysed to discover underlying reasons for it. Challenging behaviour can be seen as communication and the need to understand a person's behaviour from the perspective of the person with dementia is fundamental. (p.78)

Again, this demonstrates clear links between a person's experiences and their life history. 'Hallucinations' or 'voices' are rarely seen as potential messengers bringing important information about the person's life history or a phenomenon to be explored to consider their relevance to the person.

Alternative explanations

In Cumbria, drawing on the work of Marius Romme and Sandra Escher, the Hearing Voices Movement and the work of Ron Coleman and Karen Taylor, we have developed a more 'discovery'-based approach to exploring the experience and understanding of voices in people living with dementia.

Alternative explanations for voice hearing in people living with dementia could be:

- reaction to loss – voices may provide comfort (research has shown that bereaved people may commonly hear voices)
- reaction to change – voices may provide positive experience, rather than always being negative or described as a 'symptom'
- reaction to disconnected circumstances, memories or feelings – voices may cause distress, but when they are explored there is a clear connection with the person's life history that may be evident, such as difficult/traumatic events in the person's life, and so forth. But the identity of the voices or what they represent may be overlooked.

> *Learning point 2*
>
> Depending on your own background and experience, it may be helpful to think about the following points:
>
> - What is your understanding around why a person may be hearing voices? Do you feel this may be a result of biological illness, a response to trauma, or other psychological or social reasons?
> - Where a person is experiencing voices and begins to develop dementia, does this change the nature of their voice-hearing experience?
> - How might health professionals involved in diagnosing the dementia react to the presence of underlying voice hearing, and do you think this may affect their diagnosis?

Understanding origins and identity

It is essential that the person's voice-hearing experience is seen within the context of their life and social circumstances, rather than as the direct consequence of a biological illness, even if they only started hearing voices or see visions with the beginning of their diagnosis. This also helps the person look at how they are coping with both the voice-hearing experience itself and the consequence of this on their life, as well as helping the person change their relationship with their voices.

Careful assessment based on the person's history is essential so that the health professional can begin to search for and understand the meaning of the experience for the person hearing voices. This enables the experience to make sense. One could argue that this applies to mental health problems in general. In this way, when people suffer from mental health problems like depression, anxiety, phobias, dissociative disorders, eating disorders and so forth, they do so in reaction to daily life problems. This mostly involves difficulties and traumas in the person's relationship with important other people, or in relation to social structures and rules that are very troublesome to them. They then are not able to cope with these situations and develop mental health problems as an expression of these serious difficulties (Romme & Escher, 2000).

Where a person has dementia, this may lead to a disconnection with aspects of their life. They may struggle to manage their emotions, cope with stress and anxiety and even communicate their feelings.

This makes the exploration of the origins of the person's voice hearing extremely important.

The time when the voices first start can be quite 'startling' – that is, overwhelming, frightening and confusing for the person who hears them. They may also struggle to understand their experience. It is also often a time that may cause the person's family and/or carer(s) distress. This may be due to their own underlying beliefs around hearing voices, and can often have an entirely negative effect on the person's behaviour and lower further their self-esteem. Similarly, if the person is living in a care home, the reactions of other residents and paid carers, as well as family members, can have a significant effect on the person hearing voices.

The voices the person experiences can also be an essential part of their own self-identity. The person may have heard them for many years without distress, and may have developed a unique relationship with them, their meanings and their presence in their life. Dementia can lead to a fragmenting of this relationship and a real danger that this extremely important part of the person becomes lost or is seen as a symptom of dementia, if the assessor is unaware of their history or not informed of this different way of viewing voice hearing.

It is essential, therefore, to explore the voice-hearing experience, its origins, impact and effects on the person. Once there is consent from relatives and carers, those who are in close contact with the voice hearer can also explore the person's voices. This can be vital in establishing an alternative understanding and acceptance of this experience.

Voice profiling

Ron Coleman has developed a helpful approach to 'profiling' the voice-hearing experience with anyone who hears voices, not just those with dementia. This includes developing a greater understanding of the identity, nature and relationship the person has with the voices hearing experience.

The steps outlined below help the 'supporter' to begin to develop a greater understanding, as well as conveying trust and openness to the person. The person is listened to and this helps the gentle exploration of further details.

1. What is happening at the time the person starts hearing voices? (Have there been any particular life changes, traumas, worries/fears, changes in the person's physical health?)
2. How many voices does the person hear? Is the voice male or female?
3. Does the person have an idea as to who the voice is? Does the voice relate to any events/situations that the person can remember?
4. What makes them think this?
5. Does the voice invoke strong feelings?
6. Does the person have any idea why they hear a particular voice? (Is there any relationship between the voice beginning and other events or situations?)
7. Does the person find the voice pleasant or distressing?
8. Does the voice talk to or about the person? Does the voice tell the person to do something? Does the voice ever give advice? Does the voice comment on what the person is doing or thinking? Does the voice say unpleasant things? Does the voice threaten or harm the person or anyone else in any way?

9. How does the person cope with the voice? (Does their behaviour change – for example, do they experience anger, aggression, anxiety?)
10. How do others react to this experience?

The above questions and discussions may prompt a rich understanding of the experiences that the person is having, and may also begin to shape an outline hypothesis around the person's understanding and acceptance of the experience.

Carers' experiences

Carers often have a crucial role in supporting the person living with dementia. Their knowledge may be vital in understanding the context and history of the person and enabling appropriate responses to their support needs.

But carers can also hold beliefs and attitudes based on a lack of understanding, education and knowledge of hearing voices, which can lead to maladaptive coping and responses to behaviours, and can exacerbate or even cause these behaviours.

> ### *Learning point 3*
>
> Depending on your own background and experience, it may be helpful to think about the following points:
>
> - How might the beliefs and attitudes of caregivers affect the experience of voice hearing in the person living with dementia? Do you think this could impact on the person's self-esteem? Do you think that this could lead in itself to differing behaviours?
> - What opportunities for positive involvement and greater understanding do you think there may be for caregivers?

In their report *Always a Last Resort* (2008), the All Party Parliamentary Group on Dementia found evidence of widespread use of antipsychotics for people with dementia in care homes. This was due to the following:

- a response to the assumed behavioural and psychological symptoms of dementia, which can be an expression of unmet needs – for example, due to a poor environment in a care home
- inadequate leadership, lack of dementia care training for care home staff and low staffing levels.

Working with carers is crucial in developing a more positive approach. Carers may be able to explain any history of triggers, experiences/behaviour, strengths, and may be able to help the person with dementia reconnect to feelings and memories.

Carers may also help with a knowledge of life history/events and understanding of the person's stress and coping mechanisms. In addition, their knowledge and understanding of the family, culture and values may provide hugely significant resources.

Gaining knowledge and acceptance

The use of a structured interview with the carer to properly engage with them and seek to understand their position is a valued approach to help build understanding and acceptance:

1. How do you react when the person is hearing voices?
2. What happens when you react in this way and how does this make you feel?
3. What do you think is causing the person to hear voices?
4. Does the person's behaviour change when they are hearing their voice? Does this form a pattern?
5. How do you react to this?
6. Do you think that the person's behaviour is part of their illness, or to do with them hearing voices?
7. Could there be another explanation for this?

This offers further support to the argument that we need to review our approaches, and bring a more person-centred and enquiring attitude when a person is hearing voices. In turn, this can often dispel myths (such as voices being meaningless symptoms of biological illnesses and in need of medical treatment), enable better practical support in managing distress and offer alternative, non-medication-based interventions.

Lived examples

Taking forward the approaches described above in Cumbria has demonstrated the value of an alternative approach to the orthodox medical response of medication. This has included educating informal carers, care staff and NHS staff in assessment and intervention techniques, which has led to improved outcomes for a number of people living with dementia and experiencing voice hearing. Some examples of this approach are described below. The personal details have been changed to protect individuals' identities.

Lilly

Lilly was an elderly lady with vascular dementia, who was living in a care home. She was hearing voices and becoming increasingly distressed by the experience. Her relationship with her son and grandchildren was also being affected by her compulsion to talk about her voices. She also had a very negative relationship with care staff in the home.

Lilly believed that she was being watched by her care staff and the voices, and that the voices were in control of the numerous cameras she believed were situated around her room. She had stopped going out of her room and fought off her carers when they tried to help her.

Lilly had been seen by her GP, who had prescribed diazepam. When this proved ineffective, she had also been seen by the local mental health team, who offered an alternative approach.

Having met Lilly over a number of sessions and spent time working through her voice profile, it was clear that she had experienced several significant traumas in her life. In her younger days, she had worked as a secretary for a very well-known organisation. She had an extremely busy working life and was involved in managing numerous high-profile social events. She married and had one son. After Lilly and her husband retired, the couple moved to the Lake District to be closer to their son and his family.

Not long after this, Lilly developed severe osteoarthritis, which began to limit her physical abilities. Shortly after they moved, Lily's husband sadly passed away. Lilly then developed dementia and, because of this and her worsening physical health, decided to move into a care home. Her mental and physical health continued to deteriorate to the point that she could no longer walk and was totally reliant on care staff for all aspects of daily living. Her distressing voices appeared to develop over a period of three months.

From her voice profile assessment with Lilly, it became clear to us that the voice she was hearing was in fact that of her husband. His voice, however, was not controlling or distressing. Rather, it was other people's reaction to the voice that Lilly found upsetting. Her husband's voice and 'presence' was protective for her. On further discussion, it became clear that the onset of Lilly's voice hearing also coincided with her growing despair that she was totally reliant on care staff, that she felt useless and unable to enjoy anything in life.

Care staff found her often aggressive and spent as little time with her as possible, so as not to reinforce her beliefs around her voices and her increasingly paranoid thoughts.

Once we understood more about Lilly's life story and the onset, content, identity and focus of her voices, we were able to formulate an alternative approach. This hypothesised that Lilly had become 'detached' from her identity. No one knew of her amazing life and attributes; her only interactions were with people when they were trying to do things 'to her'. Her life had reduced to a bubble within her room, and her isolation was perpetuated by her distress and increasing despair. We had to reconnect to Lilly.

The approach used was to first of all to make space and time when Lilly could talk freely about her voices. The mental health nurse gained an acceptance with Lilly regarding the identity of her voices, and worked to improve her self-esteem. This included working with her on her own beliefs about voice hearing, which helped to dispel the myths that some care staff held. We created a timetable for staff when they would sit with Lilly and talk with her about her voice hearing. At other times she agreed she would not respond to her voices.

We also learned from Lilly's son and granddaughter that she had a lifelong love of poetry and reading. Lilly agreed she would write some poems. As she could not write, due to her physical health issues, we provided Lilly with a digital dictaphone. Her poems were then emailed to her granddaughter, who typed them up and brought them in. Lilly loved this. Her attention started to drift from spending time with her voices to writing her poems. She started also leaving her room and interacting with other residents.

After a further six weeks, Lilly started writing her memoirs. As she was keen to be more sociable, her son bought her an electric wheelchair and she was leaving her room daily, and leaving the care home weekly with her granddaughter. She only heard the voice of her husband at night, wishing her good night. Lilly had reconnected.

This approach was also used with several other people living with dementia and experiencing voices. The outcomes were similar and are highlighted in the further anonymised examples below.

Mrs Burton

Mrs Burton had been placed in a care home following a diagnosis of dementia and a gradual decline in her ability to care safely for herself. After several months, the care home was struggling to manage her needs. In particular, she was very anxious and was extremely reluctant to come out of her room. This caused her great distress, to the point that she was aggressive towards carers. Carers also reported that she was hearing voices and they felt they could no longer manage her needs. On working with Mrs Burton and her family, it was established, using voice profiling, that the voice she was hearing was that of an old school friend. In fact, she found great comfort in hearing this voice. The school friend had helped her many years back when she was bullied at school. It turned out that Mrs Burton's experience of the care home had made her feel like she had when she was bullied. By understanding this, it became clear that the problem was not her voices but the way the care staff were dealing with her anxiety. Some education, support and role modelling around alternatives greatly improved Mrs Burton's anxiety.

Miss Dorian

Miss Dorian would often become very aggressive when carers tried to support her with her personal care. This was especially the case when Miss Dorian had been incontinent. It could often provoke great distress and result in Miss Dorian spending long periods crying and screaming. At the same time, care staff noticed Miss Dorian was responding to voices. Miss Dorian was unable to effectively communicate what she was experiencing. However, on completing a voice profile with the help of Miss Dorian's family, it became apparent that she was responding to previous feelings of how her critical father had made her feel. As a child, she would be scorned and verbally abused by her father if she made a mess in any way. It was clear that the voice she was responding to was that of her father and she was reacting to care staff out of fear. Understanding this altered the way care staff interacted with her. Rather than seeing her as someone who was distressed, with 'challenging' behaviour, staff were aware of the importance to her of being clean and tidy and also of the need to support her incontinence in a way that helped prevent such stressors.

Mrs Xavier

Mrs Xavier had become more and more isolated in her room. She would strike out at carers who approached her, and care staff were struggling to cope with her care needs. Mrs Xavier would be aggressive when she was helped with her personal care, and was clearly responding to voices she was hearing. She would report these voices to her family when they visited and refuse to talk about anything else. She told them she was being victimised by gangsters and they were out to get her; that they were listening in on her and would have her thrown out. On voice profiling with Mrs Xavier, it was found that, some 30 years previously, she had been evicted from her home due to fires caused by a gang of youths seeking drugs from a drug dealer who lived above Mrs Xavier. The voice profile also revealed that Mrs Xavier could hear care staff talking outside her room before they entered. She had thought these voices were the 'gangsters'. Then, as her anxiety escalated, care staff would often call for more support, further escalating Mrs Xavier's distress as other staff came in to help. An alternative, more person-centred approach was tried, with one or two carers at the most spending time with Mrs Xavier before they supported her personal care needs. This reduced her anxiety and reduced the times when she heard any gangsters. Here too, further exploration revealed that her behaviour was not due to an 'unconnected' biological symptom; rather, the experiences had clear meaning in the context of Mrs Xavier's life history. Understanding this led to a greater level of acceptance among care staff and alternative ways to support her.

Conclusion

This alternative approach to gaining an understanding of the voice-hearing experience has led to significantly improved outcomes and quality of life for numerous people living with dementia in Cumbria, and also for their families.

While we do not dismiss voices or visions as biological symptoms of dementia, our person-centred approach allows a better understanding of the potential dementia has to disconnect a person from their identify and offers an alternative to pharmacological interventions to support the person and return their quality of life.

Further reading

Baker, P. (1996). *Can you hear me?* Handsell Publishing.

Coleman, R. & Smith, M. (2001). *Coping with voices and visions.* Hearing Voices Network Manchester.

Douglas, S., James, I. & Ballard, C. (2004). Non-pharmacological interventions in dementia. *Advances in Psychiatric Treatment, 10,* 171–177

Fossey, J., Ballard, C., Juszczak, E., James, I., Adler, N., Jacoby, R. & Howard, R. (2006). Effect of enhanced psychosocial care on antipsychotic use in nursing home residents with severe dementia. *British Medical Journal, 332*(7544), 756–761.

Kitwood, T. & Benson, S. (1995). *The new culture of dementia care*. Bradford Dementia Group.

Marriot, A., Donaldson, C., Tarrier, N. & Burns, A. (2000). Effectiveness of cognitive-behavioural family intervention in reducing the burden of care in carers of patients with Alzheimer's Disease. *British Journal of Psychiatry 176*, 557–562.

Nelson, H., Thrasher, S. & Barnes, T.R.E. (1991). Practical ways of alleviating auditory hallucinations. *British Medical Journal, 302*(6772), 327.

Slade, P.D. (1972). The effects of desensitisation on auditory hallucinations. *Behaviour Research and Therapy, 10*, 85–91.

References

All-Party Parliamentary Group on Dementia. (2008). *Always a last resort*. Alzheimer's Society. www.alzheimers.org.uk/downloads

Banerjee, S. (2009). *The use of antipsychotic medication for people with dementia: Time for action. A report for the Minister of State for Care Services*. Department of Health.

Brooker, D. (2007). *Person-centred dementia care*. Jessica Kingsley Publishers.

Coleman, R. (1999). *Recovery: An alien concept?* Handsell Publishing.

Coleman, R. (2011). *Recovery: An alien concept?* (2nd ed.). P&P Press.

Coleman, R. & Smith, M. (1997). *Working with voices: From victim to victor*. Handsell Publishing.

Coleman, R. & Smith, M. (2003). *Working with voices II: Victim to victor*. P&P Press.

Finkel S.I., Costa e Silva J., Cohen, G., Miller, S. & Sartorius, N. (1996). Behavioral and psychological signs and symptoms of dementia: a consensus statement on current knowledge and implications for research and treatment. *International Psychogeriatrics, 8*(Suppl.3), 497–500.

Macaulay, S. (2018). The broken lens of BPSD: Why we need to rethink the way we label the behaviour of people who live with Alzheimer's Disease. *Journal of the American Medical Directors Association, 19*(2), 177–180.

Romme, M. & Escher, S. (2000). *Making sense of voices*. Mind Publications.

22 How cognitive behaviour therapy can help people who are distressed by hearing voices

Mark Hayward

Hearing the voice of someone or something that doesn't seem to be physically present can be very frightening. If you believe the voice is very powerful, has bad intentions towards you and knows everything about you, the fear may be intolerable. But is this the whole story? Cognitive behaviour therapy (CBT) suggests that our minds can take short-cuts and only pay attention to the evidence that supports our beliefs. By deliberately looking for more of the available evidence, we can re-evaluate our beliefs about the power, intentions and truthfulness of our voices and see our assets and strengths more clearly. This chapter invites you to play the 'curious detective' and develop skills to question the evidence and re-evaluate your beliefs about yourself and your voices more accurately.

When do voices become distressing?

We know that voice hearing *per se* is not always a distressing experience. So, if you hear voices, what are the factors that can increase the likelihood of this experience becoming distressing, and can you do anything to influence these factors?

We know from research that there are at least four factors that may play a role in the cause and maintenance of voice-related distress: adversity and trauma (particularly during childhood); beliefs about the self (significantly influenced by childhood experience); beliefs about the voices, and the way you relate to the voices. Psychological therapy (or 'talking therapy') can help you to explore the relevance and experience of each of these factors for your voice-hearing experience, with a view to reducing the influence of these factors on (at least) the maintenance of any distress. Some of these talking therapies may try to address the causal roots of these factors (for example, by revisiting and 're-scripting' the narratives around traumatic events), but this revisiting of past traumas is not necessary for the reduction of distress. Indeed, you may not be aware of any traumatic routes to your voice-hearing experiences, and/or you may not wish to revisit them.

Our focus in this chapter will be on CBT – a talking therapy that was originally developed for the treatment of emotional problems (e.g. depression and anxiety) and helps people to 'ask questions' of any thoughts and beliefs that may be maintaining their distress. CBT has been adapted for use with people distressed by hearing voices and we will explore how it works by focusing on the factors that it seeks to modify.

Beliefs about self

If you are distressed by hearing voices, the beliefs you hold about yourself are likely to be very negative: for example, I am useless, worthless, unlovable and so forth. These negative beliefs are likely to accurately reflect past experiences of adversity and lack of opportunity/achievement. They will also be very strongly held, resistant to change and cause low self-esteem. Consequently, when the voice(s) says that you are useless, worthless and unlovable, it *feels* true and cannot be disputed. Furthermore, the distress that results from experiencing low self-esteem and hearing critical and derogatory voices will limit your ability to fully engage with activities and relationships that may provide evidence to the contrary. So, a negative and reinforcing cycle is established whereby negative beliefs about the self are strengthened by your actions and behaviours.

> *Learning point 1*
>
> The beliefs you have about yourself can influence the amount of distress caused by your voices. These beliefs are phrased as 'I am . . .' statements, and can be both positive and negative. If you have low self-esteem you will most likely have more negative beliefs.
>
> - What beliefs do you have about yourself?

Beliefs about voices

The negative impact of your voices may be maintained by the beliefs you have about the power and control they seem to have. Voices can seem powerful because they seem to know everything about you (including experiences that may have caused you to feel ashamed and you want to keep private). You may also have some evidence to suggest that your voices have made bad things happen in the past and lots of evidence to suggest they can control you and your behaviour. The voices may also be linked to people and relationships from the past where you have felt powerless and controlled. Consequently, it's not surprising that you may sometimes feel you have to obey the voices and do as they say – for example, harm yourself or not do something you want to do. Like the negative cycle described above, if you do what the voices say, you will be strengthening your beliefs about them and not generating any evidence to suggest that their power and control may be limited.

> *Learning point 2*
>
> The beliefs you have about your voices can also influence the amount of distress caused by voices.
>
> - What beliefs do you have about your voices?

Relating to voices

If you are distressed by hearing voices, you are also likely to experience difficult relationships – and one of these difficult relationships will be with the voices. Relationships with the voices can remain difficult if you respond passively and/or aggressively to them. These responses are natural and instinctive, and are driven by the fight-flight mechanism in your nervous system that helps keep you safe when you are in a threatened situation. However, these natural responses can also stop you changing how you relate to other people – and to the voices. If you respond passively to voices that seem very powerful, you will generate further evidence that tells you that you are weak; if you respond aggressively to the voices, they may respond with aggression and force you to submit. As described above, it's possible for your responses to the voices to sometimes make things worse.

> *Learning point 3*
>
> The ways in which you respond to your voices can influence the impact they have on you.
>
> - How do you respond to your voices when they are talking – passively, aggressively or assertively?

Are my beliefs completely accurate (all of the time)?

CBT seeks to break the negative cycles described above by encouraging you to ask questions about your beliefs and experiences. These questions are intended to evaluate the accuracy of your beliefs: are you really as useless and worthless as you feel and as voices say you are? Do the voices have complete power and control over you all the time?

But why should you seek to re-evaluate your beliefs when you hold them so strongly and *know* they are true?

It can be helpful to re-evaluate the accuracy of your beliefs because beliefs are not facts – even though this isn't how it feels. Our minds like stability, so once a belief is developed (even an unhelpful one), it uses what is called 'confirmation bias' to maintain that stability. This bias draws your attention to information and experience that support your existing beliefs. For example, if you make a mistake, you will focus on the evidence that you have made a mistake, as it *fits with* your belief that you are useless. However, if you do something well, you will tend to ignore, minimise or forget this piece of evidence because it *does not fit* with your belief that you are useless.

Playing the curious detective

Contrary to what is often said, CBT is not about positive thinking. Rather, CBT invites you to be aware of the confirmation bias and look beyond your usual gaze to notice and consider all of the available evidence. This will not come naturally to you and will require effort. You need to play the *curious detective* and continue searching until you have identified *all of the evidence* – positive and negative – for you to review. The pieces of evidence may come from the distant past (e.g. you managed to pass your driving test first time when you were younger) or the present (e.g. you managed to get to your therapy session today, despite the voices telling you not to go) – but sometimes the positive evidence will be difficult to spot as the confirmation bias will be working overtime to prevent you finding it. This is where the support of a CBT therapist can be useful – to help you to continue the search, and to search beyond the negative evidence, even when you want to stop.

What does your evidence say?

After gathering some evidence, it's time for a review. The review needs to consider all of the evidence that you have identified, not just the evidence that contradicts the unhelpful belief. The aim is to arrive at a balanced conclusion that more accurately reflects the evidence. You may have begun the search for evidence by believing that you are useless and worthless with 100% conviction. If you have identified one or two pieces of evidence to the contrary, this may have reduced your level of conviction a little (say, to 95%). If you have identified many pieces of contrary evidence, the level of conviction may have reduced considerably (say, to 50%). It's important to note that all of the identified evidence has come from having another look at your experience and gathering further evidence that was there already but was not visible, due to the influence of the confirmation bias.

> *Learning point 4*
>
> Your mind will want to maintain the beliefs that you have about yourself and your voices – even if these beliefs are unhelpful. This is typical of the way our minds work; they don't like change. You will need to look thoroughly to find any evidence that does not support your beliefs.
>
> - When you look thoroughly, what evidence do you see?

How can I relate differently to my voices?

We've considered how CBT can help you to re-evaluate the accuracy of your beliefs. Next, we need to look at how you can use these beliefs if, as a result of the re-evaluation, they have been modified in any way. As mentioned earlier, your natural reaction to voices that are threatening you or putting you down may be, understandably, to respond passively or aggressively. An alternative option, although it may not come so instinctively, would be to respond assertively – to stand up for yourself but in a way that is respectful of the voices. If you now believe that you are not completely useless and worthless all the time, you can present and evidence this different view to your voices. You can practise this in role-plays with your CBT therapist. Initially, you may focus on the words you use to express your different view ('I hear what you say… I do feel useless some of the time… but I'm starting to see myself a bit differently'); then pay attention to your non-verbal communication (to help you look and feel assertive); then pay attention to presenting the evidence that supports your different view ('I was complimented by my boss last week…'), and finally, find a way to leave the conversation when you have expressed your view (move to another room and using a coping strategy to take your attention away from the voices). The voices may not change what they say; what's important is that you *behave differently,* in a way that reflects your changing beliefs about yourself and the voices.

> *Learning point 5*
>
> Your instinctive response to your voices is likely to be either passive or aggressive. That is how your nervous system is programmed to respond when you are feeling threatened.
>
> - When you try to respond assertively, in a respectful way, what happens? How do you feel about yourself?

Putting learning into practice

Working with a CBT therapist can help you to re-evaluate your beliefs about yourself and your voices and teach you how to stand up for yourself and articulate any different beliefs that you may have developed. Playing the curious detective and being assertive are skills that can be used in many aspects of your life – for example, you can also be assertive with your colleague who bullies you at work. However, like any new skills, these skills will need to be used regularly, in your daily life, if they are to make a real difference. The ongoing support of other people will be helpful in this respect – possibly including people who have been through similar experiences. It will also be helpful to use these skills to work towards a goal that you value. You can do this gradually, in small steps, paying attention to the evidence that you gather as each step is achieved. This evidence can be used to support a more positive belief about yourself – for example, that you are competent and capable.

Beware the sabotaging voice!

The voices may try to sabotage your attempts to engage with therapy and help yourself. This is not surprising, as the balance of power and control may shift if you engage fully with therapy; the voices may have much to lose. The sabotage may take the form of the voices threatening to harm you if you attend the therapy sessions, trying to distract you during the therapy sessions and/or belittling the content of therapy and your therapist. You can use your new skills to evaluate these statements – have voices been able to harm you in the past when you haven't obeyed them? What are your own views about the content of therapy and the skills of your therapist?

Summary

We have identified and explored three factors that can lead to voice hearing becoming a distressing experience: beliefs about yourself, beliefs about your voices, and the way that you relate to voices. CBT is a talking therapy that can help you to learn how to evaluate the accuracy of these beliefs and respond assertively to the voices. These skills can help you to:

- **stop** – try not to react to voices as you usually do, as this reaction may not be helping.
- **question** – ask some questions about your experience. Do the voices have all the power and control? Can they make bad things happen? Do they speak the truth? Do you have some control?
- **choose** – how you want to respond to the voices after you have taken a step back to re-evaluate some of your beliefs about yourself and the voices.

The learning points from this chapter encouraged you to:

- identify and re-evaluate a negative belief you may hold about yourself. When you looked thoroughly at your experience, did you find any evidence that did not support this belief?
- identify and re-evaluate a belief you may hold about your voices. When you looked thoroughly at your experience, did you find any evidence that did not support this belief?
- review the way you relate to the voices. Do you tend to relate by giving in or fighting back? Can you develop the alternative response of relating assertively and standing up for yourself while being respectful of the voices?

Research and evidence base

There is evidence from a number of research trials to suggest that CBT for distressing voices is more beneficial than getting no additional treatments (van der Gaag et al., 2014). However, there is less benefit when the effects of CBT treatment are compared with simpler forms of support, such as befriending or counselling (Jones et al., 2018). Researchers have also studied the benefit of targeting CBT more specifically at some of the factors that can maintain distress, and this seems to show that it helps (Lincoln & Peters, 2019). Our research group has developed a form of CBT that targets all three of the factors described above, called Guided Intervention for Voices (GiVE). It is based on our workbook (Hazell et al., 2018a) and self-help book, *Overcoming Distressing Voices* (Hayward et al., 2018) and contains modules on 'Me' (beliefs about self), 'My Voices' (beliefs about voices) and 'My Relationships' (relating to voices). GiVE was found to be very beneficial when evaluated in a small trial (Hazell et al., 2018b) and a larger trial is currently in process.[1]

References

Hayward, M., Strauss, C. & Kingdon, D. (2018). *Overcoming distressing voices* (2nd ed.). Robinson.

Hazell, C., Hayward, M., Cavanagh, K., Jones, A.-Marie. & Strauss, C. (2018a). Guided self-help cognitive-behaviour Intervention for VoicEs (GiVE): Results from a pilot randomised controlled trial in a transdiagnostic sample. *Schizophrenia Research, 195,* 441447.

Hazell, C., Hayward, M., Strauss, C. & Kingdon, D. (2018b). *An introduction to self-help for distressing voices*. Robinson.

Jones, C., Hacker, D., Meaden, A., Cormac, I., Irving, C.B., Xia, J., Zhao, S., Shi, C. & Chen, J. (2018). Cognitive behavioural therapy plus standard care versus standard care plus other psychosocial treatments for people with schizophrenia. *Cochrane Database of Systematic Reviews, 11.*

Lincoln, T.M. & Peters, E. (2019). A systematic review and discussion of symptom specific cognitive behavioural approaches to delusions and hallucinations. *Schizophrenia Research, 203,* 66–79.

van der Gaag, M., Valmaggia, L.R. & Smit, F. (2014). The effects of individually tailored formulation-based cognitive behavioural therapy in auditory hallucinations and delusions: A meta-analysis. *Schizophrenia Research, 156,* 30–37.

---

1. GiVE2 – Increasing access to CBT for psychosis patients: A feasibility, randomized controlled trial evaluating brief, targeted CBT for distressing voices delivered by assistant psychologists. https://doi.org/10.1186/ISRCTN16166070

23 Recovery-oriented cognitive therapy and distressing voices

Aaron Brinen

The voice-hearing experience has been interpreted in many ways – spiritual, supernatural, personal, normal and pathological. In the medical field, voice hearing has traditionally been interpreted as pathological and labelled as 'auditory hallucinations' and a target for eradication. The explanation given to people who seek help with their voices from the psychiatric services is a biological one and the intervention prescribed (primarily medication) is also biological. The best course of treatment is thought to be to educate the person in the biology of these symptoms and attempt to medicate the voices away.

This approach neither respects the person's personal experience nor instills much hope. Some practitioners go so far as to consider voices to be disordered thinking. The approach also creates an adversarial nature to the treatment, as many people who hear voices have relationships with these experiences that predate treatment, and do not believe the voices are an illness and that they need to be 'cured'. Moreover, this approach (education and medication) has little evidence to substantiate the claims for its effectiveness (Lincoln et al., 2007; Morrison et al., 2012).

The cognitive model of distressing voices regards the experience as an understandable reaction by the person that resembles any other normal reaction. In fact, with the right formulation, the experience makes complete sense. For more than 20 years, researchers have developed and studied psychosocial models of psychotic symptoms, with hearing voices being one of them. Distressing voices (Hayward et al., 2018) have received equal attention and study. The cognitive model of hearing voices looks to the person's beliefs about the voices and resulting behavioural reaction for an explanation. It rejects a purely biological explanation (Beck et al., 2020).

Recovery-oriented cognitive therapy (CT-R) was developed by Aaron T. Beck and his team (of which I was one) at the University of Pennsylvania (Beck et al., 2020). The approach was developed for people least likely to engage with and benefit from psychosocial treatments for psychosis. CT-R is well suited for those struggling with distressing voices, because the treatment focuses on the person's personal aspirations (family, career, home) and the CT-R practitioner collaborates in their pursuit. With a competing focus on the distressing voices, the practitioner and the person who hears the voices can reduce the negative impact of the voice-hearing experience, correct unhelpful beliefs and adjust behaviours that maintain the experience. In time, they can correct beliefs about the voices and develop new behaviours in line with the new belief system.

> ### Learning point 1
>
> - Try completing a task (going to the shops or completing a form, for example) while a friend talks to you on your mobile through your headphones. How difficult is it to complete the task? Is it the talking that makes it difficult? What would make it easier? Imagine if the person talking to you never hung up. This can approximate voice hearing.
>
> - Imagine giving an important presentation and being in a group text chain. How nervous would you be about being interrupted during the presentation? Would you check to see if your phone was on 'Do not disturb'? Would that make it harder to concentrate? More or less frustrating? Voice hearing can feel like this experience.

People with no illness or disability hear voices (Johns et al., 2014). Many people go about their lives while regularly experiencing hallucinations but never have any dysfunction. The content of what the voices say (friendly vs unfriendly, critical vs complimentary) is not found to be the main predictor of functioning. Given that this is the case, then the phenomenon of hearing voices cannot be the obstacle to pursuing a desired life. It suggests that something else is blocking the person's ability to live life to the full – the way that they react to their voices.

Beck's (1979) cognitive model proposes that our experiences come from what we tell ourselves about a situation, and not the situation itself. If we abandon a purely biological explanation of the voice-hearing experience, it can be thought of as a situation (a person hears a voice). With this model, we can make sense of when the symptoms get worse and better, what behaviours influence the voice hearing, and what motivations drive these behaviours. Once we consider these beliefs, we can develop a strategy to inoculate against the voices that are obstructing progress and living. The following are four specific beliefs associated with voice hearing.

Control: A person who thinks they have no control over when the voices come and go has increased anxiety. The uncertainty related to the voice hearing increases the likelihood of the person avoiding going out and interacting with others, and this increases their isolation. The problem with this behaviour is that isolation can lead to increased voice hearing, which confirms the person's conclusion that they have no control over when the voices come and go. In addition, the perceived uncontrollability of the voices is stressful, stress increases the likelihood of hearing voices, and distressing voices can be quite stressful. This continues the cycle of stress, voice hearing and isolation. This belief is found to be most associated with dysfunction in people who hear voices, and it differentiates voice hearers without a psychiatric diagnosis from those who are diagnosed with a disorder.

Credibility: Some people hear a voice and believe that the voice is telling the truth. The content might include a warning (the authorities are coming for you, you are going to be killed), disparaging remarks (no one likes you, you are stupid), or another statement that is believed. In response, the person listens for or attends to the voice in an attempt not to miss the warning or miss the negative messages. When someone believes they will hear a voice, they are more likely to hear that voice. However, people do not usually listen for a message that they do not assume they will hear. When the person *catches* the voice's message, they feel a sense of relief from the anxiety that they might miss the warning. The feeling of relief is conflated with comfort that comes from hearing a credible ally. The person concludes that, had they not monitored the messages, they would have missed the important warning – and so the *listening* behaviour is more likely to occur.

Power: Voices can sometimes make threats to cause harm or create a supernatural disaster or other frightening outcome or force the voice hearer to do something they don't want to do. In these situations, the person believes that the voices have the power to follow through on their threats. In these cases, the person will either comply with the demands of the voices or try to do something to neutralise the threatened danger. For example, if a voice says, 'Don't leave your house or I will destroy Philadelphia,' the person will stay at home. Philadelphia is not destroyed and so they conclude: 'If I hadn't stayed home, Philadelphia would be gone, and it would all be my fault.' Or the person might spend all day repeating a prayer to ward off the bad spirit. They then conclude: 'Had I not said the Hail Mary all day, Philadelphia would have been destroyed.' Also, while they are saying their prayer aloud, they cannot hear the voices. This reduction in the voice hearing is then perceived as evidence that it lessens the danger and so it reinforces the compensatory behaviours.

External: Ironically, there is, to our knowledge, no evidence to suggest that the belief that the voice is external to the person is linked with dysfunction, yet it is frequently a target for intervention. This can elicit defensiveness in people and reduce engagement with treatment. Clinically, a small group of people who hear voices continue the behaviour of preparing for an external threat (a source of stress), even after recovery. Here too, this belief is not a valuable target for intervention, unless the person pursues the topic or shows an entrenched pattern of preparing for the return of persecutors (and increased stress).

These beliefs, particularly control, credibility and power, provide a framework for understanding the presence, maintenance and distress of voice hearing. Beliefs provide a pragmatic target for intervention, while honouring the experience.

> ### Learning point 2
> - Is there an obstacle you are currently struggling with (medical condition, anxiety, procrastination) or a past obstacle? Can you search on the internet for a good explanation about the problem? Did reading and understanding the problem fix the problem? Are you closer to solving the problem now? What does this tell you about how psychoeducation can be a useful intervention?
> - Think of a time when you were extremely angry. How did you overcome the anger? How did you deal with the intrusive thoughts? Would those apply to distressing voices?

Having arrived at a formulation (a hypothesis about the reason for a particular mental health problem based on the person's life circumstances) for distressing voices, the clinician's attention turns towards treatment. Many clinicians are drawn to *challenging* the belief or teaching the voice hearer skills to 'cope' with the voices. Missing from these approaches to 'treatment' is a strategy for change based on an understanding of the voice-hearing formulation. An approach that privileges treatment of symptoms over personal aspirations risks activating a series of beliefs related to the person seeing themselves as defective. These beliefs are frequently accompanied by a lack of motivation, which can create fertile ground for increased voice hearing. CT-R extends the benefits of cognitive behavioural therapy for psychosis (CBTp) to people who traditionally do not benefit from psychosocial treatments (Beck et al., 2020). The approach centres on supporting people to pursue their personal aspirations. Obstacles, like distressing voices, are addressed as they interfere with progress towards the desired life. The clinician and person's focus on aspirations activates a set of beliefs related to hope and capability. Instead of focusing on problems, CT-R capitalises on the times a person is activated and engaged in personally meaningful endeavours. This activation provides an opportunity to test out alternative routines and beliefs.

CT-R providers use the times when people are most adaptive to change, and interactions that are not 'clinical'. Such times usually coincide with enjoyable or meaningful activities (listening to music, going for a walk, eating a snack) or conversations (talking about recipes, sports or pets). In those times, the person can seem completely absent of symptoms or in a better space for adaption. Approaching the person this way activates a set of beliefs related to being valued and connected, which is incompatible with maladaptive beliefs. Further, many of these engagements are incompatible with hearing voices. For example, talking about favourite recipes uses two voice-dampening factors:

1. It increases positive affect and reduces uncontrolled stress
2. It reduces the voice-hearing experience.

The combination of inoculating voice hearing (engaging in a behaviour/activity that stops the voice-hearing experience) and activating efficacy beliefs increases a person's ability to access mental resources and provides an opportunity to elicit aspirations.

With increased mental resources, the practitioner and person focus on future aspirations. The 'big picture' view of life provides the person with a competing focus to the distressing voices and motivation to attempt to face the distressing experience. Aspirations speak to the fundamental desires that drive behaviour. Facing and working through distressing voices requires courage and strength. Aspirations provide that motivation.

Consider these two 'goals' – which one would provide motivation to face distressing voices?

1. Take medicine as prescribed and shower daily.
2. Teach my son to make homemade pasta.

The first goal is clinical and the second is aspirational. Considering that many people have problems with motivation and distressing voices do not typically engender a fighting attitude, the aspirations need to provide a powerful reason for change. Furthermore, as the person envisions the desired future, a body of evidence grows that contradicts many of the demeaning statements heard from the voices. With an increased motivation, the person develops action steps to realise the aspiration.

Action is a core element of the CT-R protocol and provides four main benefits. First, by creating a schedule of activities, the person is able to plan times when they are less vulnerable to being distracted by the voices (for example, when listening to music or practising mindfulness). The person gets a bit of a 'break' from the distressing voices. Second, that they are able to plan such activities provides evidence that they are in control, not the voices, and undermines the credibility of the voices and their power to follow through on their threats. Third, the activity schedule is an opportunity to take steps towards achieving their hopes and goals. Finally, this 'treatment' is no different from what anyone might do to maintain their mental wellness, which itself is evidence that the voice hearer is just like anyone else. I have drawn many a person's attention to the fact that they are recovering from psychosis by simply living life.

While the main thrust of CT-R focuses on increasing productive activity towards aspirations, the larger CBTp cannon provides a wide variety of interventions to draw on when the distressing voices interfere with a person's attempts to move forward. A main intervention type involves refocusing attention away from the voice-hearing experience towards aspirations or other productive activity. Any time the person focuses their attention away from the voice-hearing experience, engages their mind and speaks, the voice-hearing experience is lessened. These times provide a respite from voice hearing and evidence that the person can control the experience. Examples include:

- talking to another person
- listening to music
- mindfulness
- naming items around the room.

Each of these activities is best used to refocus attention towards a desired activity. Some will think the purpose is distraction. Refocusing provides forward momentum and hope for an individual. With the person having a different experience as a result of the CT-R protocol, they can learn new lessons and correct beliefs in order to sustain recovery.

> ### Learning point 3
> - Imagine you start taking medication for high blood pressure. If you stop taking the medication, the underlying problem returns. Coping skills are similar. As long as you use them (take the medicine), they help. When you stop using them, the problem returns because whatever is underlying the problem has not changed.
> - If you change your diet and exercise routine and get into good health, the high blood pressure is likely to reduce, even if you stop the medicine. The same is true for voices; they get better when you correct the underlying problem, beliefs, behaviours and unhelpful routines.

The CT-R protocol creates an experience rich with opportunities to correct the person's beliefs about the voices and wider beliefs about the self, the world, others and the future. Regardless of the intervention used by the practitioner and the voice hearer, the effect is temporary unless the beliefs are corrected. Like psychotropic medicines, the interventions only work as long as the person continues to use the skill. For example, a person who is taught a coping skill to stop the voice-hearing experience will gain the benefit as long as they continue to use the coping skill when the voice emerges. The problem inherent in this approach is that these experiences can seem unpredictable and bring up strong emotions during episodes. These make it hard for the person to remember to use their coping skills when needed, leaving them susceptible to voice hearing.

An alternative approach to treatment involves using these successful experiences to check the accuracy or helpfulness of the belief. As the person notices the unhelpfulness of the thinking, they can start acting differently and see the impact of this on their distress or productivity. For example, a person stays at home because they believe the voices control when they come and go. They check the helpfulness of the thought and notice that, when alone, they are always inundated with the voices. So, self-isolating because they think that the voices will come unexpectedly and embarrass them isn't helping them feel better. But if they go out and interact with others, they will start noticing that the voices lessen when they are around others. They notice the following:

1. I chose to go out and the voices went down.
2. When I stay home the voices are louder.
3. I could have chosen to stay home, but chose to go out anyway.
4. If going out leads to lower voices and I choose to go out, I have some ability to control the voices.

As the person learns that they have control over the voices, they change their behaviour and start going out more, because they know that this will lead to reduced voice hearing. The success reinforces the idea that they have control over the voices. Just as the distressing voices are maintained and empowered by the negative cycle, this positive cycle maintains the improvement and inoculates the person from reverting to the old belief about needing to avoid others because the voice has control.

The process of drawing these conclusions progresses from observational to empirical. Initially, the provider and the person notice the changes, such as the times when the voices are lessened. Once they notice the change, they start making note of the reliability of the outcome (whenever I talk, the voices are less). Over time, hypotheses are generated as to new possibilities (perhaps avoiding others is making my voices worse and I can control them) and tests are developed (setting times to go out and talk with people). The behaviours over time are changed in response to the new 'rule' about the voice hearing. In time, the provider shifts the discussion towards more central themes related to the self, others, the world and the future.

Conclusion

CT-R for distressing voices shifts the traditional psychological treatment from a focus on an illness with a biological cause to one of recovery. While the notions of internal strengths and wholeness have been around since the middle of the last century, focusing on recovery and thriving is difficult in the face of the mystery that distressing voices pose. CT-R provides a systematic approach to drawing the person away from the distressing experience, refocusing their attention from the voices and permanently disrupting the voice hearing as an obstacle to living. As the person corrects their beliefs about the distressing voices, they develop new routines that reinforce the adaptive beliefs. Realising these personal aspirations corrects core beliefs about personal value and strength. At the end of treatment, some people no longer hear voices, while others continue to hear voices but do not imbue them with any power or meaning. A CBTp study of people who followed through on command hallucinations (Birchwood et al., 2014) has indeed found this to be the case: at the end of treatment, not all people stopped hearing their voices and some continued to hear commands, but they no longer believed the voices had any power, so they did not care.

CT-R takes a pragmatic approach to voice hearing. It considers the maintenance, distress and dysfunction associated with voice hearing as an understandable and logical reaction to a frightening experience. CT-R does not challenge the interpretation of the voice hearing as spiritual or personal. In CT-R, voice hearing is solely regarded as an obstacle in the way of a person's progress towards their desired life. In this way, CT-R and other good CBTp are compatible with and can be used with other approaches to voice hearing. CT-R aims to honour the person's experience and help them to achieve their desired life.

References

Beck, A.T. (1979). *Cognitive therapy and the emotional disorders.* Plume Publishing.

Beck, A.T., Grant, P.M., Inverso, E., Brinen, A.P. & Perivoliotis, D. (2020). *Recovery-oriented cognitive therapy for serious mental health conditions.* Guilford Press.

Birchwood, M., Michail, M., Meaden, A., Tarrier, N., Lewis, S., Wykes, T., Davies, L., Dunn, G., & Peters, E. (2014). Cognitive behaviour therapy to prevent harmful compliance with command hallucinations (COMMAND): a randomised controlled trial. *Lancet Psychiatry, 1*(1), 23–33. https://doi.org/10.1016/S2215-0366(14)70247-0

Hayward, M., Straus, C., & Kindon, D. (2018). *Overcoming distress in voices* (2nd ed.). Robinson.

Johns, L.C., Kompus, K., Connell, M., Humpston, C., Lincoln, T.M., Longden, E., Preti, A., Alderson-Day, B., Badcock, J.C., Cella, M., Fernyhough, C., McCarthy-Jones, S., Peters, E., Raballo, A., Scott, J., Siddi, S., Sommer, I.E. & Laroi, F. (2014). Auditory verbal hallucinations in people with and without a need for care. *Schizophrenia Bulletin, 40*(4), S255–S264.

Lincoln, T.M., Lüllmann, E. & Rief, W. (2007). Correlates and long-term consequences of poor insight in patients with schizophrenia: A systematic review. *Schizophrenia Bulletin, 33*(6), 1324–1342. https://doi.org/10.1093/schbul/sbm002

Morrison, A.P., Hutton, P., Shiers, D. & Turkington, D. (2012). Antipsychotics: Is it time to introduce patient choice? *British Journal of Psychiatry, 201*, 83–84.

24 AVATAR therapy: a digital therapy to help people with distressing voices

Mar Rus-Calafell and Tom Craig

> The thing that frightened me the most is that I couldn't see what they looked like when they were shouting at me. (Quote from anonymous voice hearer)

What is AVATAR therapy?

Recent studies using phenomenological approaches have shown that voices are often experienced as having distinguishable characteristics and distinct identities, such as relatives, celebrities, religious beings or deities (Beavan, 2011; McCarthy-Jones & Resnick, 2014; Nayani & David, 1996; Woods et al., 2016). Certain basic elements of voice hearing have been proposed to occur across the psychosis continuum: their content is personally meaningful to the person, they have an emotional impact, the person establishes a personal relationship with the voice, and the voice is experienced as very real (Beavan, 2011). Wilkinson and Bell (2016) have recently highlighted the importance of exploring the representation of agents in voice hearing (that is, specific social beings with beliefs, desires and intentions) in order to accurately describe and fully understand the person's experience, which is bound up in how voice hearers and clinicians speak about hearing voices (Wilkinson & Bell, 2016). In this view, the agents regarded as the origin of the voices are understood as social beings, with the voice-hearing experience considered to be a dynamic interpersonal relationship that comes to play a central role in the person's life, often over the course of several years.

AVATAR therapy (audio-visual assisted therapy aid for refractory auditory hallucinations) is a newly developed treatment for distressing voices that adopts the understanding that voices are social beings communicating with the voice hearer. Originally created by Professor Julian Leff (Leff, 2013), it involves a three-way interaction between client, therapist and a computerised representation of their voice (the avatar). To be able to create this avatar, therapists use a special computer software that transforms the therapists' voice to match the pitch and tone of the chosen distressing voice and the voice hearer creates a visual representation of the agent thought to be the source of the voice. The voice and image are combined to produce the avatar, through which the therapist interacts with the voice hearer in this three-way conversation ('trialogue'). Where there are multiple voices, the client selects one to work with (usually the most dominant, frequent and distressing). The therapist supports the client to interact with the voice and challenge the negative things it says in order to change the relationship between them and their voice from a distressing experience to a more positive or neutral interaction. The aim is for the dialogue to evolve with the person in control of the changing relationship, and to enable an increased experience of power to generalise to the everyday voice experience. When the psychological changes are measured after AVATAR therapy, the assessment takes in all the voices (not only the one focused on in the trialogue) (Craig et al., 2018; Leff et al., 2013).

In the first session of AVATAR therapy, participants undergo a detailed assessment of the voice-hearing experience in the context of their current and previous significant relationships (Birchwood et al., 2000, 2004). It is argued that beliefs about the power of the voice are essentially a differential judgement the hearer makes about their own power (or, more usually, lack of power) in relation to the voice: i.e. a relational judgement. People who have experienced powerlessness and inferiority in social relationships are found to be more likely to report similar experiences when interacting with their voices (Birchwood et al., 2000). Therefore, this initial clinical assessment includes information about the source of the voices (e.g. gender, age, ethnicity, whether it is someone the person has met or knows, human or non-human), whether the voices seem to be part of a network (e.g. criminal gang, former work team), whether they reflect unresolved social and emotional issues and how the experience of hearing a voice is influenced by the person's cultural background and experiences earlier in life, such as childhood maltreatment, bullying and other traumatic events, low self-esteem and co-morbid depression. After this assessment, the client creates with the help of the therapist the avatar that they feel represents the source of the target voice.

The therapy system is set up in two different rooms in the same building, with two linked computers or laptops. The client sits in one room, facing the monitor on which the avatar appears. The therapist sits in the other room, facing the monitor, with a control panel that allows them to talk to the participant in their own voice or in the morphed avatar voice created for them. The therapist can see and hear everything that is appearing on the client's monitor, as well as the client's responses, and can adjust his or her therapeutic interventions (in their own voice) in response to the unfolding dialogue between the client and their avatar.

Using real-time voice conversion delivery software, the therapist voices the avatar engaging in a direct dialogue with the person, with the ultimate aim of modifying the relationship between the client and their voice. Therapy comprises six sessions of 45 minutes, of which approximately 10 to 15 minutes are spent in dialogue with the avatar. The sessions are audio-recorded and given to the client on an MP3 player for continued use at home.

The therapy proceeds through two phases. Phase 1 (typically sessions 1–3) involves the client listening to the avatar speaking the typical content of the client's voices, while the therapist encourages the client to respond assertively: for example, telling the avatar that they are no longer prepared to accept these threats and insults and challenging any apparent 'misconceptions' the avatar seems to have. In phase 2 (typically sessions 4–6), the dialogue gradually evolves in the light of this assertive responding and a clinical formulation (hypotheses discussed with the therapist about reasons for the voices when considering the person's life circumstances and the relationship between the participant and their voice). This phase typically incorporates a shared reflection with the therapist on the autobiographical context, meaning-making, and experiences of trauma and powerlessness. The avatar gives way and acknowledges the strengths and good qualities of the client, saying: 'Yes, you are certainly a strong person… So what now?'

To plan the transition between phases, which normally defines the moment in which the client is willing and prepared to resolve or move forward in the relationship, the therapist may discuss this in supervision with the wider AVATAR clinical team. During these supervision sessions, actual recordings of the sessions may be listened to in order to plan the transition in advance and elaborate a plan that can be agreed with the client. Spontaneity and ability to improvise are important qualities for therapists willing to deliver AVATAR therapy. There can be moments in the dialogue between the client and the avatar voice where unplanned reactions, or even revelations that the person has not yet shared with the therapist, such as the painful memories of a sexual abuse, will arise, which may be because the client is embarrassed and ashamed to talk about them with other living people. For example, Bridgette,[1] a young woman who took part in the AVATAR randomised controlled trial (Craig et al., 2018), spontaneously talked with the avatar in session 2 about the painful memories of a sexual abuse she suffered when she was a child. Bridgette did not talk about it when being assessed by the therapist at the beginning of the therapy. During the session's debriefing, Bridgette said that she only talked about it with her voice as she felt embarrassed and ashamed when talking about it with other people.

Learning point 1
- What do you think are the main psychological challenges when creating a visual representation and audio analogy of a distressing voice? What, in your opinion, are the main advantages of using digital technology to access the voice and recreate a dialogue with them?

AVATAR therapy as a relational approach

AVATAR therapy is one of a new wave of psychological therapies that adopt an explicitly dialogical and relational approach to reducing the distress caused by

---
1. Bridgette is a pseudonym and her story has been anonymised

negative voices. These approaches focus on the relationship between the voice hearer and the voices and do not specifically seek to erase the experience of hearing the voice. They target particular aspects of that relationship and also seek to improve the client's sense of their own power within the relationship. Apart from AVATAR therapy, the two main relational therapies that have recently shown encouraging results to improve distressing voices are relating rherapy (Hayward et al., 2009, 2017; see also Chapter 25 in this book) and Talking with Voices (Corstens et al., 2012; see also Chapters 1, 18 and 19 of this book).

Relating therapy (Hayward et al., 2009) applies Birtchnell's interpersonal model to the voice and hearer relationship, identifying key interpersonal dimensions of power and proximity (Birtchnell, 1996). Therapy consists of approximately 16 sessions and starts with the discussion of similarities in terms of power and proximity between the person's relationship with their voice and other social relationships. The therapist then encourages the person to explore themes within their relational history, their experience of their relationships with voices and interpersonal relating within their family and social environment. Finally, the therapy moves on to explore different ways of relating to the voice using a variety of techniques, including assertiveness training, role-play and empty chair work, with the aim of increasing the person's sense of control within the relationship.

In Talking with Voices, Dirk Corstens and colleagues (2012) draw on a therapeutic approach more commonly associated with psychoanalytic approaches in which the personality is conceived as comprising a number of alternative selves, each with their own perceptions and reactions to the world. The voices heard by clients can be related to in a similar way to how it is possible to relate to these selves, who want to be heard and may have important things to say to or about the client, perhaps relating to some emotional crisis in their life. The therapeutic process will normally form part of a wider engagement with the Making Sense of Voices approach (Romme & Escher, 2000), and involves asking the person to concentrate on a chosen voice and locate it in the room. The facilitator (they do not need to be a therapist) then engages in a dialogue with the voice, which is spoken by the voice hearer as an intermediary. The aim is to explore and change the relationship so that the person and voice come to a better mutual understanding, the person regains control and the voice may even transition from 'a tormentor to an encouraging companion' (Corstens et al., 2012).

AVATAR therapy focuses on the relationship between the voice hearer and their most distressing or dominant voice by offering a new therapeutic context that allows a 'face-to-face' dialogue with a representation of the voice. Digital technology allows the person to give a physical representation to their personified but disembodied voice. The embodiment of the voice is enhanced by the use of direct verbatim statements from the voice and enactment of the ascribed character and background of the voice. It offers a unique way for therapists to understand how voice hearers interact with a realistic representation of their voice. Furthermore, the use of technology facilitates two important facets of AVATAR therapy: 1) the incorporation of a tangible 'self' or 'other' representation, helping to differentiate between the two agents of the relationship; 2) improvement of the interactivity, realism and impact of the dialogue between the person and the voice (Rus-Calafell et al., 2020).

The continuous exposure to the experience of seeing and hearing the voice over therapy sessions, along with the modification of the relationship with the voice, may be contributing to the reduction of the voice's associated distress and to the disconfirmation of maladaptive beliefs about the voice. One may argue that the same technique could be applied by using the voice hearer's imaginative capacity (without any technological support). By providing both visual and audio stimuli to the participant, we are encouraging clients to face their voices in a 'safe space'. Learning to face this potentially terrifying presence and overcoming the initial fear reaction in a safe and supported way can be a crucial step towards changing the relationship to a voice. This allows the therapist and the client to focus on key emotional processes, such as the client's dysfunctional beliefs about the voice and shifting the experience to feelings of empowerment and enhanced self-esteem, while having a real-time dialogue with the avatar (Ward et al., 2020). It has recently been demonstrated that the interaction between the virtual embodiment of the 'voice as avatar' (i.e. the client's perception that the avatar is a realistic simulation of the experience of hearing and relating to their voice) and reduction of anxiety are associated with an improvement in the severity and frequency of the voices (Rus-Calafell et al., 2020).

Learning point 2
- Following Rus-Calafell's findings (2020), would you say it is better to have a conversation with the voice 'face-to-face'? If yes, why? Would it be enough to do it only using audio settings (i.e. like having a phone conversation)?

Using technology to improve distressing voices

Technology is used in a very novel way in AVATAR therapy. Research has shown that voice hearers often identify their voices as being those of people known to them or famous people. McCarthy-Jones and colleagues found that around 70% of voice hearers reported that the voices they heard were like those of people who had spoken to them in the past (McCarthy-Jones et al., 2012). This implies that often the voice is clearly understood as a representation of an abstraction, in the form of a person or entity. The approach used in AVATAR therapy allows the voice hearer to access and visualise this abstract, non-physical entity. You could define it as a *virtual embodiment* of the experience. This visualisation of the voice may facilitate two essential processes in the AVATAR therapy: 1) the validation of the experience, and 2) the flow of dialogue with the voice through the sessions while modifying the nature of the relationship between the voice and the voice hearer. This virtual embodiment of the experience is fully achieved by matching the voice of the avatar to the current voice, which adds even more realism to the experience and seems to be a key aspect of the therapy. In this sense, AVATAR therapy offers a unique opportunity to work relationally through real-time dialogue with an avatar created by the hearer as a representation of their voice.

> ### Learning point 3
> - Virtual reality and other technologies are currently used to enhance the effects of psychological therapies. Would you like to see more of them available through statutory mental health services, like the NHS in the UK? What do you think are the main advantages and disadvantages of using this technology?

Evidence for AVATAR therapy

Three main studies have investigated the efficacy of AVATAR therapy. They include two pilot studies, one using the original software created by Mark Huckvale and colleagues at University College London (UCL) (see Leff et al., 2013 for details), and another based on the approach developed by Professor Leff but using a different, independently developed immersive system to deliver the therapy (a virtual reality technology using a special headset that allows the person to experience being fully immersed in a computer-generated environment within which the avatar appears) (du Sert et al., 2018).

The study by Leff and colleagues (2013) analysed the effects of AVATAR therapy with a group of 24 voice hearers who had experienced a longstanding single or dominant persecutory voice. It found highly clinically significant reductions in the frequency, distress, omnipotence and malevolence of the voice at 12 weeks (Leff et al., 2013). The therapy was provided for a maximum of seven sessions, each lasting 30 minutes. Very similar 12-week outcome results were found by du Sert and colleagues in their pilot study with 19 participants comparing immersive AVATAR therapy (seven weekly sessions) and treatment as usual (defined as antipsychotic medication and usual meetings with their clinicians) (du Sert et al., 2018).

A third study, a randomised controlled trial involving 150 participants, has taken the work of Leff and colleagues (2013) one step further. The participants were all diagnosed with long-standing psychosis and had been hearing distressing voices for at least 12 months. They were randomised to receive either the AVATAR therapy or an intensive supportive counselling intervention (Craig et al., 2018). The intention-to-treat analysis (i.e. including the data on everyone who consented to take part in the study and who was randomised to one of the two treatments, regardless of what treatment (if any) they received) showed that AVATAR therapy was significantly superior to supportive counselling at 12 weeks in reducing the severity, frequency and associated distress of the voices, reducing beliefs about the omnipotence of the voices and improving participants' acceptance of their voices as part of their everyday life . These gains were maintained at 24-week follow-up for the AVATAR therapy group, but the supportive counselling group had continued to improve, so the difference in outcomes at 24 weeks between the two groups, while still apparent, was no longer large enough to reach statistical significance (i.e. to be able to be confidently interpreted as a benefit for AVATAR therapy over and above that of supportive counselling). Future work on this project will focus on further personalising and optimising therapy delivery and evaluating its effectiveness with a view to dissemination. The authors are also working on a report based on a qualitative investigation of people's experience of taking part in AVATAR therapy and an exploration of their views on voice embodiment and emotional reactions (e.g. shame, anger or guilt) during therapy.

The future of AVATAR therapy

Although three clinical trials to date support the short-term effectiveness of AVATAR therapy, its long-term benefits are not known. More studies, including long-term follow-up assessments as well as the evaluation of booster 'top-up' sessions to enhance the therapy effects, should be conducted. Whether both AVATAR therapy and supportive counselling would outperform treatment as usual also remains to be answered, as this option was not included in the RCT by Craig and colleagues (2018).

Research is also needed to explore the effects of each of the phases of AVATAR therapy separately: a more simplistic approach of just the phase one focus on reducing fearfulness (the client listens to what the voices say through the avatar and responds assertively) could be enough for some people, while a more complex approach that also includes the clinical formulation as described for phase 2 could be needed for other types of experiences (e.g. where voices are thought to be associated with prior traumatic experiences).

One of the biggest challenges facing AVATAR therapy is its implementation in public and private mental health services. Up to this point, the therapy has been delivered by skilled therapists with high expertise in the psychological treatment of psychosis (often with prior expertise in CBT for psychosis (CBTp) and previous experience of using talking therapy with people hearing negative distressing voices and associated emotional processes), which limits the implementation of the therapy in other settings or its delivery by the wider mental health workforce. It is possible that a simplified approach that focuses on the first phase of the therapy (essentially managing anxiety and improving self-esteem) would be enough for many clients and could be delivered by a wider workforce with appropriate training. This is a question being addressed in our ongoing research.

However, even so, therapy delivery requires skill, sensitivity, training and supervision. The voice hearer's understanding, existing support and readiness for this approach should also be assessed and regularly reviewed (Ward et al., 2020). Other specific challenges related to the use of technology, such as switching between speaking as therapist and avatar in real-time and ethical considerations regarding the verbalising of specific distressing content, should also be considered by those therapists willing to learn the apprach.

Conclusion

AVATAR therapy is a new psychological approach to working with people seeking help for negative distressing voices. Focusing on the relationship between the client and the voice, it offers a unique, personalised and tailored interactive experience to the voice hearer. Its efficacy has been tested in three research studies (two pilot studies and one randomised controlled study). Although preliminary evidence supports its acceptability and effectiveness on reducing severity, frequency and distress related to negative voices, larger studies are required to replicate these findings before it can be rolled out more widely. Other important aspects, such as specific training and supervision, along with the acquisition of the specific software, will also need to be addressed if therapists are to deliver AVATAR therapy in the future.

Acknowledgements

The AVATAR clinical trial was funded by a Wellcome Trust Translation Award (number 09827).

References

Beavan, V. (2011). Towards a definition of 'hearing voices': A phenomenological approach. *Psychosis: Psychological, social and integrative approaches, 3*(1), 63–73.

Birchwood, M., Gilbert, P., Gilbert, J., Trower, P., Meaden, A., Hay, J., Murray, E. &d Miles, J.N. (2004). Interpersonal and role-related schema influence the relationship with the dominant 'voice' in schizophrenia: A comparison of three models. *Psychological Medicine 34*, 1571–1580.

Birchwood, M., Meaden, A., Trower, P., Gilbert, P. & Plaistow, J. (2000). The power and omnipotence of voices: Subordination and entrapment by voices and significant others. *Psychological Medicine, 30*(2), 337–344.

Birtchnell, J. (1996). *How humans relate: A new interpersonal theory.* Psychology Press.

Corstens, D., Longden, E. & May, R. (2012). Talking with voices: Exploring what is expressed by the voices people hear. *Psychosis: Psychological, social and integrative approaches, 4*(2), 95–104.

Craig, T.K., Rus-Calafell, M., Ward, T., Leff, J.P., Huckvale, M., Howarth, E., Emsley, R. & Garety, P.A. (2018). AVATAR therapy for auditory verbal hallucinations in people with psychosis: A single-blind, randomised controlled trial. *Lancet Psychiatry, 5*(1), 31–40.

du Sert, O.P., Potvin, S., Lipp, O., Dellazizzo, L., Laurelli, M., Breton, R., Lalonde, P., Phraxayavong, K., O'Connor, K., Pelletier, J.F., Boukhalfi, T., Renaud, P. & Dumais, A . (2018). Virtual reality therapy for refractory auditory verbal hallucinations in schizophrenia: A pilot clinical trial. *Schizophrenia Research, 197*, 176–181.

Hayward, M., Jones, A.M., Bogen-Johnston, L., Thomas, N. & Strauss, C . (2017). Relating therapy for distressing auditory hallucinations: A pilot randomized controlled trial. *Schizophrenia Research, 183,* 137–142.

Hayward, M., Overton, J., Dorey, T. & Denney, J. (2009). Relating therapy for people who hear voices: A case series. *Clinical Psychology & Psychotherapy, 16*(3), 216–227.

Leff, J. (2013). Computer-assisted therapy for medication-resistant auditory hallucinations. *British Journal of Psychiatry, 203*(4), 313–313.

Leff, J., Williams, G., Huckvale, M.A., Arbuthnot, M. & Leff, A.P. (2013). Computer-assisted therapy for medication-resistant auditory hallucinations: Proof-of-concept study. *British Journal of Psychiatry, 202,* 428–433.

McCarthy-Jones, S. & Resnick, P.J. (2014). Listening to voices: the use of phenomenology to differentiate malingered from genuine auditory verbal hallucinations. *International Journal of Law and Psychiatry, 37,* 183–189.

McCarthy-Jones, S., Trauer, T., Mackinnon, A., Sims, E., Thomas, N. & Copolov, D.L. (2012). A new phenomenological survey of auditory hallucinations: Evidence for subtypes and implications for theory and practice. *Schizophrenia Bulletin, 40*(1), 231–235.

Nayani, T.H. & David, A.S. (1996). The auditory hallucination: A phenomenological survey. *Psychological Medicine, 26*(1), 177–189.

Romme, M. & Escher, S. (2000). *Making sense of voices.* Mind Publications.

Rus-Calafell, M., Ward, T., Zhang, X.C., Edwards, C., Garety, P. &, Craig, T.K. (2020). The role of sense of voice presence and anxiety reduction in AVATAR therapy. *Journal of Clinical Medicine 9*(9), 2748. doi: 10.3390/jcm9092748

Ward, T., Rus-Calafell, M., Ramadhan, Z., Soumelidou, O., Fornells-Ambrojo, M., Garety, P. & Craig, TK. (2020). AVATAR therapy for distressing voices: A comprehensive account of therapeutic targets. *Schizophrenia Bulletin, 46,* 1038–1044.

Wilkinson, S. & Bell, V. (2016). The representation of agents in auditory verbal hallucinations. *Mind and Language, 31*(1), 104–126.

Woods, A., Jones, N., Alderson-Day, B., Callard, F. & Fernyhough, C. (2016). Experiences of hearing voices: Analysis of a novel phenomenological survey. *Lancet Psychiatry, 2,* 323–331.

25 Relating therapy for voices: learning how to respond assertively in difficult relationships

Mark Hayward, Sheila Evenden and Angie Culham

Voices can make comments that are very personal, critical and threatening. These comments can be difficult to ignore, and we can be drawn into responding instinctively – for example, by giving in, trying to get away or fighting back. Sometimes these instinctive responses can be helpful and give us a bit of peace in the short term; but in the long term, these responses may not change the negative views we have of ourselves and our views of the voices as powerful and all-knowing. Relating therapy teaches voice hearers how to respond to voices in a different way – through being assertive.

This chapter will draw on the lived experiences of the authors to offer some insights into the challenges and benefits of relating therapy and trying to respond assertively in difficult relationships. Sheila and Angie draw on lived experience of hearing distressing voices and receiving relating therapy. Mark draws on experience of delivering relating therapy.

Do people have relationships with the voices they hear?

Relationships are a part of our everyday lives. We have relationships with our families, friends, colleagues, peers and possibly with spiritual entities too. When these relationships are two way and involve mutual trust and respect, they can be positive and a source of pleasure and support. However, relationships can sometimes be difficult and make us feel bullied, manipulated and intruded upon. In these circumstances, we might give in, try to get away or fight back.

Does this description of relationships also apply to the voices that some people hear? Research studies suggest that most people who hear voices do have two-way conversations with the voices (McCarthy-Jones et al., 2014), so there seems to be some sort of relational exchange going on. If these conversations are respectful and helpful, there may be a sense of companionship and a positive relationship. Within these positive relationships, voice hearers have reported the importance of getting closer to and engaging with voices and relating to them in a strong and assertive manner (Jackson et al., 2011). But voices can often be abusive, critical and bullying, and can cause a lot of distress by forcing the voice hearer into a submissive role where their needs and views are neglected. In these circumstances, the relating might feel one-directional (from the voice) and this may not seem to be a relationship in the true sense of the word (Chin et al., 2009). What can voice hearers do to become more active in these circumstances and ensure they stand up for their needs and views?

Before we explore ways of becoming more active when relating to voices, two further findings from research studies are noteworthy. First, relationships with voices may not spontaneously change over time (Hartigan et al., 2014). Consequently, voice hearers may need some assistance to change the way they relate to voices. Second, the way that voice hearers relate to their voices seems to be quite similar to the way they relate to people in their social environments (Birchwood et al., 2000; Hayward, 2003). If relationships with voices are difficult, this may reflect difficulties with relationships across the board. Support may therefore be needed to relate differently in all difficult relationships, both with voices and with other people.

> *Learning point 1*
>
> People who hear voices can experience difficult relationships with their voices. These difficulties can also be experienced with some people in their social environments. Support may be needed to help voice hearers respond differently in all difficult relationships.

Supporting voice hearers to relate differently

A number of psychological therapies are being developed to try to help voice hearers respond differently. These therapies share a common goal of supporting voice hearers to have a guided experience of engaging and conversing with voices in an assertive manner, but they approach this goal in different ways. Some therapies use digital technology to support a conversation with a visual representation of the voice (see Chapter 24 on AVATAR therapy; Craig et al., 2017); other therapies try to have 'live' conversations with voices (see Chapters 18 and 19 on experience focused counselling and Voice Dialogue, or Talking with Voices, in particular; Corstens et al., 2012), and yet other therapies use traditional role-plays to bring to life these conversations with voices (Hayward et al., 2017). These various therapies are at different stages of development and evaluation and it's too soon to compare their effectiveness. They may all be found to be effective, potentially creating choices for voice hearers about the therapy that might best suit them. This chapter will focus on relating therapy (Hayward et al., 2017), which uses role-plays to support voice hearers to relate differently to their voices. Some of the techniques from relating therapy can be integrated into cognitive behaviour therapy (CBT) when learning about assertiveness skills (see Chapter 22). This chapter will explore the content and experience of relating therapy when offered as a full course of therapy.

Relating therapy – the basics

Relating therapy is based on a set of ideas that are guided by some of the research evidence described above:

- The way that voice hearers relate to distressing voices is likely to reflect the ways they respond in difficult social relationships, both past and present. This suggests that curiosity should extend to all difficult relationships across time.
- Voice hearers tend to respond to distressing voices either passively (keeping their needs and views to themselves) or aggressively (forcefully pushing their needs and views onto others). Both forms of responding are intuitive and natural in the face of a threatening voice and are hard-wired as the 'fight or flight response'. However, both responses have the potential to perpetuate difficult relationships by maintaining low self-esteem (passive response) and/or provoking aggression (aggressive response).
- Assertive responding may offer an alternative way to relate to distressing voices – the voice hearer can have the esteeming experience of standing up for their needs and views in a respectful manner that is less likely to provoke an aggressive response.

Before considering these ideas in more detail, let's explore the relationship to which a significant proportion of change is attributable in psychological therapy – the therapeutic relationship. Sheila is one of the co-authors of this chapter; she received relating therapy from Mark and was interviewed by a lived-experience researcher as we prepared for the writing of this chapter. Sheila's experience of relating therapy offers some insights into the importance of the therapeutic relationship.

Sheila: At the start of any therapeutic relationship, you don't know HOW or IF you are going to be able to form a working bond with your therapist – or indeed, if they will be able to bond with you – but for me, once I felt emotionally safe with the therapist, then I knew I could put 100% effort into it.

Interviewer: Yep. I suppose, another question then… I'm just wondering how it might have been challenging for you if it wasn't someone that you got on with?

Sheila: I wouldn't have opened up so much, I know that. If I hadn't felt comfortable in opening my soul to him, I wouldn't haven't opened up so much and I wouldn't have said as much about myself as I did, if I hadn't had that trust, because you're opening a Pandora's box aren't you, when you start dealing with people's emotions and going into them. You don't know what's going to be let out, so it was a trust I had in him.

Interviewer: So that's a key?

Sheila: That is a key, the fact that, you know, you can tell when you haven't. I've been able to tell over the years when I've seen somebody that's not really interested at all, and you think, why should I bother. But you could see with him, that he was interested in me as a person; in that hour of an appointment, I could tell that he was focused on me, not just thinking what he was having for dinner at night. You know, you could tell there was the actual interest in what he was doing, and that came over and in fact, some of the elements that I didn't like, like the role-play, which I hated, I don't think I would have done it if it wasn't somebody who I had confidence in.

Sheila's experience reminds us that a trusting therapeutic relationship is a fundamentally important foundation for exploring difficult relationships. A positive experience of the therapeutic relationship is key to all beneficial psychological therapy, but is arguably more pivotal in the context of the private and subjective experience of voice hearing. Research studies have helped us to appreciate the challenges that can be faced by voice hearers seeking to disclose their experience as they can be deterred by voices making threats and feelings of shame and concern about how others will respond (Bogen-Johnston et al., 2019). These difficulties can be compounded by the concerns of the therapist, as they too may have reservations about talking about voice-hearing experiences (Bogen-Johnston et al., 2020).

> *Learning point 2*
>
> Learning to respond assertively in difficult relationships may be built on a trusting therapeutic relationship. The relationship between therapist and voice hearer will offer an experience of and a model for healthy relating.

Relating therapy – getting started

Relating therapy is typically offered over 16 sessions.[1] This length allows time for the therapeutic relationship to develop and also enables the voice hearer's past and current relationships with voices and other people to be explored. The initial sessions of therapy are dedicated to exploring all relationships and noticing the relating patterns of the voice hearer. This relationship 'map' for the voice hearer can include experiences of both positive and difficult relationships.

After the therapist and voice hearer have developed a relationship map, the therapy focuses on a specific difficult relationship, often a relationship with a distressing voice. A specific conversation with the voice is explored in detail and the verbal, emotional and behavioural responses of the voice hearer are collaboratively categorised as passive, assertive or aggressive (see Figure 25.1). These ways of responding are acknowledged as 'natural' in the face of a threatening

---

1. The current evidence for the effectiveness of relating therapy has been generated from therapy offered face to face. Our experience during the 2020/21 Covid-19 pandemic suggests that it is also feasible to offer relating therapy remotely by videocall and phone.

other. Responding assertively is offered as an alternative, but it is a response that will be unnatural, and therefore will require effort to learn and use.

Figure 25.1: the relating categories of relating therapy

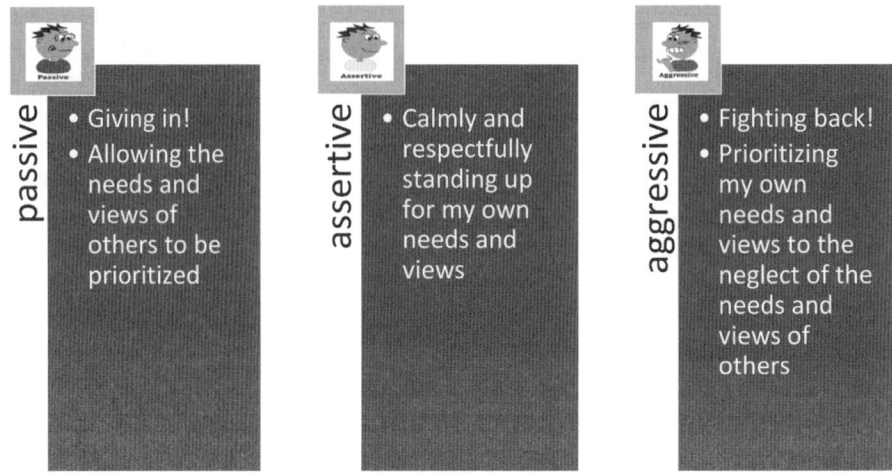

Assertive relating involves a voice hearer standing up for their own needs and views, while respecting the differing views of the voice. This work may require the voice hearer to initially clarify their own view and separate it from the view of the voice. For example, if the voice says, 'You are useless and worthless,' the voice hearer may need to explore the accuracy of this view. The voice hearer may believe this view to be accurate to some extent, at least historically, but may currently have a slightly different view. Separating the views of the voice hearer and the voice is a vital first step before trying to stand up for the different view.

Relating therapy acknowledges that responding assertively in difficult relationships can be very challenging. Consequently, the skill of relating assertively is broken down into the following components, which are focused on one at a time:

- verbal – using words that respectfully convey your view, without criticising the view of the other
- non-verbal –- using your body language to communicate in a strong manner that is consistent with the words spoken
- remaining assertive – drawing on evidence from your experience to support your view and help you to mean it
- leaving a conversation – on your own terms, when your view has been sufficiently foregrounded.

An assertive response within the selected conversation will be collaboratively created and written into a script. When the script is ready, it can be brought to life and 'experienced' through role-plays.

> *Learning point 3*
>
> Responding passively and/or aggressively in difficult relationships is quite natural. Learning to express and stand up for our views in an assertive manner can be quite unnatural and challenging.

Bringing assertiveness to life

Experiential exercises can 'bring the voice into the therapy room' and deepen the learning experience. In relating therapy, role-plays involve the use of an extra chair that represents the voice. Either the voice hearer or the therapist will sit in the chair and speak the comments of the voice from the script. Whoever sits in the voice hearer's chair will speak the voice hearer's assertive response in the script. The role-plays are initially brief as they are likely to be an unusual experience. Angie, another of the co-authors of this chapter, also received relating therapy from Mark and was interviewed by a lived-experience researcher as we prepared for the writing of this chapter. She describes her initial experience of the role-plays:

Interviewer: How did it make you feel when [therapist] was pretending to be your voices, as you said?

Angie: It was a bit awkward to start with because I hadn't really heard my voices coming from somebody else, so that, that did seem strange and I felt a bit uncomfortable with it and all my voices, when [therapist] was doing that, my voices didn't like it and I was struggling a little bit but, yeah, I just learnt how to not let them have their own way.

The aim of the initial role-plays is to offer the voice hearer an experience of standing up for their view while being respectful of the differing view of the voice. This may be difficult at first, as being assertive is so 'unnatural' to the voice hearer. The voice hearer may struggle to acknowledge the negative emotions generated by the comments of the voice and it can help to 'own' these feelings: for example, 'I have felt useless and worthless in the past and this upsets me, but I am developing a different view.' The voice hearer may also struggle to believe their own view. As the role-plays progress, the voice hearer is invited to explore and present the evidence ('facts') from their experience that supports their view. This presenting of the facts can help the voice hearer to mean what they say and to remain assertive. As the role-plays become longer, there will be a time when the voice hearer feels as if they have got their view across and wants to leave the conversation. The voices may not change in any way, so the voice hearer needs to develop an exit strategy that will enable them to end their participation in the conversation. Again, this can be difficult when the voices are continuing to talk about emotive issues, and it may need lots of practice in role-plays.

While initial role-plays often involve the voice hearer role-playing themselves (while the therapist takes the role of the voice), it can also be helpful for the voice hearer to take the role of the voice, as Angie explains:

Angie: When I was telling him [therapist] what my voices were saying [by role-playing the voice], it felt strange. In a way, it made the voices a bit more real, but it also taught me that, although the voices say that they can do things, that they can control things, it taught me that they couldn't, because I was talking about them and they couldn't do anything, you know, and they did a lot of threatening, but by actually sticking with it and talking about what the voices were saying to [the therapist], it sort of dulls down their power, if that makes sense.

The role of the difficult 'other' in the role-plays is not exclusive to the voice(s). Most voice hearers have difficult relationships in their social environments and the role-plays can be used to 'bring to life' an assertive response to one of these people. The aim here is to generalise the principles being learned to all difficult relationships.

Throughout the process of role-playing, much of the learning is generated and captured during the reflections that follow each role-play. This reflective space offers the voice hearer an opportunity to notice particular aspects of the experience of trying to be assertive: what went well and what could be done differently next time? This process of 'reflect, re-set and repeat' can facilitate learning at a slow and iterative pace that is accessible to all voice hearers.

> *Learning point 4*
>
> Learning to respond assertively in difficult relationships can be supported by trying to 'act' assertively during role-plays. These role-plays can offer an experience of using assertive words and body language, using evidence to help us to remain assertive, and leaving a conversation when we have got our point across.

What difference does it make?

Relating therapy has most recently been evaluated in a randomised controlled trial that compared voice hearers who had received a course of relating therapy from an experienced therapist with a control group of voice hearers who did not receive relating therapy. The voice hearers who received the therapy experienced a larger reduction in voice-related distress than the control group, and this reduction was maintained three months later (Hayward et al., 2017). Interviews with some of the voice hearers suggested that changes were noticed primarily in themselves (and less so in the voices): they felt stronger, were able to stand up for themselves and were more connected with other people (Hayward et al., 2018).

Angie explains the changes she experienced following a course of relating therapy:

Angie: It's definitely helped because I'm not by nature a very assertive person and I think I was, sort of, letting the voices rule. The only time I still struggle really with the voices is in the morning when I wake up. Sometimes I still struggle with that, but as a whole it has really helped and it's made me feel like I'm in charge of the voices and not the other way round. I feel more in control and not so frightened really, because it's quite frightening when you've got voices saying horrible things.

Angie's reflections remind us that relating therapy is not a panacea. At the conclusion of therapy, the voices are still likely to be active and the assertiveness skills of the voice hearer may not be fully formed. Consequently, the voice hearer may need ongoing support to facilitate further learning and the integration of assertiveness skills into their everyday life. Angie comments on the support that she received at the conclusion of therapy:

Angie: When the sessions were finished, we made an appointment for [therapist], myself and [nurse] to get together and talk about what we'd worked on, so [nurse] could carry on some of the work that we'd been doing. So, that was a great help because it gave [nurse] the chance to understand what we'd done and how we'd done it and how she could help me, so that was very worthwhile.

> *Learning point 5*
>
> Developing assertiveness skills and learning to use them in difficult relationships can take a long time. Ongoing practice and support will be needed to further develop and sustain the emerging skills.

The last (and artistic) words are left to Sheila and Angie, who have each described their experience of relating therapy in a poem:

A poem written by Sheila

The voices I hear used to fill me with dread,
I truly believed I was 'sick in the head'.
I'm 60 years old now – most treatments I'd tried,
had given up hope and at times wished I'd died.
I'd learned of research through my CMHT,
my first thought was that they'd have no use for me.
With nothing to lose though I gave them my name,
from that day 'til this my life's not been the same.
The therapy offered was something brand new,
my therapist caring, he taught me to view,
the voices in ways that gave me some control,
to tame them, not stop them completely – my goal.

They're not fully silenced – they're still part of me,
but they've loosened their grip – at last I am free,
to savour life's pleasures – to finally be,
at peace with the person I feared – which was me.

A poem written by Angie

Relating therapy – something new to me
I wanted to give it a try and see.
I decided to be positive, to learn as much as I could
Relating therapy – turns out it's really good.
Some of it I found quite tough,
but the therapist knew his stuff.
Learning to stand up to the voices,
realising I have choices.
Did I want them to rule my mind,
or learn and see what skills I could find?

As the weeks went by, I felt calmer,
understood the voices could do no harm.
It was a struggle, difficult at first,
But I did learn how to cope with voices at their worst.
Thank you so much for helping me cope
and for giving voice hearers hope.

References

Birchwood, M., Meaden, A., Trower, P., Gilbert, P. & Plaistow, J. (2000). The power and omnipotence of voices: Subordination and entrapment by voices and significant others. *Psychological Medicine, 30*, 337–344.

Bogen-Johnston, L., de Visser, R., Strauss, C., Berry, K. & Hayward, M. (2019). 'That little doorway where I could suddenly start shouting out': Barriers and enablers to the disclosure of distressing voices. *Journal of Health Psychology, 24*, 1307–1317.

Bogen-Johnston, L., de Visser, R., Strauss, C. & Hayward, M. (2020). A qualitative study exploring how practitioners within early intervention in psychosis services engage with service users' experiences of voice hearing? *Journal of Psychiatric and Mental Health Nursing, 27*, 607–615.

Chin, J., Hayward, M. & Drinnan, A. (2009). Relating to voices: Exploring the relevance of this concept to people who hear voices. *Psychology and Psychotherapy: Theory, research and practice, 82*, 1–17.

Corstens, D., Longden, E. & May, R. (2012). Talking with voices: Exploring what is expressed by the voices people hear. *Psychosis, 4*, 95–104.

Craig, T.K.J., Rus-Calafell, R., Ward, T., Leff, J.P., Huckvale, M., Howarth, E. & Garety, P. (2017). AVATAR therapy for auditory verbal hallucinations in people with psychosis: A single-blind, randomized controlled trial. *Lancet Psychiatry, 5*, 31–40.

Hartigan, N., McCarthy-Jones, S. & Hayward, M. (2014). Hear today, not gone tomorrow? An exploratory longitudinal study of auditory verbal hallucinations ('hearing voices'). *Behavioural & Cognitive Psychotherapy, 42*, 117–123.

Hayward, M. (2003). Interpersonal relating and voice hearing: To what extent does relating to the voice reflect social relating? *Psychology and Psychotherapy: Theory, research and practice, 76*, 369–383.

Hayward, M., Bogen-Johnston, L. & Deamer, F. (2018). Relating therapy for distressing voices: Who, or what, is changing? *Psychosis, 10*, 132–141.

Hayward, M., Jones, A-M., Bogen-Johnston, L., Thomas, N. & Strauss, C. (2017). Relating therapy for distressing auditory hallucinations: A pilot randomized controlled trial. *Schizophrenia Research, 183*, 137–142.

Jackson, L., Hayward, M. & Cooke, A. (2011). Developing positive relationships with voices: A preliminary grounded theory. *International Journal of Social Psychiatry, 57*, 487–495.

McCarthy-Jones, S., Trauer, T., Mackinnon, A., Sims, E., Thomas, N. & Copolov, D.L. (2014). A new phenomenological survey of auditory hallucinations: Evidence for subtypes and implications for theory and practice. *Schizophrenia Bulletin, 40*, 231–235.

26 Meaning-making in voice hearing
Nicola Barclay, Guy Dodgson and Anna Luce

We are all clinical psychologists working in Early Intervention in Psychosis (EIP) services in the UK. In this chapter, we will provide an overview of some of the information ('psychoeducation') we share and conversations we have with clients/those experiencing troubling voice hearing. Our aim in our therapeutic work is to develop a stance of joint curiosity and shared understanding where previously there has been loneliness, fear and doubt – or terrifying certainty. Since human brains, internal worlds and experiences are so complex and can be understood in many different ways, we are not seeking one single 'truth'. However, we do feel that most experiences can be understood and made sense of, and that different disciplines (arts and sciences) and perspectives can helpfully contribute.

We start from a position that human experiences (including psychotic-like experiences) occur on continuums (Baumeister et al., 2017). It tends to be when we are 'stuck' or pushed to extremes that difficulties arise, and possibly we might 'meet the criteria' for certain medical diagnoses. Thus, under a particular set of circumstances (for example, severe sleep deprivation or isolation), any one of us might experience voice hearing (Anderson et al., 2021) – or what may sometimes be diagnosed as psychosis. Thus, these experiences fall within the realm of 'normal' human experience, although occurring relatively infrequently. We are interested in generating some curiosity and doubt about, or less frightening or threatening alternative explanations for, these phenomena, and we draw on a range of theoretical models and research evidence to find a tentative explanation that 'fits' well enough to be helpful to the person so they can get on with their life. The ideas presented here are just that – ideas that can be explored and discussed and don't have to be imposed or accepted. We invite those we work with, and readers, to be curious about how the human mind works and the influence that life experiences, emotions and our current situations have on how we perceive and interpret the world and construct 'reality'.

Curiosity about mental distress

We often use an adapted stress-vulnerability model (Zubin & Spring, 1977), or 'stress bucket'[1] (Brabban & Turkington, 2002), as a starting point for developing understanding about how a person may have begun to experience difficulties with their mental health, including voice hearing and/or psychosis. This model proposes that, given sufficient life stress or difficulties, all humans begin to experience distress or mental (and physical) health difficulties. It acknowledges that each person has unique biology, physical and mental abilities, life experiences, family and support systems, and opportunities and skills that influence their capacity to manage stress ('vulnerability'/size of the 'bucket' and 'coping' abilities). In our experience, 'unhelpful' coping strategies frequently include avoiding or trying to ignore or deny; use of illicit substances or alcohol; withdrawing from others or lashing out; sustained hypervigilance; excessive worrying or engaging in self-blame or self-criticism. Developing a range of heathier ways of coping with stress and distress is a key task for our clients, as it is for all human beings throughout our lives.

This model is thus normalising, non-stigmatising, and helps generate hope – for, if we can identify and reduce the stresses, improve our coping skills/support networks and increase our resilience, we can reduce the likelihood that a person will become overwhelmed again in future. This way of understanding how things may have become difficult for someone is often met by the individual with relief and brings increased self-compassion and a curiosity about what may be helpful in the future.

> *Learning point 1*
>
> You can use the stress-vulnerability model/bucket to think about your own experiences of becoming overwhelmed, distressed, and/or first beginning to hear voices.
>
> - What 'stressors' (water in the bucket) are you able to identify happening in your life beforehand? (Remember, even positive experiences such as holidays or moving in with someone make demands on our energy so can be 'stressors', and loneliness and boredom are also highly stressful for humans.)
> - What did you do to try to cope with these demands, and what was most effective?
> - Looking back, do you think that some of your coping strategies might have inadvertently increased your stress levels over time?

---

1. www.youtube.com/watch?v=ld5JypUYT-o

Curiosity about hallucinatory experiences

We use the term 'hallucinations' to describe the phenomenon when our senses are activated (we see, hear, feel, taste or smell something) without there being an obvious external cause. In fact, hallucinatory experiences can be hugely varied (from low murmuring to screaming; sporadic words to an ongoing narrative; feelings of being touched or bugs crawling under the skin; seeing faces, shapes or animals; smelling rotting flesh, and so forth), can change over time, and can be multi-sensory (Lim et al., 2016). Here, we focus on voice hearing; however, we propose that similar processes may be involved with other sensory experiences. Essentially, it is about the brain misinterpreting or misidentifying internal experiences as coming from outside ourselves, or over-estimating/misidentifying threat.

Voice hearing is something human brains do!

Below are some key ideas that we find helpful to discuss with people who are troubled by their voices.

- Hearing voices is something that human minds seem to do relatively easily – and have done throughout history – but which have been understood in different ways at different times (Corstens et al., 2012; Fernyhough, 2017; Perry, 2012; Durham University's Hearing the Voice research programme[2]).
- As with all human experience, we view voice hearing as on a continuum, with most of us having at least some (mild) sense of these experiences: for example, thinking we can hear the phone vibrate or someone calling our name, or sensing that others might be talking about us.
- Some studies estimate that up to 25% of people experience voice hearing at some point in their lives (van Os et al., 2001), but most don't ever have contact with mental health services or receive a medical diagnosis.
- Voice hearing experiences can be very varied (loud/quiet, young/old, 'posh'/with an accent, recognised/unknown, long or short sentences or single words). They can be experienced as occurring inside or outside the head, near or far, from any direction (Nayani & David, 1996), and they differ between cultures (Luhrmann et al., 2015).
- Certain experiences and bodily states are associated with an increased likelihood of hearing voices, including sleep deprivation, bereavement, dissociation and taking certain drugs.[3] In particular, there is a clear, stepwise relationship between early adversity and interpersonal trauma and voice hearing and psychosis (bullying, abuse, neglect, discrimination, separation, loss) (Shevlin et al., 2007), although voice hearing may also occur when no trauma history is reported (Luhrmann et al., 2019).

---

2. www.dur.ac.uk/hearingthevoice/
3. In McCarthy-Jones' excellent book (2017), the chapter 'Breast pumps from hell' highlights this issue well.

- The environment and wider social context in which we live also increases or decreases our likelihood of hearing voices or being diagnosed with psychosis. For example, living in urban environments (van Os et al., 2001), or being in a minoritised ethnic group (Boydell et al., 2001), as well as high levels of societal inequality, are all associated with increased risk (Johnson et al., 2015).
- Increased likelihood of voice hearing can 'run in families', although the degree to which it is a genetic heritability is contested, and likely relatively low compared with other shared (e.g., environmental, social, parenting, dietary and so forth) factors (Read et al., 2013).
- Voice hearing has often been linked to creativity: for example, many writers have described hearing voices, including Charles Dickens, Virginia Woolf, David Mitchell and Hilary Mantel.
- It is thought that often our physical, cognitive and emotional responses to, or attempts to cope with, voice-hearing experiences inadvertently keep them going (e.g. feeling highly anxious and not sleeping, withdrawing from others, listening out for more voices, dissociating, using alcohol or drugs) (Garety et al., 2001).
- Hallucinatory experiences, including voice hearing, can occur with many health conditions (infection and delirium) and mental health difficulties (including psychosis, bereavement, depression, 'personality disorders', childhood trauma, dementia and so forth), and – most often – *with no mental health problem at all* (Vilhauer & Sharma, 2018).
- It is when these experiences/voices are very frightening or upsetting and feel uncontrollable or overwhelming that people tend to struggle and seek help.
- Thus, it seems that it is *the relationship* we have to our voice-hearing experiences, or the interpretation of what the experience means, that influences how distressed we feel and how we respond (Chadwick & Birchwood, 1994; Morrison, 2001).

Human beings are essentially 'meaning-makers': we search for meaning in the experiences we have on a daily basis. When something out of the ordinary occurs, our brain tries to make sense of it as best it can. This might be by seeing how it fits with experiences we have already had and what we have learned from the world around us, or using our capacity to imagine possibilities to see if we can make sense of it. Hearing a voice for the first time is often outside of our ordinary experiences, and our brain does its best to help us to understand what is happening. Sometimes, this can leave us with a very frightening explanation and struggling to generate any other possible ways of understanding what is happening for us. People can get stuck in unhelpful, self-reinforcing patterns of thinking or feeling (usually high distress, strong 'negative' emotions and withdrawal from others). EIP services aim to reduce fears, unstick this process, and help the voice hearer find more helpful ways of coping with distress and difficulties.

Applying Clarke's (1986) cognitive model for panic disorder can be helpful here. This suggests that it is the 'catastrophic misinterpretation' of an internal sensation that is the driver of the severe anxiety or panic attack that follows, rather than the sensation itself. For example, a person may experience heart palpitations and make a 'catastrophic misinterpretation' that this sensation is the sign of a heart attack (the life-threatening catastrophe), which then sends their threat-response system into overdrive and sets up a vicious cycle driven by fear. When we apply this same understanding to voice hearing, we can begin to make sense of what it is about the experience of voices that is so distressing for that individual, such as: 'I'm going mad'; 'If the voices are saying I should hurt someone, that must mean I really want to hurt other people'; 'I have to hurt myself'; 'I have to agree or go along with what they say or something bad will happen'. We then try to help people challenge or find alternatives to the catastrophic interpretation, such as: 'Voice hearing is a common human experience'; 'I must be really stressed out'; 'I don't like these voices, but they can't hurt me or control me, and they don't mean I'm going mad... I can cope'.

> ### Case study (anonymised)
>
> James first heard a voice when he was alone at home, trying to get to sleep. The voice told him that he was useless. James was very frightened, as this was a new experience for him and he didn't know what it meant. From his understanding of voice hearing (from family and the media), he thought it meant that he was 'going crazy'. The idea of going crazy (a 'catastrophic misinterpretation') was very frightening for him, his difficulties with sleeping got worse and he began to look out anxiously for other signs that he was going crazy (hypervigilance). He felt unable to talk to his friends about what was happening, and cut himself off socially, spending his time alone in his room.

We try to help people to improve their relationship to their voice-hearing experiences through inviting curiosity, having conversations about the experiences and offering psychoeducation (like the ideas above) to develop non-'catastrophic' interpretations/explanations for these experiences. For James, the experience of hearing voices both acted as a stressor ('I am going crazy') and reduced effective coping (unhelpful coping strategies included increased withdrawal, isolation and hypervigilance), creating a vicious cycle that made further voice-hearing experiences more likely (and even more frightening).

> ### Learning point 2
>
> If you can remember, think back to your own first voice-hearing experience. If you do not experience voices, think about how you might respond.
>
> - What was your first idea/explanation about what was happening, if you had one?
> - What were your emotional responses?

- How do you think commonly held views and media stories about mental health problems and hearing voices in particular might have influenced your own response?

Curiosity about our complex and contrary brains

In our discussions with clients, we find it helpful to begin by sharing some ideas about the human brain and its threat system and responses. We discuss how our threat system is an ancient, unsophisticated, but highly effective part of the brain, originally developed to respond to immediate, physical threat. It is always running in the background, and when it detects threat, it can take over the functioning of the brain and body in quite an alarming way (remember what we said about panic attacks). It prepares us to respond with 'fight or flight'; our heart and breathing rates increase (getting oxygen to the organs), and the body is flushed with chemical changes to enable it to react fast. There are changes in our senses: for example, our hearing and vision become sharper and more focused. Importantly, changes in thinking also occur: the brain takes short-cuts to respond quickly and efficiently to threat, but at the cost of accuracy. Thus, anxious brains are more likely to make mistakes and over-estimate the degree of threat ('Better safe than sorry'). Brains 'jump to conclusions', with little evidence, and are 'primed' to only take on board evidence that confirms what is feared, so anything that looks/sounds even slightly like a threat is processed as one. This gets worse when there is more background noise (in crowded, busy places, shops and so on). Anxious brains are also less able to consider alternatives, or to take the time to do a reality check. Despite human evolution and our large 'thinking' brain, these basic fear responses still operate automatically, outside of our conscious control, and can hijack our thinking brain and our body.

Some of the difficulties we experience as modern humans are because we only have this one threat system to respond with. When anxiety is related to social threat (that is, being judged negatively by others), academic performance or financial threats (money worries), the body reacts as if this is an immediate life-threatening situation. However, the 'fight or flight' preparation in the body and short-cuts in thinking are often very unhelpful for solving these types of problems. Growing up or living in violent or unpredictable situations can mean that our threat systems need to stay on 'red alert' to survive, and it can be difficult to switch this off, even when we have left this situation. Last, our own thoughts can activate our threat system. For example, a worry about my work performance, a memory of my painful break-up, my concern about how I fit into my social group or my worry about what the types of thoughts or feelings I am having might mean about me can all activate my threat system.

The brain has a third – normal, healthy and automatic – response to threat and trauma, which kicks in when 'fight or flight' are not an option. This is known as 'freeze or flop' (or 'playing dead' in animals), when we feel too overwhelmed and powerless to do anything at all except submit, and we may also dissociate. Dissociation enables the mind to cut off from horrific or overwhelming experiences while they are happening, and also to hide from/block related memories, feelings or body sensations experienced during such events. It is like a power switch that turns off all or parts of the event, but it can also mean that the event (and associated feelings) becomes detached from other memories and information to which it would usually be joined (that is, it doesn't get fully assimilated into our memory of past events). Freeze and dissociative responses often develop in childhood (since children are small, powerless and have little control), or during prolonged traumatic experiences such as physical or sexual assault.

Once our brains have learned to respond to threat in this way (and it seems to have kept us safe), our threat systems are more likely to respond in the same way when detecting threat again (even social threat). Common dissociative experiences include derealisation (which includes feeling as though the world around us is unreal; seeing objects changing in shape, size or colour; feeling as if other people are robots, even though rationally we know they are not) and depersonalisation (feeling as though we are watching ourselves in a film or looking at ourselves from the outside; feeling as if we are just observing our emotions; feeling disconnected from parts of our bodies or emotions; feeling as if we are floating away; feeling unsure of the boundaries between ourselves and other people). If we don't understand what is happening, these types of experiences can be very frightening.

Thinking about our thinking

In EIP, we have noticed that many people appear to be frightened by their own thoughts, possibly because they believe that thoughts should be ordered and controlled or that they represent something fundamental about ourselves. This is not our understanding. We use ideas from mindfulness, noticing how thoughts come and go and acknowledging our wandering 'monkey minds'. We are particularly interested in the concept of *intrusive thoughts* – thoughts that pop into our heads that we don't want, haven't planned for or don't expect. In fact, it's quite common for people to have thoughts that go against their real beliefs and attitudes, or that feel very strange to them. Having 'horrible' or 'weird' thoughts is a normal part of life and doesn't say anything bad about us: thoughts are just thoughts, they're not actions or wishes. It actually makes sense that our brains actively imagine the worst-case scenario, or generate ideas or images that we would usually find very upsetting. It's part of the brain's attempts to keep us safe by being prepared for the worst.

Purdon & Clark (1992) asked healthy young people about the types of intrusive thoughts they had. Forty-nine percent of men (and 31% of women) admitted to thinking about breaking wind in public; around half (54% men, 46% women) said they had intrusive thoughts of hitting an animal or a person with a car; 16% and 19% (male, female) suddenly thought about cutting off a finger, and 44% of men and 37% of women inadvertently thought about kissing an authority figure. We hope this shows how common some weird, wonderful (violent or sexual) thoughts are among healthy adults – and of course these are the ones they felt comfortable admitting to. Last, think about any horror writer – they make money out of imagining the most unpleasant things, but (to our knowledge) none of them act out these ideas.

We use an analogy of our brains being like a 'pan of soup' in which all our memories, TV programmes we've seen, dreams, facts we've learned, thoughts and ideas, conversations and so forth are mixed up and floating about. It makes sense that, if we have witnessed abuse and violence, our 'pan' will have more violent and abusive ideas/images/sounds floating around in it. Most of these generally don't stay in our conscious mind unless we try to think about them or something triggers a memory. The surface of the soup is what we are actively thinking about at any one time. Some thoughts, generally those that make us feel anxious, angry, sad or other strong emotions, tend to pop up to the surface and into our minds unbidden, even when we don't want to think about them. Because they have an emotional impact ('heat'), the brain 'decides' they must be important and repeatedly brings them back into our consciousness. In addition, because these thoughts (and associated emotions) are unpleasant to us, we often actively try to push them out of our minds (this is called 'thought suppression'). Unfortunately, trying really hard not to think about something just makes that thought pop up more often and more strongly (try the 'pink elephant' experiment[4]).

Our emotional state also influences the type of thoughts we have, so when we feel very angry or upset, we can have quite extreme thoughts (e.g. 'I want to kill so and so'; 'I should just hurt myself'). Similarly, when we feel suspicious or under threat from others, our thoughts can represent this (e.g. 'What the f**k are they looking at?'). So, it is a part of life to have weird, violent, unpleasant thoughts – what is important is how we relate to them and make sense of them, as this can increase or decrease the emotional 'heat' (making them more or less likely to recur). For example, 'mindfulness' practice promotes a different way to relate to our internal worlds: gently noticing thoughts in a non-judgemental manner (so reducing strong emotional reactions to them), and then disengaging from them/ letting them go/pass by. Becoming mentally absorbed in something different can also help (called 'distraction').

> *Learning point 3*
>
> Reflecting on these ideas about brains, threat systems, and thoughts above:
>
> - Do these ideas help you make sense of some of your own experiences? What might they be?
> - Can you think of times when your own thoughts might be activating your threat system?

---

4. https://psych-n-life.blogspot.com/2008/10/dont-think-about-pink-elephant.html

- Have you noticed any connection between voice hearing and feeling threatened (physically, socially, or emotionally – including through self-attack/criticism)?
- If you have tended to try to suppress or avoid difficult thoughts or you notice that you judge yourself harshly for having certain types of thoughts, might you try some 'mindfulness' exercises or use distraction?
- If you have tended to try to suppress difficult thoughts or judge yourself harshly for having certain types of thoughts, might you try 'mindfulness of thoughts' or using distraction?

Different 'types' of voice hearing

Researchers and psychologists have been exploring voice hearing a lot more in recent years and wondering if there are meaningfully different 'types' (for example, whether they are experienced as occurring inside or outside the head, which has now been discredited (Copolov et al., 2004)). Our current understanding, which voice hearers seem to find helpful and is supported by the scientific evidence to date, is that there may be three main types of voice hearing: hypervigilance-based voice hearing, 'inner speech' voice hearing and memory-based voices. People can experience any of these at different times. We find the distinctions helpful, as they appear to cover the range of human experiences that brains produce, help us and our clients make sense of what may be going on, and offer ideas about what to attempt first to try to make these experiences less frightening or overwhelming. These distinctions may also help us understand how voices develop over time, as some subtypes may be a stage in the development of 'inner speech' voices (type 2 below).

1. Hypervigilance-based voice hearing

One common 'type' of voice-hearing experience appears to be linked with our threat system, as it occurs particularly when we are very anxious, feel under imminent threat and are actively scanning our environment. We call these 'hypervigilance hallucinations' (Dodgson & Gordon, 2009). These occur when people are feeling highly anxious (including socially anxious or self-conscious) and tend to be brief utterances or noises (for example, hearing your name being called, derogatory words, banging sounds). They generally occur in environments with a lot of background noise or poor sound quality (for example, busy shopping centres or flats where you can hear your neighbours through the wall). How we make sense of the world depends on the sensory data that we receive, but it is also strongly influenced by our expectations of how the world is.

As mentioned earlier, the human perceptual system frequently makes mistakes, misses information and mishears and misinterprets: for example, think about visual illusions, or times when you mishear song lyrics. Our perceptual system is even more likely to make mistakes when we are anxious or afraid, as this is part of our evolved threat detection and survival mechanism. The more background noise there is or the poorer the quality of sound (for example, a crowded pub, mumbling from people in the next room, noisy electrical equipment), the more mistakes and 'false alarms' our perceptual systems make. When we are anxious, we become 'hypervigilant' and our attention system actively scans background noise or listens out for possible threats, which often concern (or confirm) our own fears or insecurities (for example, that others think we are ugly, boring, stupid or fat). The 'better safe than sorry' setting means that anything that appears at all similar to threat is assumed to be an actual threat, therefore increasing the number of mistakes (false alarms). These seem to confirm our fears, and a vicious cycle is established ('People definitely are talking about me'). When we have been anxious for long periods of time, it can be difficult to 'step down' from this. It's like a soldier coming back from active service in a war zone and jumping at sudden noises from the street; these anxious ways of thinking, repetitive worrying and being hypervigilant become 'cognitive habits' that can be difficult to drop.

2. 'Inner speech' voice hearing

A second 'type' of voice hearing (estimated to explain around 80% of voice-hearing experiences (Jones & Fernyhough, 2007; McCarthy-Jones, 2017) is thought to occur when we mistake an internal process (our own thoughts, or 'inner speech') as coming from outside (as audible 'voices'). Although some experiments have shown that the same part of the brain is activated when people are experiencing hearing voices and when inner speech occurs (Allen et al., 2007), there are other studies that do not confirm this hypothesis.

If this hypothesis does indeed turn out to be correct in the future, then we think there are four reasons that currently make sense to us as to why people may start to not recognise their own thoughts as thoughts and begin to hear them as voices. The first is that voice hearing often begins (and tends to get worse) when people are in an extremely emotional state, or under strain, which may alter brain and thinking processes. You may notice that voice hearing gets worse when you are feeling stressed, angry or emotionally agitated/excited, and is not present (or is less present) when you are relaxed and calm or focused on something.

A second reason is that voice hearing is often *intrusive* (which we discussed earlier): thoughts/ideas that we don't want, plan or expect seem to pop into our heads. Related to this is reason number three: that the content of the thoughts (voices) is unacceptable, frightening or disgusting to the person in some way. However, as we have seen, people often have thoughts that go against their real beliefs and attitudes, or that feel very strange to them. Unfortunately, the more frightening or upsetting thoughts are, the more easily and often they can pop into our minds – and the less 'coming from within us' they feel to be.

The fourth reason people might not recognise their voices as their own thoughts is that voices often do not sound like their own (inner) voice. However, brains are able to 'play' different sounds/voices to themselves in a part of the brain called the 'phonological loop'. When you recall some dialogue from a favourite film or a catchphrase from a cartoon character or have a song stuck in your head, you 'hear' this in the original performer's voice, not usually as your own voice. Importantly, the 'phonological loop' doesn't only play back what you have heard, it can also create new sounds or speech. Many of us finish arguments in our heads, playing both sides and always making sure we win. Also remember Beethoven, who must have used this part of the brain to compose whole symphonies when he lost his hearing.

One theory about inner speech voices (and many other visual and sensory hallucinations) is that they happen to people who have a 'source-monitoring problem', which means they are more likely to be confused about whether an experience comes from within their own mind/body or from the outside environment (see Griffin & Fletcher, 2017). It may be that a person makes a mistake about where the 'source' of a voice is coming from (e.g. outside of themselves, rather than their own mind). This may be a controversial idea, though, as it seems to imply that some people have some kind of deficit in their source monitoring that leads to them hearing voices.

3. Memory-based voices

As mentioned earlier, and as Romme and Escher (e.g. 1989) highlighted, many voice-hearing experiences appear to be linked with traumatic past experiences, particularly being bullied or abused. A third 'type' of voice-hearing experience, called 'memory-based' voices, has therefore been proposed (Jones, 2010). For some people, the links between voices with past experience are obvious, while for others the connection is less clear. There may be several reasons why people don't recognise a voice as being related to past experiences or memory. First, as in post-traumatic stress disorder (PTSD), the memory or voice may intrude into our awareness without any context. Often traumatic memories don't have a 'time stamp', so it can be hard for us to recognise where the experience is coming from. Second, the voice may say different things to the person you are remembering or may not sound like them. This is because memory is tricky and imprecise; it is not an accurate, unbiased 'recording' of what happened, but our interpretation or impression of what happened (Williams et al., 2008). Third, when we are overwhelmed or feeling cut-off/dissociated, it can be difficult for our thinking brain to make sense of what is going on or recognise where something is coming from. Last of all, many of our memories are laid down in very early life (before we have speech or language), while we are extremely anxious or dissociated, or involve physical sensations/impressions, and can therefore feel unrecognisable or separate to us when we are older (Eacott, 1999).

Clients find they are most likely to experience these types of voices when they are either feeling 'too much'/hyper-arousal (distressed, fight/flight), or 'too little'/hypo-arousal (feeling cut off, numb or distanced, dissociative); both are survival responses we spoke about earlier.

The evidence for the relationships between trauma, dissociation and voice hearing is now overwhelming (Pilton et al., 2015; Varese et al., 2012), and promising interventions are being developed and trialled. For example, Varese and colleagues (2020) have results from a study showing that, if dissociation is reduced by using grounding strategies within a CBT approach, the frequency and intensity of voice hearing is reduced. Trauma-focused work (as for PTSD) has also been shown to make sense of these intrusions into experience and can be used to process difficult memories so that they do not keep intruding, and also to recalibrate our over-sensitive threat system.

> *Learning point 4*
>
> Reflecting on the hypotheses of these proposed three 'types' (or processes) leading to voice hearing:
>
> - Do you think any of your voice-hearing experiences map onto any of these subtypes?
> - Do the voices represent your own worst fears or negative beliefs about yourself? Do they remind you of what others have said to or about you? Do they express something that is difficult for you to express in other ways or that is difficult for you to make sense of?
> - Have they changed over time?

Managing voice hearing

While traditionally clinicians may have focused on eliminating voice-hearing experiences (especially for those diagnosed with psychosis), our position is that voice hearing itself is not always problematic. Voices cause difficulties when our relationship to them, or our interpretation of these experiences, causes us high levels of emotional distress (fear, shame, anger), and/or they prevent us living a rewarding life. Our main aim is therefore to take the 'heat' out of the experience of hearing a voice by providing non-threatening, non-blaming and normalising explanations for how we – as humans – may come to have such experiences, thus challenging any 'catastrophic interpretations', and to try to increase the person's sense of control. This involves psychoeducation about the links between traumatic and stressful life events and mental health difficulties and how our brains and threat systems work (and sometimes don't work so well in modern life), and introducing the proposed different 'types' of voice hearing where this feels helpful. Working with our clients, we aim to create an understanding that they find helpful and feel is a fair 'fit' with their experiences. A second and equally important focus for intervention is to improve clients' relationship with themselves and their (inner) experiences, towards a more compassionate, accepting and generally kinder self-stance. Paul Gilbert's compassionate-mind ideas and practices,[5] and 'compassion for voices' work,[6] alongside improving self-care and re-connecting with hobbies and interests, friends and family, may be particularly helpful.

---

5. https://compassionatemind.co.uk/
6. www.youtube.com/watch?v=VRqI4lxuXAw

There are many methods and techniques a person can use to help them live with and manage their voices. They include:

- psychoeducation about how brains work, the impact of trauma, and how frequent voice hearing is, so that the experiences of voices are less scary
- using distraction to break the vicious cycle of thought suppression and hypervigilance by gently moving the attention towards other stimuli (enjoyable or absorbing activities)
- reducing avoidance and isolation by re-engaging with activities and social life/community
- understanding dissociation and managing this with 'grounding' techniques
- using emotional regulation skills and/or compassionate mindfulness
- talking therapies (such as those introduced in this book, but also CBT, family/systemic therapy, and trauma-focused therapy may be good to consider)
- considering medication
- attending to your self-care needs – adopting healthier sleep patterns, eating regularly and healthily, taking exercise and so forth
- connecting with other voice hearers and voice-hearing perspectives.[7]

Generally with managing voice hearing or other unusual sensory experiences, the less fear or anxiety we have around these experiences and the calmer and better rested we are, the less we will experience them. Finding healthy ways to manage stress, low mood or difficult emotions (such as anger, fear or shame) is vitally important, and involves trying out a variety of things at different times. Some ideas include going out for a walk or taking up an absorbing hobby; dancing or listening to music; talking with friends, family or a therapist; doing calming breathing exercises, relaxation or mindfulness practices; writing our feelings down, or talking kindly to ourselves. A significant part of overcoming difficult feelings is related to ensuring that we are being kind to our mind and body, which includes building in time for exercise and relaxation, taking care of our physical health (having enough sleep and eating healthily), and making sure we have plenty of social contact and are involved in enjoyable, fun and meaningful activities.

We can try to change our relationship to voices – learn to calmly notice them, then move our attention elsewhere, rather than pushing them away, going along with them, or getting emotionally involved with them. Thoughts (voices) can't hurt us, don't represent reality, come and go, and have no power over us – we don't have to believe them or go along with them. Many people feel that voices have something important to tell us about our past or about our internal worlds. Their import lies not necessarily in what they say (as their words often reflect our own worst fears or bullying experiences), but what they tell us about our unexpressed

---

7. www.hearing-voices.org/

emotions, traumatic experiences or attempts to keep ourselves safe (see, for example, the work of your local, regional or national Hearing Voices Network, or Eleanor Longden's TED talk, *The Voices in My Head*[8]).

If we are doing something we enjoy or that takes a lot of attention, we are less likely to hear the voices. This is called *distraction* and may include, for example, listening to music, having a conversation, or doing an absorbing puzzle when the voices become intrusive. Other ideas might include going out and doing something active or sociable, reading a book, watching a TV programme/film, playing a game and so forth. The more mentally absorbing an activity is, the better the distraction. Some people find that reading to themselves, 'hearing' music in their heads, listening to music through headphones or humming out loud can reduce voice hearing when it is happening (this blocks the 'phonological loop'). Sitting alone in a room when you are feeling low or anxious is generally the least helpful thing to be doing (although it might be the thing our mind and body urge us to do) – so try not to give in to the urge to withdraw. Instead, stay connected with others or do something distracting, pleasurable or self-soothing with your time.

> *Learning point 5*
>
> Reflecting on your own experiences of living with, coping with, or managing voice-hearing experiences:
>
> - What ways of coping have you found that help you to live well with your voices?
> - Are there things you have tried that were unhelpful?
> - What is your current relationship with your voices, and has this changed over time?
> - Have you found learning from and/or talking to other voice hearers helpful? In what ways?

Conclusion

There are a variety of ways of understanding and managing voice hearing (as the other chapters in this book explain). We have shared here some possible explanations that some of our clients have found helpful. These ideas are not uniquely ours or copyrighted – we have drawn on ideas from a huge number of sources, researchers, clinicians, clients and co-workers and our understanding will continue to develop as new evidence emerges, clients teach us more and our thinking evolves.

As we wrote at the start of this chapter, we offer these as alternative explanations, not as 'truths'. It is our hope that they will help voice hearers develop less frightening interpretations or more positive and meaningful relationships with their voices, in

---

8. www.youtube.com/watch?v=syjEN3peCJw

whatever forms these may take. We have found that reducing the emotional 'heat' in relation to voice hearing and developing new ways of relating to the voices can often reduce the frequency or intensity of distressing voices. Some clients are very clear that they want the voices to go away; others can live well with their voices, and we respect both these positions. It is our sincere hope that our clients can get on with living their lives, with or without hearing voices.

References

Allen, P., Aleman, A. & McGuire, P.K. (2007). Inner speech models of auditory verbal hallucinations: Evidence from behavioural and neuroimaging studies. *International Review of Psychiatry, 19*(4): 407–415.

Anderson, A., Hartley, S. & Bucci, S. (2021). A systematic review of the experimental induction of auditory perceptual experiences. *Journal of Behavior Therapy and Experimental Psychiatry , 71*, 101635. doi: 10.1016/j.jbtep.2020.101635

Baumeister, D., Sedgwick, O., Howes, O. & Pet, E. (2017). Auditory verbal hallucinations and continuum models of psychosis: A systematic review of the healthy voice-hearer literature. *Clinical Psychology Review, 51*, 125–141.

Boydell, J., van Os, J., McKenzie, K., Allardyce, J., Goel, R., McCreadie, R.G. & Murray, R.M. (2001). Incidence of schizophrenia in ethnic minorities in London: Ecological study into interactions with environment. *British Medical Journal, 323*, 1–4.

Brabban, A. & Turkington, D. (2002). The search for meaning: Detecting congruence between life events, underlying schema and psychotic symptoms. In A.P. Morrison (Ed.). *A casebook of cognitive therapy for psychosis* (pp.59–75). Brunner-Routledge.

Chadwick, P. & Birchwood, M. (1994). The omnipotence of voices: A cognitive approach to auditory hallucinations. *British Journal of Psychiatry, 164*(2), 190–201.

Clarke, D.M. (1986). A cognitive approach to panic. *Behaviour Research and Therapy, 24*(4), 461–470.

Copolov, D., Trauer, T. & Mackinnon, A. (2004). On the non-significance of internal versus external auditory hallucinations. *Schizophrenia Research, 69*(1), 1–6.

Corstens, D., Longden, E. & May, R. (2012). Talking with voices. *Psychosis: Psychological, social and integrative approaches, 4*(2), 95–104.

Dodgson, G. & Gordon, S. (2009). Avoiding false negatives: Are some auditory hallucinations an evolved design flaw? *Behavioural and Cognitive Psychotherapy, 37*(3), 325–335.

Eacott, M.J. (1999). Memory for the events of early childhood. *Current Directions in Psychological Science, 8*(2), 46–49.

Fernyhough, C. (2017). *The voices within: The history and science of how we talk to ourselves.* Profile Books.

Garety, P.A., Kuipers, E., Fowler, D., Freeman, D. & Bebbington, P.E. (2001). A cognitive model of the positive symptoms of psychosis. *Psychological Medicine, 31*, 189–195.

Griffin, J.D. & Fletcher, P.C. (2017). Predictive processing, source monitoring, and psychosis. *Annual Review of Clinical Psychology, 13*, 265–289.

Johnson, S.L., Wibbels, E. & Wilkinson, R. (2015). Economic inequality is related to cross-national prevalence of psychotic symptoms. *Social Psychiatry and Psychiatric Epidemiology, 50*, 1799–1807.

Jones, S.R. (2010). Do we need multiple models of auditory verbal hallucinations? Examining the phenomenological fit of cognitive and neurological models. *Schizophrenia Bulletin, 36*(3), 566–575.

Jones, S.R. & Fernyhough, C. (2007). Neural correlates of inner speech and auditory verbal hallucinations: A critical review and theoretical integration. *Clinical Psychology Review, 27*(2), 140–154.

Lim, A., Hoek, H.W., Deen, M.L., Blom, J.D. & GROUP Investigators (2016). Prevalence and classification of hallucinations in multiple sensory modalities in schizophrenia spectrum disorders. *Schizophrenia Research, 176*(2–3), 493–499.

Luhrmann, T.M., Alderson-Day, B., Bell, V., Bless, J.J., Corlett, P., Hugdahl, K., Jones, N., Larøi, F., Moseley, P., Padmavati, R., Peters, E., Powers, A.R. & Waters, F. (2019). Beyond trauma: A multiple pathways approach to auditory hallucinations in clinical and nonclinical populations. *Schizophrenia Bulletin, 45*(1), s24–s31.

Luhrmann, T.M., Padmavati, R., Tharoor, H. & Osei, A. (2015). Differences in voice-hearing experiences of people with psychosis in the U.S.A., India and Ghana: Interview-based study. *British Journal of Psychiatry, 206*(1), 41–44.

McCarthy-Jones, S. (2017). *Can't you hear them? The science and significance of hearing voices.* Jessica Kingsley.

Morrison, A.P. (2001). The interpretation of intrusions in psychosis: An integrative cognitive approach to hallucinations and delusions. *Behavioural and Cognitive Psychotherapy, 29*(3), 257–276.

Nayani, T.H. & David, A.S. (1996).The auditory hallucination: A phenomenological survey. *Psychological Medicine, 26*(1), 177–189

Perry, A. (2012). CAT with people who hear distressing voices. *Reformulation, 38*, 16–22.

Pilton, M., Varese, F., Berry, K. & Bucci, S. (2015). The relationship between dissociation and voices: A systematic literature review and meta-analyses. *Clinical Psychology Review, 40*, 138–155.

Purdon, C. & Clark, D. (1992). Obsessive intrusive thoughts in nonclinical subjects. Part 1: Content and relation with depressive, anxious and obsessional symptoms. *Behaviour Research and Therapy, 31*(8), 713–720.

Read. J., Bentall, R., Mosher, L. & Dillon, J. (2013). *Models of madness: Psychological, social and biological approaches to psychosis.* Routledge.

Romme, M.A.J. & Escher, A.D.M.A.C. (1989). Hearing voices. *Schizophrenia Bulletin, 15(2)*, 209–216.

Shevlin, M.D., Dorahy, M. & Adamson, G. (2007). Childhood traumas and hallucinations: An analysis of the National Comorbidity Survey. *Journal of Psychiatric Research, 41*(3–4), 222–228.

van Os, J., Hanssen, M., Bilj, R.V. & Vollebergh, W. (2001). Prevalence of psychotic disorder and community level of psychotic symptoms: An urban-rural comparison. *Archives of General Psychiatry, 58*(7), 663–668.

Varese, F., Barkus, E. & Bentall, R.P. (2012). Dissociation mediates the relationship between childhood trauma and hallucination-proneness. *Psychological Medicine, 42*(5), 1025–1036.

Varese. F., Douglas, M., Dudley, R., Bowe, S., Christodoulides, T., Common, S., Grace, T., Lumley, V., McCartney, L., Pace, S., Reeves, T., Morrison, A.T. & Turkington, D. (2020). Targeting dissociation using cognitive behavioural therapy in voice hearers with psychosis and a history of interpersonal trauma: A case series. *Psychology and Psychotherapy: Theory, research and practice, 10*: e12304. doi: 10.1111/papt.12304.

Vilhauer, R.P. & Sharma, H. (2018). Unsolicited reports of voice hearing in the general population: A study using a novel method. *Psychosis: Psychological, social and integrative approaches, 10*(3), 163–174.

Williams, H.L., Conway, M.A. & Cohen, G. (2008). *Autobiographical memory.* In G. Cohen & M.A. Conway (Eds.), *Memory in the real world* (pp.21–90). Psychology Press.

Zubin, J. & Spring, B. (1977). Vulnerability: A new view on schizophrenia. *Journal of Abnormal Psychology, 86*(2), 103–126.

27 Responding to trauma dialogically: an introduction to peer-supported Open Dialogue

Mark Hopfenbeck

Definitions of trauma vary but, very broadly, trauma refers to the existential wounds we experience when our integrity is threatened and our mental, social, emotional or spiritual wellbeing is harmed. These wounds can be fairly mild and heal quickly. They can also be the result of a single extremely painful assault on our being, or the cumulative and complex distress resulting from recurring adverse events, both of which can take a lifetime to heal, especially if sufficient support is not available in dealing with these events. These experiences can include not only acute acts of abuse and violence, but also the cumulative effects of neglect, disempowerment, invalidation, exclusion and isolation resulting from prolonged exposure to relational injury and social injustice through the violation of trust, rejection, betrayal, bullying, chronic stress, bereavement, racism, sexism, oppression, discrimination, unemployment, poverty and homelessness (Gómez et al., 2016; Silva et al., 2016; Isobel, et al., 2019).

These hurtful life events can lead to mental and emotional coping strategies based on the need to protect oneself, but these same survival strategies may lead to intense loneliness, alienation, anxiety, shame, powerlessness and despair. These experiences can often result in social withdrawal and the loss of relationships that could confirm our self-worth and ground our experiences in a shared reality (Allen et al., 1997). Through vicious cycles of avoidance, hypervigilance, rumination, guilt and self-blame, one can become absorbed in one's own fears, doubts and anxieties, leading to a feeling of being shattered, trapped and abandoned (Bogle & Boden, 2019). Voice hearing can be a part of a complex response to these adverse events:

> The observation that trauma can play a significant role in the onset and maintenance of voice hearing is one of the most striking and important

developments in the recent study of psychosis (Luhrmann et al., 2019, p.24).

> *Learning point 1*
> - How do you understand trauma?
> - Have you ever experienced something like trauma?
> - Have you ever felt threatened or powerless?
> - How did that make you feel?
> - How did you respond?
> - How do you cope with your experiences of trauma?

Trauma-informed care

Understanding hearing voices as a means of coping with and surviving trauma rather than as a symptom of a mental illness may help us better understand and support voice hearers (McEnteggart, et al., 2017). At the core of a trauma-informed approach to hearing voices is a shift of perspective from 'What's wrong with you?' to a compassionate exploration of 'What happened to you?' A trauma-informed approach acknowledges that trauma is a subjective experience; the gravity of similar experiences can be very different between individuals and not everyone may identify as being a survivor of trauma, yet the principles can help anyone experiencing emotional distress, including voice hearers (Sweeney et al., 2018).

Recently, the US-based Substance Abuse and Mental Health Services Administration (SAMHSA) (2014) identified six key principles to guide a trauma-informed approach to mental health care:

1. promoting a sense of physical and interpersonal safety
2. building and maintaining trust through transparency
3. establishing hope and enhancing collaboration through peer support and mutual self-help
4. facilitating collaboration and mutuality through the meaningful sharing of power and decision-making
5. fostering individuals' strengths and recovery through empowerment, voice, choice and self-advocacy
6. offering services that are responsive to the diverse needs of the individuals served by recognising and addressing cultural, historical, and gender issues.

A similar understanding of trauma can be found in the Power Threat Meaning Framework, developed by psychologists in the UK in collaboration with people with lived experience of mental health difficulty and mental health service use, as an alternative to psychiatric diagnosis (Johnstone & Boyle, 2018).

Learning point 2
- If you are a service provider, is the system you work in trauma informed? If not, how might you make it more trauma informed?
- If you are a service user, do you feel you are receiving trauma-informed care? If not, do you know where you might be able to receive such care?
- Do you know of any peer-support or self-help groups, such as the Hearing Voices Network, in your local community?

Learning point 3
- Did anything happen to you when you first started hearing voices?
- Do your voices remind you of anyone in your life, past or present?
- What do you think your voices are trying to tell you?
- Would any of your voices like to talk to anyone in your social, family or support network?

Peer-supported Open Dialogue (POD)

Peer-supported Open Dialogue (POD) is an adaption of the Open Dialogue approach to psychosis developed in the mental health system in Western Lapland, Finland, in the 1980s. Open Dialogue grew out of 'need-adapted treatment', developed by professor of psychiatry Yrjö Alanen as a form of systemic-psychodynamic family therapy (Alanen, 2009). Behind the work was a multidisciplinary team, including clinical psychologist and family therapist Jaakko Seikkula, now professor emeritus at the University of Jyväskylä, Finland. They found that it was often possible to avoid both medication and hospitalisation when the team responded immediately to the person in crisis. Meetings were organised around the wishes of the person in crisis and arranged in familiar places where the person felt safe, often in the person's own home. People considered important and helpful in the person's social network were invited to participate in these 'network meetings', which could occur daily during the crisis. The primary goal was not to make a diagnosis, prescribe neuroleptics or relieve symptoms, but to create a dialogical space where all voices could be expressed and responded to in order to find words for whatever the person in crisis and the people from their network were experiencing. The person in crisis was then better able to cope with whatever they were experiencing, often avoided a hospital admission, and could return sooner to their life (Seikkula & Arnkil, 2006).

POD has been developed in UK mental health crisis services over the past six years (Razzaque & Stockmann, 2016) as an integration of Open Dialogue with values-based practice, person-centred care and, most importantly, peer support (Hopfenbeck, 2015). In POD, all the community-based multidisciplinary teams include peer workers with lived experience of mental distress, who participate in POD network meetings as integral members, on an equal basis. The benefits for service users from peer workers' support have been shown to include improved quality of life, decreased social isolation and increased sense of empowerment, confidence, autonomy, self-efficacy, self-management, belonging and hopefulness (Gillard & Holley, 2014; Murphy & Higgins, 2018).

It is also important to remember that there is no one-size-fits-all approach to helping people who hear distressing voices. Some will prefer to take medication; others will choose not to. Some will want to develop a relationship with their voices; others hate their voices and may not feel comfortable engaging with them. In recognition of this, Open Dialogue is not so much an isolated intervention as 'an approach which integrates other approaches' (Lakeman, 2014). Within an Open Dialogue framework, other interventions such as CBT, EMDR, supported employment and medication and even a trauma-informed, hearing voices-specific approach, as introduced in other chapters of this book, can be suggested and coordinated, based on the person's wants and needs and what is available.

There are seven primary principles of the Open Dialogue approach that developed organically during the 1990s in response to what was found to contribute to positive outcomes (Seikkula & Olson, 2003; Seikkula & Arnkil, 2006, Seikkula & Alakare, 2019). These principles are as follows:

1. *Immediate response*. Providing help in the form of a network meeting within 24 hours of first contact provides a unique opportunity to engage with the person in crisis and their social network. This first meeting and subsequent meetings are based on the needs of the person in crisis, and they are asked who they would like to bring into the meeting. If it is a friend or relative who is making contact with the OD team, they are asked who the person in crisis might want to be there with them in addition to the OD team. Even if the person is experiencing an acute psychotic episode, there is no need to wait. By responding immediately, it is often easier to create a space for difficult issues related to the psychotic experience to emerge that have not previously been expressed or shared. The meeting is not planned ahead of time and the meeting begins with an open question such as, 'How should we use this time together?' By responding early and creating a safe and open atmosphere, while listening and reflecting on whatever comes up in the conversation, it is hoped that hospital admission and potential retraumatisation can be avoided.

2. *Including the social network*. It is important that the person in crisis does not feel isolated and alone. Network meetings should be safe places where the person at the centre of concern feels supported and accepted. Therefore, it is important that the person in crisis is allowed to invite those persons that they trust and feel

supported by. Very often this will be the family of the person. However, the person may not feel safe with family due to a history of relational trauma, so friends, work colleagues, neighbours or other professionals can be invited too. This basic idea was already first expressed by Speck and Rueveni, back in 1969, in their article 'Network therapy: A developing concept':

> By simply gathering the network together in one place at one time with the purpose of forming a tighter organization of relationships, potent therapeutic potentials are set in motion. (1969, p.182)

Each member of the network represents a unique perspective and contribution, and once they are brought together, it is important that all the voices are heard. The person in crisis will be invited to share what they are experiencing, including any voices they may be hearing. If the person chooses to share these experiences, the voices can then become part of the dialogue between the network members.

3. *Flexibility and mobility*. The meetings are organised according to the specific and changing needs of the person in crisis. The core principle is that meetings can be arranged any time, anywhere, with anyone, to discuss anything. Very often the meetings will be arranged in the person's home and, if it is considered helpful, they can occur as often as daily during the initial crisis period. This represents a radically person-centred approach that supports the self-determination and autonomy of the person at the centre and helps them to reclaim agency in the context of their daily life (von Peter et al., 2019).

4. *Responsibility*. In Open Dialogue, whichever staff member is contacted first takes responsibility for organising the first meeting, including putting together the multidisciplinary team that will attend. Providing a sense of 'You have come to the right place, you are not alone and we can help' is an important first response for a person and network in crisis. The team attending the first meeting will then be responsible for creating an integrated, co-ordinated network of care, inviting other services and professionals into the network meetings as needed.

5. *Psychological continuity*. This team will have consistent contact with the network for as long as they are in need of help from services, which for some may include inpatient care. Healing from complex trauma can often take a considerable amount of time, from months to years, and there is a need for patience and a willingness to progress at a pace that is tolerable in order for that healing to occur. Open Dialogue teams provide this long-term continuity where trustful, human relationships may be built up over time and the network does not need to be anxious about the person being discharged too early or transferred to a separate specialist team after a given amount of time, as is often the case in routine mental health services where Open Dialogue is not practised.

6. *Tolerating uncertainty*. Experiencing a crisis and emotional distress means living with uncertainty, which can at times seem overwhelming. This can often lead to a desire for simple explanations and rapid solutions to remove that uncertainty. In the Open Dialogue approach, however, there is an explicit intention to acknowledge that uncertainty is normal and to keep multiple possibilities and perspectives open. Part of this is moving forward slowly with any major decisions, such as medication, and allowing time for the person to find the words and language for whatever they are experiencing, as well as facilitating a collective process of meaning-making originating from the person and the network. Being present with this kind of uncertainty is often very challenging, but by creating an open space where all voices (including the inner voices of the voice hearer) can be respected and heard, a different sense of safety can be cultivated – a safety based on being accepted and listened to without judgement. This can occur when the practitioners can arrange network meetings on a daily basis if necessary, allowing for the expression of powerful and often painful emotions, making room for contradictory and conflicting perspectives and responding compassionately to the person's and network's needs so as to develop a sense of mutual trust.

7. *Dialogism*. One of the major differences between traditional approaches and Open Dialogue is that Open Dialogue practitioners don't lead the meeting as experts; they follow the words that are spoken, using the network's language, and often repeating verbatim what has been said. The emphasis is not on interpretation or mutual agreement but an honest sharing of unique individual perspectives. According to Seikkula and Trimble (2005, p.462):

> The drama of the process lies not in some brilliant intervention by the professional, but in the emotional exchange among network members, including the professionals, who together construct or restore a caring personal community.

This relies on the core attitudes of authenticity and transparency, embodying the psychiatric system survivors' motto, 'Nothing about us, without us'. In Open Dialogue, all conversations 'about' the person at the centre of concern occur with the person present, and preferably in the network meetings. These conversations often occur as part of a reflection where the practitioners share their thoughts and emotions while the rest of the network listens and responds (Andersen, 1995).

Creating a genuine and spontaneous dialogue between people isn't easy (Olson et al., 2014), especially for the person who has experienced trauma. Putting words to painful emotional experiences can often seem unbearable, but by being present in the moment (Stern, 2004) and responding to whatever is said with authentic human warmth, it is possible for the network to create mutual understandings, reshape identities and rebuild relationships. According to Wharne (2018), voices can be considered 'a form of communication which others need to hear so that relationships can be improved' (p.399). Helping voice hearers re-establish and develop relationships with people in their social network can help them to change their relationships with their voices as they learn to reconnect with themselves, navigate their own vulnerabilities and become more assertive regarding their own needs (Hayward et al., 2014). Hope is created in spaces where it is safe to speak and listen and where all voices can be heard, providing opportunities for reconciliation and healing (Clarke, 2016).

Learning point 4
- Who can help and support you with what most worries you at the moment?
- Who in your network knows you are hearing voices?
- Whom in your network can you trust and talk with?

Learning point 5
- Can you remember a time when you have felt listened to?
- What did that feel like?
- What did the person do that made you feel like you were listened to and heard?

What is the evidence?

The benefits of open dialogues in network meetings are difficult to document, as are other such community-based, psychosocial interventions. An evaluation conducted by Seikkula and colleagues (2001a, 2001b) found very positive results, with fewer symptoms, reduced use of medication and the large majority returning to work or education. A follow-up study (Aaltonen et al., 2011; Seikkula et al., 2011) went through the same data 10 years later and their results correspond to a great extent with the findings from 2001. Despite some limitations with the studies' methodology, Open Dialogue is considered to be one of the most promising psychosocial interventions for people experiencing psychosis (Turkington & Lebert, 2017).

A recent review of the evidence has also concluded that there is a vital need for more extensive evaluations of the efficacy of Open Dialogue, using more robust research methods (Freeman et al., 2019). This is now under way. The first randomised controlled trial (RCT) of Open Dialogue, ODDESSI (Open Dialogue: Development and Evaluation of a Social Network Intervention for Severe Mental Illness) has recently started in the UK, and an international research collaboration, HOPEnDialogue, was launched in 2019.

While we await the results of these studies, it is equally important to recognise the significance of Open Dialogue as a means by which to foster human rights in mental health care practice and fulfil public policy in relation to person-centred care, service user participation, network involvement and mental health recovery (Lakeman, 2014; von Peter et al., 2019).

Conclusion

The voices people experience have their own histories and reasons for being what they are. Responding to trauma dialogically means providing an opportunity for those voices to be heard by the network of relationships that we are a part of. Reaching out and opening up to one's network can be difficult in a time of crisis, and yet we are all part of a larger web of relationships that we depend upon. Involving and trusting the people who care about you can be the first step towards resolving the distress you may be feeling. Sometimes it can be as simple as bringing together your friends and supporters and creating a safe space where painful memories, hidden fears and unspoken voices can be shared and explored with curiosity and respect. And even though it may be a relatively simple idea, it is not always easy to put into practice. Take your time and, when you're ready, start the dialogue.

References

Aaltonen, J., Seikkula, J. & Lehtinen, K. (2011). The comprehensive Open-Dialogue approach (II). Long-term stability of acute psychosis outcomes in advanced community care: The Western Lapland project. *Psychosis*, *3*(3), 1–13.

Alanen, Y.O. (2009). Towards a more humanistic psychiatry: Development of need-adapted treatment of schizophrenia group psychoses. *Psychosis,* 1(2), 156–166.

Allen, J.G., Coyne, L. & Console, D.A. (1997). Dissociative detachment relates to psychotic symptoms and personality decompensation. *Comprehensive Psychiatry*, *38*(6), 327–334.

Andersen, T. (1995). Reflecting processes: Acts of informing and forming. In S. Friedman (Ed.), *The Reflecting Team in Action* (pp.11–37). Guilford.

Bogle, S. & Boden, Z. (2019). 'It was like a lightning bolt hitting my world': Feeling shattered in a first crisis in psychosis. *Qualitative Research in Psychology*; doi.org/10.1080/14780887.2019.1631418

Clarke, L. (2016). Embracing polyphony: Voices, improvisation, and the Hearing Voices Network. *Intersectionalities: A global journal of social work analysis, research, polity, and practice*, *5*(2), 1–11.

Freeman, A., Tribe, R., Stott, J. & Pilling, S. (2019). Open Dialogue: A review of the evidence. *Psychiatric Services*, *70*(1), 46–59.

Gillard, S. & Holley, J. (2014). Peer workers in mental health services: Literature overview. *Advances in Psychiatric Treatment*, *20*, 286–292.

Gómez, J.M., Lewis, J., Noll, L.K., Smidt, A.M. & Birrell, P.J. (2016). Shifting the focus: Nonpathologizing approaches to healing from betrayal trauma through an emphasis on relational care. *Journal of Trauma & Dissociation*, *17*(2), 165–185.

Hayward, M., Berry, K., McCarthy-Jones, S., Strauss, C. & Thomas, N. (2014). Beyond the omnipotence of voices: Further developing a relational approach to auditory hallucinations. *Psychosis*, *6*(3), 242–252.

Hopfenbeck, M. (2015). Peer-supported Open Dialogue. *Context, 138*, 29–31.

Isobel, S., Goodyear, M. & Foster, K. (2019). Psychological trauma in the context of familial relationships: A concept analysis. *Trauma, Violence, & Abuse, 20*(4). https://doi.org/10.1177/1524838017726424

Johnstone, L. & Boyle, M., with Cromby, J., Dillon, J., Harper, D., Kinderman, P., Longden, E., Pilgrim, D. & Read, J. (2018). *The Power Threat Meaning Framework: Towards the identification of patterns in emotional distress, unusual experiences and troubled or troubling behaviour, as an alternative to functional psychiatric diagnosis*. British Psychological Society.

Lakeman, R. (2014). The Finnish Open Dialogue approach to crisis intervention in psychosis: A review. *Psychotherapy in Australia, 20*(3), 26–33.

Luhrmann, T.M., Alderson-Day, B., Bell, V., Bless, J.J., Corlett, P., Hugdahl, K., Jones, N., Larøi, F., Moseley, P., Padmavati, R., Peters, E., Powers, A.R. & Waters, F. (2019). Beyond trauma: A multiple pathways approach to auditory hallucinations in clinical and nonclinical populations. *Schizophrenia Bulletin, 45*(Suppl 1), S24–S31.

McEnteggart, C., Barnes-Holmes, Y., Dillon, J., Egger, J. & Oliver, J. (2017). Hearing voices, dissociation, and the self: A functional-analytic perspective. *Journal of Trauma & Dissociation, 18*(4), 575–594.

Murphy, R. & Higgins, A. (2018). The complex terrain of peer support in mental health: What does it all mean? *Journal of Psychiatric Mental Health Nursing, 25*, 441–448.

Olson, M., Seikkula, J. & Ziedonis, D. (2014). *The key elements of dialogic practice in Open Dialogue*. University of Massachusetts Medical School.

Razzaque, R. & Stockmann, T. (2016). An introduction to peer-supported Open Dialogue in mental healthcare. *BJPsych Advances, 22*(5), 348–356.

Seikkula, J. & Alakare, B. (2019). Open dialogues principles and dialogical meetings for psychosis. In J. Pereira, J. Gonçalves & V Bizzari (Eds.), *The neurobiology- psychotherapy-pharmacology intervention triangle* (pp.127–140). Vernon Press.

Seikkula, J. & Arnkil, T.E. (2006). *Dialogical meetings in social networks*. Karnac Books.

Seikkula, J. & Olson, M. (2003). The Open Dialogue approach to acute psychosis: Its poetics and micropolitics. *Family Process, 42*, 403–418.

Seikkula. J. & Trimble, D. (2005). Healing elements of therapeutic conversation: Dialogue as an embodiment of love. *Family Process, 44*, 461–475.

Seikkula, J., Alakare, B. & Aaltonen, J. (2001a). Open Dialogue in psychosis I: An introduction and case illustration. *Journal of Constructivist Psychology, 14*(4), 247–265.

Seikkula, J., Alakare, B. & Aaltonen, J. (2001b). Open Dialogue in psychosis I: A comparison of good and poor outcome cases. *Journal of Constructivist Psychology, 14*(4), 267–284.

Seikkula, J., Alakare, B. & Aaltonen, J. (2011). The comprehensive open-dialogue approach in Western Lapland: II. Long-term stability of acute psychosis outcomes in advanced community care. *Psychosis, 3*(3), 192–204.

Silva, M., Loureiro, A. & Cardoso, G. (2016). Social determinants of mental health: A review of the evidence. *European Journal of Psychiatry, 30*(4), 259–292.

Speck, R. & Rueveni, U. (1969). Network therapy: A developing concept. *Family Process, 8*, 182–191.

Stern, D.N. (2004). *The present moment in psychotherapy and everyday life*. W.W. Norton & Co.

Substance Abuse and Mental Health Services Administration. (2014). *SAMHSA's concept of trauma and guidance for a trauma-informed approach*. HHS Publication No.(SMA) 14-4884. Substance Abuse and Mental Health Services Administration.

Sweeney, A., Filson, B., Kennedy, A., Collinson, L. & Gillard, S. (2018). A paradigm shift: Relationships in trauma-informed mental health services. *BJPsych Advances*, *24*(5), 319–333.

Turkington, D. & Lebert, L. (2017). Psychological treatments for schizophrenia spectrum disorder: What is around the corner? *BJPsych Advances, 23*(1), 16–23.

von Peter, S., Aderhold, V., Cubellis, L., Bergström, T., Stastny, P., Seikkula, J. & Pura, D. (2019). Open Dialogue as a human rights-aligned approach. *Frontiers in Psychiatry*, *10,* 387. https://doi.org/10.3389/fpsyt.2019.00387

Wharne, S. (2018). 'On being an auditory hallucination': A reflection on theory, practice, existential philosophy, and hearing voices. *The Humanistic Psychologist, 46*(4), 399–411.

28 A psychodynamic understanding of voice hearing

Christine Cox

Many people experience hearing voices in everyday life without feeling unduly disturbed by them. Unusual experiences such as the hearing of voices discussed here are generally associated with mental illness, but they can occur in everyday life for many people not considered to be ill. For example, it is not uncommon for the recently bereaved to hear the voice of the dead person. From my work with veterans, I also know it not to be unusual, for example, to hear the voices of comrades when re-living the acute trauma of being on active service in the battlefield.

What the voices say affects the voice hearer's reactions, emotions and feelings. Sharing the experience with another person provides a different point of view. Sometimes doing so leads to relief; at other times, it may increase distress. But a conversation with an empathic listener can provide a benign container for the distress. Hence the quality of interpersonal relationships becomes essential to being able to live with and understand these voices.

Psychodynamic understanding offers a way into understanding the complexity of the voice-hearing experience.

This approach to understanding the experience of a voice or voices in the mind revolves around the acceptance of a complex inner world in which both conscious and unconscious thoughts and feelings are constantly on the move. This is true for everyone, whether or not you consider yourself, or are thought of by others, to be a voice hearer.

Fleeting thoughts or feelings may move rapidly in the moment, following a shift in mood or the experience of an emotion, and then move to another fleeting thought and emotion. The line between a dream or fantasy world and the real world is constantly shifting. The nature of one's consciousness is constantly being challenged. Voices and conversations, daydreams, night-time dreams and nightmares produce unbidden thoughts, ideas and emotions that come and go.

The aim of this chapter is to show how understanding the principles of psychodynamic theory, and object-relations theory in particular, can help us to understand how and why some people hear voices and are distressed by them, and what the voices signify. It does not attempt to suggest that voices can or should be removed from a person's mental life but that they may be able to react differently to them if they have a greater understanding of their meaning. Psychodynamic theory is interested in meanings and they will be different for every individual.

To my knowledge, there is no research on the effectiveness of the psychodynamic understanding of voice hearing. This is due to the model's subjective nature and its reliance on an individualised therapeutic relationship, which is extremely difficult to quantify. From discussions over many years with practising psychodynamic and psychoanalytic therapists, I have come to appreciate that using understanding of psychodynamic theory, and object-relations theory in particular, allows containment of and insight into the voices and their meaning. Hopefully, opportunities for research into this mode of understanding and treatment can be initiated in the coming years.

Learning point 1
- Have you experienced hearing a voice or conversation in your head?
- How do you feel about it?
- Are you comfortable with sharing it with someone else?

Psychodynamic theory

Psychodynamic theory begins by looking at the normal development of an infant with its mother and other relationships. When there is an understanding of normal, ordinary patterns of development, it is easier to understand when things go wrong. Greater perspective and empathy for the pathological becomes possible.

In understanding mental life, psychodynamic theory helps us accept the experience of the present. It tries to understand its context and sees if and how that person's experience of the present relates to their past experiences. Accepting and understanding feelings and experiences can reduce the anxiety provoked when they recur. This can be achieved by regular conversations in a safe environment with the complete attention of the listener. In psychodynamic therapy, this would be with a trained counsellor or therapist.

A psychodynamic approach to therapy aims to understand and make conscious the contrasting and often conflicting parts of the self (Howard, 2018, pp.9–11). This requires a willingness to observe one's changing states of mind and emotions without judgement. It also requires a desire and willingness to express and explore them. A capacity for mentalisation is necessary: both the voice hearer and their listener need to be interested and curious and prepared to suspend judgement of their thoughts and feelings. Exploring meanings without always needing to know answers thus becomes possible. So mentalisation is a vital component of the voice hearer's capacity to understand their voices and learn to manage them (Bateman & Fonagy, 2012, pp.3–5).

> **Learning point 2**
> - Are you curious about how your mind works?
> - Can you suspend judgement of your thoughts so you can wonder what they might mean?

Conversations in the head are part of a normal mental state and we all experience them, whether or not we consider ourselves, or are considered by others, to be ill. For example, telling oneself to 'hurry up' or 'Don't be so stupid' is common, as is a more soothing inner voice that encourages and supports. Within psychodynamic theory, we would generally assume that this is a self-generated way of speaking to ourselves; we do not regard it as the sound and actual presence of another, as the voice hearer does.

Voice hearers have a particular challenge in that these conversations are perceived to be actually happening in the present moment and located in sounds that are only audible to them and are frequently attached to the sense of the presence of another.

This is generally the situation when the voice hearer is currently troubled by hearing the voices. When not currently troubled by the voices, their inner self-generated conversations may be responding to conscious and unconscious experiences, thoughts and feelings, as happens most of the time for the majority of people. This understanding of one's inner dialogue is common to other psychological therapies as well as psychodynamic therapy (Jacobs, 1986, pp.8–10).

Developing conscious awareness and recognition of patterns in the movements of thoughts and feelings can highlight their significance so that their unconscious meaning can be explored (Mollon, 2000, pp.56–64).

For the voice hearer who is troubled by currently hearing one or more voices, the line between conscious awareness and unconscious experience is compromised and the voices take on a more concrete state, in which they are perceived as coming from real people.

For example, the voice hearer who says that the voices are talking about them to each other outside their front door may be unable in that moment to distinguish between the conversation they hear and the external reality of the situation. So, suggesting that they check outside the front door to see if anyone is there produces confusion. The voice hearer knows that there are no real people there and yet they also know that they are hearing the voices of these people, so s/he has to assume they must be there. In that moment, there is a blurring of their external and internal realities. This produces intense anxiety.

Describing these voices as 'symptoms' rather than being currently troubled by internal events frames the voice hearer within the medical model of understanding unusual experiences in the mind, which may limit the possibilities for exploring other ways of understanding their experiences. Psychodynamic theory can offer a different way of understanding these mental events.

> *Learning point 3*
> - If you describe yourself as a voice hearer, do you experience a difference between the external voices you hear and other internal conversations, such as telling yourself to 'hurry up'?
> - How do you understand the difference between the two?
> - Do you feel anxious if you are questioned about the reality of your voices?
> - If so, how do you manage that anxiety?

Objects and object-relations theory

Everyone has an impulse to relate to others and this can be observed from the moment of birth when the new-born infant seeks the gaze of the mother, or other care-giver. A history for the baby is already being formed; indeed, it was from the moment of conception or before. The baby takes in this relationship with its mind and body, thus starting to build its inner emotional world.

This is not problematic when the baby's experiences are sustaining and rewarding. However, when they cause discomfort and distress, the baby feels them to be bad and wants to get rid of them. Its developing mind manages this by splitting the good from the bad and putting the bad out of reach, repressing it and its associations.

This is the basis of object-relations theory, and particularly the version developed in Britain in the years after the First World War, which has been influential on the thinking of psychodynamic practitioners since that time (Scharff & Scharff, 1998, pp.41–44). Freud first used the word 'object' to describe an instinctual move towards a need-satisfying and tension-relieving place within the psyche. The usefulness of the terminology continues to be questioned but, failing any satisfactory alternative, the word 'object' continues to be used.

Fairbairn (1952/1994, pp.5–8) realised that objects do not exist in isolation but relate to each other, hence 'object-relations'. These object-relations represent the parents and other significant individuals on which, in early life, the child builds its ideas about itself and develops its ways of relating to others. Fairbairn took this further to observe that the process of taking in and internalising these influences gives rise to the formation of internal object-relations. Hence the child develops an inner world that contains versions of its experiences of significant people in its external world. The process of coming to terms with the goodness or badness of these external and internal objects gives rise to the internal-world process of splitting and repression.

Learning point 4
- Do you recognise that your ideas about yourself now are based on the early experiences you had with significant people, especially parents, in your early childhood?
- How much do these relationships continue to influence the way that you think about yourself?

Repression, splitting and projection

Repression is an unconscious process that tries to find a place for unwanted emotions that are either held onto – repressed – sometimes for a life-time, or projected out. The well-known Rorschach, or ink-blot, test is a simple example of projection – the same ink blot will be seen to represent many different things by different people, according to what form their unconscious inner world projects into it (Concise Medical Dictionary, 2010). In object-relations, a person may project unwanted parts of their self into other people without being aware of so doing.

Learning point 5
- You can replicate the Rorschach test by randomly choosing a photograph in a paper or magazine and describing what you see in it and the feelings it stirs in you.
- This is the experience of unconscious projection and is likely to reflect aspects of your current state of mind and inner world.

Melanie Klein, particularly through her work with young children, developed an understanding of the way the mind splits off unwanted thoughts and feelings. The child projects them into a likely container, frequently the mother or other significant carer. This person then, in the child's mind, takes on the characteristics of their unwanted parts (Klein, 1932, p.153) and contains them for them. Klein started to emphasise the importance of understanding the first years of life as a time when the blueprint for future development is laid down, and this beginning was built upon by later analysts.

> Michaela,[1] age five, is angry with her mother for leaving her at school today when she has a cold and wants to stay at home with her. She is unable to find acceptable ways of expressing her feelings, for fear of reprisal should she hurt her mother, so she splits off the difficult feelings and deposits them (projects them) in her mind into her schoolteacher, who upset her earlier in the day

---

1. Michaela and Robert are pseudonyms and the details of their stories have been completely anonymised.

> by reprimanding her for being noisy in the class. She can then justify to herself the angry feelings for her teacher and allow herself to hate her, while continuing to keep her mother untouched by her anger. Therefore, she can continue to feel safe with her mother. Her internal object-relations are kept manageable by splitting the good from the bad, the love from the hate.

Integrating conflicting emotions within the Self is a continuous developmental task. This starts at the very beginning of life. The child depends on being helped by its mother, or other primary care-giver, to manage the confusing and fragmenting feelings in its inner world. In infancy, the child locates the feelings in its body – it cries to show its distress and is comforted when literally held and cared for. This helps the child to keep itself whole and located safely in its body. When this experience is successful, the child can start to develop its own sense of a Self that is separate to that of its mother. The child feels contained and is therefore able to learn to contain itself (Winnicott, 1945/1987, pp.145–156).

> *Learning point 6*
> - Can you identify a similar experience to Michaela's in your early life?
> - Do you sometimes get angry with someone else rather than with the person who has really upset you?
> - Do you recognise that this is the mind splitting the emotion in two and projecting it out in two directions as a way of managing it?

Attachment and loss

Freud described the effects of the loss of the object of attachment – that is, the mother or other attachment figure – and related the subsequent sadness and distress to the process of mourning. If mourning happens without too much interruption, it resolves over time. However, coming to terms with loss and mourning requires an acceptance that the object was not perfect and was disappointing. This acceptance of non-perfection is an important part of the mourning process. Without it, feelings of anger, guilt and shame towards both the lost person and oneself can continue to be problematic and can take a long time to resolve. This is what Freud described as melancholia (Freud, 1917/2006, pp.311–312).

> Michaela has to come to terms with the fact that her mother is not, in her eyes, a perfect mother. This loss is a universal experience that everyone has to negotiate in their own way. However, loss is also an experience within the internal world, and this often proves problematic. How does she come to terms with the loss of the object-mother when it feels as if a part of herself, in her inner world, has been lost? This is particularly difficult when the lost part of the self has been idealised

and was supposed to be perfect. Michaela wanted her mother to be perfect and to meet all her needs in the ways that would best satisfy her. Her mother has disappointed her, so she has to mourn that loss. Moreover, she also has to mourn the part of herself that has internalised an idea of a perfect mother and made it her own. As her own internalised perfect object-mother has also failed her, she has that loss to manage too. She feels she has disappointed herself. The way she does this is to employ various defence mechanisms.

Learning point 7
- Do you recognise Michaela's feelings for her mother?
- Can you identify a similar process in your own life?
- How do you resolve it?

Freud's structural theory and defence mechanisms

In 1923, Freud described the workings of the mind as being tripartite: id, ego and superego (Freud, 1923, pp.443–445). Simply put, the ego is the self, the id holds the unconscious, instinctual impulses, and the superego is the controlling and moralistic part of the self.

Conflict arises from the continuous inter-relating of these parts of the internal world. There is constant anxiety-driven striving to manage the feelings that have been aroused. Various types of defence mechanisms develop in order to keep a semblance of order.

Repression, splitting and projection are unconscious defence mechanisms that act in a primitive fashion. When the ego develops a more observing stance, then more sophisticated defence mechanisms such as denial, suppression and rationalisation may be used. Anna Freud (1936/1993, pp.29–30) gives a picture of the ego as developing this capacity to observe. Being able to observe one's thoughts is vital if the experiences of the mind are to be kept in a manageable place.

The superego plays a dominant role in the development of an inner conversation. It keeps an overview of the struggle between the id and the ego, but also adds a voice of its own. If the child's relationship with its parents and care-givers has so far been relatively benign, this voice can moderate and criticise with an overall sense of reinforcing the strength of the ego and sense of self and need not be problematic. However, once the child begins to internalise too many negative messages from its care-givers, the superego can take on a highly critical and moralistic tone. This increases fear and anxiety.

Michaela may continue to act out her distress and frustration with her mother and her teacher by expressing her anger even more noisily and becoming even more disruptive in her class at school, which is likely to lead to more criticism. She is likely to internalise this and reinforce her critical and punitive superego.

The unconscious emotional conversations taking place in the internal world can start to dominate, leading to fear and inhibition. These conflicts may then be projected out into the child's external world through difficult behavioural patterns, as Michaela shows in the classroom.

Learning point 8
- Do you recognise your superego?
- Can you see when it is being unhelpful by being unnecessarily critical of yourself?

If the child's behaviour is understood by its care-givers as having meaning, its behaviour patterns and distress can be contained and the tensions in its inner world reduced. Bion (1962, pp.306–10) emphasised the importance of the mother being able to tolerate the child's hatred and destructive impulses. If she hears the baby's distress, she can accept the angry projections and hold onto them. By understanding them, she detoxifies them. The baby unconsciously perceives this understanding and is relieved of its anger and hatred. It can then continue to feel securely contained by its mother.

If, however, the mother and child consistently fail to manage this unconscious process in their relationship, there is greater likelihood that problems in the child's inner world will develop as it grows. This may include, for some people, the development of illnesses with psychotic elements and beliefs and behaviours that are regarded by many psychotherapy and psychiatric professionals as symptoms of major psychotic illness, such as schizophrenia.

The developmental model in object-relations theory and voice hearing

Robert, age 23, is a postgraduate student in mathematics who is looking for work. His parents divorced when he was 12 years old and, as he changed to secondary school, he was bullied because of his short height and because he was intellectually ahead of his peers. He gradually withdrew from relationships with others, both in the family and at school, and there was no particular person to whom he could relate easily. He felt himself to be different from others and was conscious of altered states of mind when under stress. He started to think that people were talking about him. He managed the transition from school to university by devoting himself to intellectual work. However, the conversations in his mind became louder and more troublesome to him.

> When his father died suddenly, when Robert was in his final year at university, the voices he heard talking about him became louder and more insistent. They were only critical and voiced all his faults and problems in harsh tones. He felt the voices to be present in the room or just outside. He became afraid that he was going mad, and eventually decided to seek help.

When a voice hearer hears internal voices as external and real and not just as voices in the inner world, then mental conflict takes on a different quality. The voice hearer becomes preoccupied with their sound and believes that this is a real event in the present moment. Their anxiety and fear grow.

The boundary between the inner world of the mind and the conscious experience of the moment is breached and what might have remained an internal-world conversation between parts of the self becomes an externalised conversation happening in the moment. Although the voice hearer thinks this is outside of themselves, it is in fact still within their mind. But they have split off the experience from the whole mind and made it into an object in its own right. This fragmentation may lead to psychosis when the ego's relation to reality is lost and delusions develop. The relationship with the past is lost and constructing a coherent narrative becomes difficult (Bollas, 2015, pp.103–110).

The focus of the voices is usually on something being said about or done to the voice hearer. This can be understood from a psychodynamic perspective as containing unacceptable ideas about the self that have been split off and projected into the critical voice. This is paranoia, in which the critical voices are reflecting back the unacceptable parts of the self.

> In psychodynamic counselling, Robert was encouraged to speculate on the content of the conversations the voices were having about him. This revealed ideas and assumptions about himself that he had developed since childhood, which were without exception all negative and to do with perceived failings and fear that he had caused harm to others.
>
> The paranoid thoughts he heard in the voices could be safely expressed to the therapist and taken seriously. Exploring the experiences of his childhood revealed many instances of feeling put down by his parents and teachers, reinforced by the bullying at school. His relationship with his father had been particularly rivalrous and contained much mutual hatred. His anger, envy, guilt and shame had no acceptable outlet and became repressed. He tried to compensate by working hard at school in order to gain affirmation. This succeeded to some extent, until the added stress of working for his final examinations. He was determined to prove himself by achieving a first-class degree. When, at this point, his father died suddenly of a heart attack, Robert's inner-world conflicts became overwhelming and the voices that had been hovering on the perimeter of his consciousness became real in his mind. They seemed to be acting as an attempt to give back life to the father.

> The therapist understood this as fragmentation of Robert's internal objects that his mind tried to manage by creating the voices (Steiner, 1993, pp.67–69). When the fantasy of being responsible for his father's death started to dominate, the voices told him it was all his fault, and he would be punished forever. There was no space in Robert's mind for him to think about or express both his sadness and his anger at his father's sudden death. The distinction between the reality of the loss of his father through death and the fantasy of his responsibility became catastrophically blurred, leading to psychosis (Bion, 1959, pp.108–109).
>
> The therapist was able to help Robert understand the function the voices were performing for him. They had a defensive purpose that allowed him to remove them from his inner world, externalise them and give them their own reality, thus giving him some distance from them. They also protected him from potentially acting out his hatred of his father by hurting other people or himself in the place of his father (Ogden, 1992, pp.84–87).
>
> Therapy allowed Robert to feel and then try to understand the anger, rage and fear he felt both for the reality of his disappointing father and the voices that were tormenting him. This could happen once Robert allowed himself to let the therapist know about his anger and disappointment with her for not being perfect and discover that she could accept and contain it without retaliating. He slowly began to recognise that the voices were representing unacceptable split-off parts of himself that he had somehow to come to terms with and re-integrate.

Mourning the idealised Self

Most people struggle with acceptable and unacceptable ideas about the Self. This is necessary in order to develop a balanced sense of self-esteem and appreciate one's abilities and achievements. An unhealthy self-preoccupation with successes and failures, however, leads to a fear of either abject failure or, at the other end of the narcissistic spectrum, a grandiose expectation of attaining spectacular success. This latter becomes an idealised version of the Self. Trying to maintain the fantasy of a perfect Self can become unbearable. If this is a dominant force in the inner world of a voice hearer, the messages attributed to the voices can become rigid and carry an authority that the voice hearer strongly believes to be true.

The superego becomes harsh and punitive and this internal saboteur (Fairbairn, 1954/1994, pp.44–45) refuses to allow growth and development.

> At their loudest, Robert's voices told him he was a complete failure, would never be any good in the world, would be a mental patient all his life and was also the murderer of his father. At their quietest, they criticised him for being mentally ill, for not looking after himself properly and for not being good enough to get on with his work, so he would never find a job.

Over time in the counselling sessions, Robert began to recognise the destructive nature of the loudest voices. With further exploration of the complex feelings he had towards his father, he began to release some of their power over him. This was the long work of mourning, both for his lost ideal Self, who had been built up defensively throughout his childhood and adolescence, and his years lost to fighting mental illness, as well as the loss of his actual father, who had been such a difficult and unhelpful parent. He began to understand his quieter voices as sabotaging his attempts to help himself. If he could change their message to an empathic and caring one, he could allow himself to improve his self-care in practical and emotional ways.

Learning point 9
- How do you manage the struggle with your own ideas about yourself?
- How do you balance the longing to be perfect with the fear that you are no good?
- What ways do you find to talk to yourself that help you manage this?

Repair and integration

Repairing the damage that is, within a psychodynamic understanding, unconsciously feared as having been inflicted on the Self by the voices, requires repeatedly realising that the voices are products of the Self. This is challenging mental work, but the understanding that they are repetitions from the past that repeat the fear of breakdown is the first step. Fear of breakdown is a fear of something that has already happened but has not been processed (Winnicott, 1974, pp.103–107). The fracture originally happened in the unintegrated state of the infant who was insufficiently helped by its parents and the environment at the time. There was then insufficient reparation in later experiences and relationships, so the unintegrated state of mind was repeated when growing up, as was the case for Robert.

Reparation can happen through insight into the emotional as well as rational experiences in the therapeutic relationship. The containment the relationship provides can foster a willingness to challenge assumptions and a desire to relinquish old patterns. The voice hearer may then discover sources of creativity in daily life that, if expressed, can help them to hold the voices in check, understand them and give them a place, while allowing growth and development to continue unimpeded.

Learning point 10
- What ways do you find to be creative in your everyday life?
- How do they help to repair hurt and restore a sense of your whole self?

Conclusion

When understanding voice hearers' experiences, it is vital to take into account the whole context in which the voices are heard. This may range from an acute, lone episode to frequent manifestations of chronic depression or psychosis. Several sources of help and care within the medical model may be needed in addition to the therapeutic conversation. Using object-relations theory to understand each voice hearer's unique experience can go some way towards containing the fear that hearing voices produces. When their potential meaning is understood, change becomes possible.

References

Bateman, A.W. & Fonagy, P. (2012). *Handbook of mentalizing in mental health practice*. American Psychiatric Publishing Inc.

Bion, W. (1959). Attacks on linking. *International Journal of Psycho-analysis, 40*, 308–316.

Bion, W. (1962). A theory of thinking. *International Journal of Psycho-analysis, 43*, 306–310.

Bollas, C.(2015). *When the sun bursts*. Yale University Press.

Concise Medical Dictionary (2010). Oxford University Press.

Fairbairn, W.R.D. (1952/1994). Psychoananalytic studies of the personality. In J.S. Grotstein & D.B. Rinsley (Eds.), *Fairbairn and the origins of object relations* (pp. 5–8). Free Association Books.

Fairbairn WRD (1954/1994). *An object-relations theory of the personality*. In: J.S. Grotstein & D.B. Rinsley (Eds.), *Fairbairn and the origins of object relations* (pp. 44-45). Free Association Books.

Freud, A. (1936/1993). *The ego and the mechanisms of defence*. Karnac Books.

Freud, S. (1917/2006). *Mourning and melancholia*. In A. Phillips (Ed.), *The Penguin Freud reader*. Penguin Books.

Freud, S. (1923/1991). *The ego and the id*. In S. Freud, *The essentials of psycho-analysis*. Penguin Books.

Howard, S. (2018). *Psychodynamic counselling in a nutshell*. Sage.

Jacobs, M. (1986). *The presenting past*. Open University Press.

Klein, M. (1932). *The psychoanalysis of children*. Hogarth Press.

Mollon, P. (2000). *The unconscious: Ideas in psychoanalysis*. Icon Books.

Ogden, T.H. (1992). *The primitive edge of experience*. Karnac Books.

Scharff, J.S. & Scharff, D.E. (1998). *Object relations individual therapy*. Karnac Books.

Steiner, J. (1993). *Psychic retreats*. Routledge.

Winnicott, D. (1945/1987). *Primitive emotional development*. In D. Winnicott, *Collected papers: Through paediatrics to psychoanalysis* (pp.145–156). Hogarth Press.

Winnicott, D. (1974). Fear of breakdown. *International Review of Psycho-analysis, 1*, 103–107.

29 Compassion-focused therapy and the courage of compassionate relating to voices

Charles Heriot-Maitland

In this chapter, I will first introduce you to some of the key ideas from compassion-focused therapy (CFT). We will then start to see how these ideas can be brought in to help voice hearers, as well as to guide ways of understanding and relating to voice-hearing experiences. The CFT approach was developed by the British psychologist Professor Paul Gilbert (Gilbert, 2009). To really understand this approach, let's first focus on this word 'compassion' itself, which can have very different meanings and associations for different people.

What does compassion mean to you?

Often, when we start our CFT training workshops, we ask people to think about the meaning of the word 'compassion' for themselves. It's interesting what a mixture of responses we hear back. A lot of the associations people come up with are things like 'kindness', 'warmth', 'caring', 'empathy' and 'love'. These words seem to convey quite a positive and helpful, friendly tone. However, we also get a lot of other words and phrases coming up that create quite a different tone: 'soft', 'fluffy', 'vulnerable', 'weak', 'naïve'. We think this is really important – the recognition that people start with very different, and often mixed, relationships and feelings with this word *compassion*. For some people, it will signal a really strong and helpful force for the good. For others, it will signal a much weaker and more vulnerable place; something that's feared and best avoided.

> *Learning point 1*
>
> What does compassion mean to you?
>
> - When you think about the word compassion, what feelings come up?
> - Do you have any concerns or worries about it? If you do, remember that's absolutely fine and normal, very understandable and something

> that's widely shared with others.
> - If it feels okay, take a minute to see if you can notice what your feelings are about this word.

The fact that there are such diverse and interesting reactions to the word 'compassion' really highlight the need for us to define exactly what we mean in the context of this chapter, and more generally in the CFT model. So below is the definition that has typically been used by Paul Gilbert, and that I use, as well as other people who are involved with developing, sharing and teaching CFT ideas.

> Compassion is a sensitivity to the suffering of self and others (and its causes) with a commitment to try and relieve it and prevent it.

The first thing to notice about this definition is that it can be divided into two main aspects: first, there's a sensitivity aspect, involving some kind of *engagement* and connection with suffering, difficulty or distress; second, there's an aspect about a commitment to do something about it, which is more about *alleviation* of the suffering. Let's explore these two aspects in a little more detail.

The first aspect of compassion, which we call the 'psychology of *engagement*', involves the ability to understand, approach and engage with the difficulty or distress. Just think about that for a minute, what that actually means – to engage with something really difficult and distressing. Now that is hard! The easier option would be to turn away. So, turning towards suffering is hard, and it takes strength and courage. Does that sound 'fluffy' or 'soft' or 'weak' to you? Absolutely not. In this definition, compassion is very much about strength and courage to move towards, tolerate and engage with something difficult and painful (whether it's your own pain or distress, or that of someone else).

The second aspect of compassion, which we call the 'psychology of *action*', involves the desire and motivation to do something about the distress, to uproot the causes, and to try and prevent them from causing more distress in the future. Again, let's just think about what that actually means. To do something helpful in the midst of distress is likely to require a fair amount of confidence, knowledge and skill. Confidence that I *can* be useful; wisdom about *how* to be useful in this particular situation, and the skills, tools or resources to actually carry this out. And even with all these qualities, it still might take some time, so this intention to be helpful is also likely to require patience, persistence and dedication.

Now that we've clarified the CFT definition of compassion and broken it down a little, how does this definition sit in relation to your initial feelings about the word? We see compassion as something quite different to some of those negative associations that are often mentioned (e.g. 'soft', 'weak' and so forth). Although these are common, they are not what we would associate with the definition we're using in this chapter. We would see compassion more as a moral courage and motivation to be helpful and supportive, involving key qualities such as wisdom, strength and caring commitment.

> *Learning point 2 – Your intuitive knowledge of compassion*
>
> Imagine you are with somebody struggling with similar things that you've struggled with. Maybe they are frightened or hearing voices that are difficult for them.
>
> - How would you like to show compassion for them? How would you like to talk to them and be with them? How would you feel towards them?
> - If you could be very compassionate to somebody you care about who is struggling, how do you think that would be for them?
>
> That's great. That's your intuitive knowledge of compassion, right there.

Why do we need compassion?

We need compassion because life is tough. It really is tough. One of the reasons for this is that we, as humans, have very *tricky brains* to contend with. Many of the patterns and systems hard-wired into our brains through evolution cause all sorts of problems for us. If you think about it, the human brain was not perfectly designed and built for our 21st-century life. Scientific evidence (from the study of fossil records) suggests that the human brain has evolved over many thousands of years, through different periods where human lifestyles, environments and dangers were very different to those we face today. Even before we evolved into humans, it is probable that what is now the human brain had been evolving for a few million years already, operating and functioning in even more diverse environments (including, most probably, under water).

Not only are our brains not perfectly designed for our lives *today*, they are also not designed for what so many of us aspire to today – happiness. Other, more powerful needs have driven and shaped brain evolution; most importantly, survival. So what I am suggesting here is that our brains are built more for survival than for happiness or wellbeing. And, in an evolutionary context, this means survival in a whole range of (historical) environments, including those with predators sniffing around for their human lunch. So, it's no wonder that today, in our Western, industrialised, 21st-century lives, we often find that our brains cause us problems. For example, very strong survival-based emotions can suddenly take hold of us, our decisions and our actions. One moment we might be sitting comfortably at home on the sofa, and the next we can be totally consumed with a powerful rage or fear, triggered by something we've seen on television. This is the brain doing its job. Even though there's no actual, real danger, the brain's job is to keep us safe and ensure our survival. It therefore sends powerful emotions through our body that are of no use to us in this precise moment, but would, in our past, have made the difference between life or death.

Essentially, our brain is not very well designed for us in *our* lives now. And that's not our fault. That's just the way it is. We're all in the same boat together with this; our brain is built in a way that is likely to cause us suffering, and that's one of the key reasons why we need compassion, for each other and for ourselves. We often think that our brains and bodies should work perfectly, and if they don't, something's gone wrong, or there's something wrong with *us*, or it's our fault in some way. But, as we'll see in this chapter, so much of the time, it's really nothing to do with us at all. It's often very much to do with our tricky human brains.

Compassion shapes our minds

According to evolutionary psychologists (who study our minds in terms of their evolutionary function), there are patterns in our mind that have not been learned or picked up by us; they are built-in patterns that we are born with. Paul Gilbert calls these 'social mentalities', which can be described as co-assemblies of motives, emotions and information-processing routines and behaviours that are hard-wired into the brain through evolution (similar, in many ways, to Carl Jung's idea of 'archetypes' (Jung, 1917/2014)). The activation of a social mentality essentially switches on and off different components of the mind, orientating it towards a specific social role as well as its reciprocal social role. Because of this, the social mentalities are fundamental to relationships. We're now going to look at some of the evolved patterns of mind organisation that might be particularly relevant for voice hearers.

An important social mentality (pattern of mind/brain organisation) in all humans is one that's focused on social rank – that is, social hierarchy in terms of who is more powerful and dominant in a group and who is weaker and subordinate. Our evolved social-rank mentality has the job of orientating our minds towards the dominant, controlling power of some people, and towards the vulnerable, weak, powerlessness of others. Understandably, our social-rank mentality will become particularly activated if we go through our own personal experiences of being in dominant- subordinate roles. For instance, if we have felt vulnerable in the presence of a powerful other, such as being bullied, hurt or abused, this would activate our social-rank mentality. With this mentality switched on, our mind would naturally be more focused on the power of others and our own powerlessness. Other aspects of this mentality might be feelings of defeat, inferiority, rejection and shame, more sensitivity to social comparison, and the use of protective strategies such as submission, depression and dissociation.

Research with voice hearers has shown that many do report difficult experiences of bullying, discrimination and abuse in their lives (Varese et al., 2012), and also that the relationships people have with their voices often mirror some of these dominant-subordinate relationships (Birchwood et al., 2000, 2004). Social-rank theory can help us understand why our person-to-person social experiences might map onto the relationships we have with our voices. When our built-in, evolved patterns become activated and accentuated through experiences, this not only shapes our minds, it also organises our relationships with people and voices (Heriot-Maitland et al., 2019).

So, a big question for this chapter is, if we are distressed by voices ourselves, or if we are helping someone who is distressed by voices, how might we *re-shape* our/

their minds away from social-rank mentalities towards patterns that are more helpful for their wellbeing? In this chapter we argue, consistent with the CFT approach, that intentionally shaping our minds with compassion (or 'compassionate mentality') will be more helpful for us and for our relationships. In the same way that 'social-rank mentality' is a hard-wired pattern that can be switched on and off by experiences, environments and so forth, 'compassionate mentality' is also hard-wired, linked to our evolved human motives for caring, attachment and affiliation. We may not recognise it right now, but there is a compassionate mind built into all of us, and in this chapter we will be exploring the various ways we can access it, cultivate it and use it to start organising our relationships with ourselves, other people and our voices.

Table 29.1 will help you identify some of the differences between the two mindsets.

Table 29.1: Social-rank-threat and compassionate-self patterns

Examples of social-rank-threat patterns	Examples of compassionate-self patterns
Words/thoughts/voices • Insulting voices ('You are useless'; 'Loser'; 'Slut') • Threatening voices ('I'm going to kill you'; 'I'm going to hurt you') • Blaming voices ('It's all your fault') *Attention/focus* • On any potential danger • Scanning for evidence that people don't like me or are against me (and ignoring evidence that they're not) • How can I keep myself safe? • Attention on the power of voice and my vulnerability *Body* • Tense, alert • Heart beating fast • Quick breathing *Behaviour* • Avoid eye contact • Stay in	*Words/thoughts/voices* • 'This is your threat system' • 'These are linked to memories of…, it makes sense why this feels so real – this was the reality back then' • 'It's not happening now'; 'It's okay'; 'You're safe'; 'You're a good person' • 'You can ride the wave of anxiety' • 'Brains are tricky'; 'It's not your fault' *Attention/focus* • Mindful – present moment • Acts of kindness • Gratitude • Imagery (safeness/compassion) *Body* • Soothing breathing • Upright, grounded posture *Behaviour* • Composed, calm • 'Fake it til you make it'

Compassion-focused therapy for voice hearers

The idea of bringing a *compassion focus* to therapy essentially means that the therapy is aiming to help someone engage their compassionate mentality as the place from which to address the difficulties they're struggling with. The claim is that, whatever emotional concerns a person would like help with in therapy, the help is more likely to be successful if these concerns are approached, understood and addressed from the compassionate mind – a mind state that organises multiple physiological processes differently to a threat mind state, which has been prepared, shaped and trained to address threat-based concerns. To describe how this unfolds in a course of therapy, I will take you through the stages of a 50-page therapy manual that we developed for a CFT research study in collaboration with people with lived experiences of voice hearing. The therapy contains five main stages:

1. establishing safeness and connection
2. learning about evolved (tricky) brains, emotional systems and multiple selves
3. understanding how my emotions and mind have become shaped
4. building the compassionate self
5. directing compassion to self, others, emotional parts and voices.

1. Establishing safeness and connection

This stage of therapy aims to create experiences of safeness, stability and groundedness in the body. This involves experimenting with certain body postures and movements to support these experiences. We practise slowing down our breathing while paying attention to sensations of slowing down in our body. People often find that slowing their breathing and practising taking smooth, even breaths can lead to feeling calmer, more settled and grounded. We can also practise focusing on images and memories of safeness (e.g. a 'safe place'), which is another way of cultivating these feelings in the body.

2. Learning about evolved (tricky) brains, emotional systems and multiple selves

In this stage of therapy, we learn about how our brains can be naturally tricky and problematic for us. This is due to evolved functions and patterns that can result in our minds getting caught in what CFT calls 'loops' – angry loops, depressive loops, self-critical loops and so forth. There might be loops about feeling others are trying to harm us, feeling judged, or feeling overwhelmed and unable to cope. The list is endless. It can be helpful to start (mindfully) noticing our own daily loops and patterns, so that, rather than being caught up in these, we can step back and become an *observer* of them instead, and maybe even a *compassionate observer*.

> ### *Learning point 3 – Your daily loops*
> - What are your typical daily loops?
> - Over the last week, can you think of times when you might have got stuck in loops?
> - Remember loops are built in, they're things we all share. It's not your fault.

In this stage, we also learn about the three major emotion systems (threat, drive, soothing) and recognise how our experiences and loops are linked to different emotion systems. For example, problematic experiences and relationships with voices are often driven by the threat system. We also learn about our 'multiple selves', which helps us to recognise, name and give identities to certain patterns (e.g. my 'anxious self', 'angry self', 'sad self', 'paranoid self' and so forth). This extends to mapping out our voices as well (e.g. 'critical voice', 'anxious voice' and so on).

3. Understanding how my emotions and mind have become shaped

The aim of this stage is to try to understand how our past experiences and relationships might have contributed to the difficulties we are now experiencing in our daily lives – for example, with paranoia and voices. In CFT, we focus on understanding the development and maintenance of the threat system by looking at i) early experiences; ii) key threats; iii) strategies (to protect ourselves from threat), and iv) unintended consequences of these strategies.

4. Building the compassionate self

The 'compassionate self' is a self-identity that acts as a container for all the various practices, postures, qualities, skills, motives and so on that are being practised. In this stage of therapy, we aim to develop the compassionate self as an embodied experience that we can 'step into' to help focus on the particular qualities/skills needed to address the struggles with voices. We can ask questions like, 'What would my compassionate self ideally be like in order to deal with this struggle?' 'Even if we feel we can't do it, what qualities would my compassionate self be drawing on to be able to do this?' When relating to voices, it might be that compassionate qualities of strength and wisdom are important: that is, strength to stand up to voices and fears, along with wisdom to understand what's driving them (from past experiences) and to determine a helpful way forward.

5. Directing compassion to self, others, emotional parts and voices

Once we have developed a compassionate self (e.g. using imagery, posture and so forth, and lots of practice) we can then 'put it to work'. This involves directing the compassionate self into the areas of life that are difficult, such as anxiety and fears ('anxious self'); losses in your life and lost opportunities ('sad self'), as well as 'psychosis'-related experiences such as voices and the parts that are feeling paranoid about rejection or harm (for example). We can aim to direct compassion to these experiences in a number of ways, using techniques such as role-plays (compassionate self-talking with another self/part/voice), chair work (switching between different chairs to embody the different parts), imagery and letter writing.

The evidence base for CFT for voice hearers

There are several small-scale studies evaluating the effectiveness of CFT for voice hearers and comparing it with other treatment. In one such study, compassionate mind training was used to help three participants with experiences of malevolent voices. This therapy focused on developing empathy and compassion for their distress and self-criticism, which was found to lead to a reduction in the malevolence of voices (Mayhew & Gilbert, 2008).

In another study, Braehler and colleagues (2013) evaluated CFT groups for 22 participants with psychosis-related experiences, including voice hearing. They found statistically significant reductions in depression associated with psychosis among the group receiving CFT, but not among the control group (who were receiving what is known as 'treatment-as-usual' – generally medication and monitoring). However, the differences between the two groups were not significant.

Evidence from a recent case series study of seven participants receiving individual CFT for psychosis (five of whom were voice hearers) showed that CFT improved measures of depression, stress, general wellbeing, voices and delusions – improvements that were maintained six to eight weeks after therapy had finished (Heriot-Maitland, 2020). One participant from this study has shared some of his therapy experiences in a book chapter co-authored with his therapist (Heriot-Maitland & Russell, 2018, p.110). He used CFT to address his relationship with distressing voices. He reflected:

> I know it's hard to accept that to love and care for these evil voices is the correct way to go. But think about it, by giving this caring love to them you are really giving yourself this love. The voices are you, they are not external, they are part of you. Be compassionate to yourself.

There are also several personal accounts in the literature from another voice hearer who has experienced CFT for psychosis (Ellerby, 2013a, 2013b, 2014a, 2014b; Kennedy & Ellerby, 2016).

These are all relatively small studies and, although they show promising indications, further research is needed before conclusions can be drawn about the effectiveness of CFT for voice hearing.

Conclusions

You may feel there is a lot to take in here. There is! And sometimes it's hard to imagine from just reading a text what the approach would actually look like in real life. This is why my colleagues and I have also produced two videos to illustrate and bring to life the ideas and approaches described above. These are freely available on YouTube via the weblinks given in the references. They are *Compassion for Voices* (Cultural Institute at King's, 2015), which is a five-minute animation overview of the main stages of CFT for voice hearing, and *Engaging with Voices* (Engaging with Voices, 2019), which is a series of 15 demonstration videos, each focusing on different aspects of the approach.

If it's still feeling like quite a lot of information, don't worry; take your time with it. Maybe come back to it later and read it again. It took me a while to get my head around this too. If there is one key idea to take away from this chapter – one key process that I would recommend as something that can be practised over and over again – it would be this: notice when the threat system pops up, name it, and then shift into a compassionate mindset (go back to Table 29.1 for some practical examples).

> *Learning point 4 – Noticing threat patterns and switching to compassion*
> - What do you notice about your threat patterns?
> - How can you prepare the body and mind for compassion?
> - If you could be your most grounded, wise and compassionate best, how would you engage with your voices? What would be the tone/expression/body language of your compassionate self in this interaction?

I'd like to close with a quote from Paul Gilbert at the end of the *Compassion for Voices* video, which reminds us about the point made at the very start of this chapter: that compassion is absolutely not soft or a weakness. At the very heart of compassion is courage – the courage to turn towards and engage with the more difficult and distressing aspects of our experience: 'Compassion is the courage to descend into the reality of human experience.'

References

Birchwood, M., Gilbert, P., Gilbert, J., Trower, P., Meaden, A., Hay, J., Murray, E. & Miles, J.N.V. (2004). Interpersonal and role-related schema influence the relationship with the dominant 'voice' in schizophrenia: A comparison of three models. *Psychological Medicine, 34*(8), 1571–1580.

Birchwood, M., Meaden, A., Trower, P., Gilbert, P. & Plaistow, J. (2000). The power and omnipotence of voices: Subordination and entrapment by voices and significant others. *Psychological Medicine, 30*(2), 337–344.

Braehler, C., Gumley, A., Harper, J., Wallace, S., Norrie, J. & Gilbert, P. (2013). Exploring change processes in compassion focused therapy in psychosis: Results of a feasibility randomized controlled trial. *British Journal of Clinical Psychology, 52*(2), 199–214.

Cultural Institute at King's. (2015). *Compassion for voices: A tale of courage and hope*. [Video]. www.youtube.com/watch?v=VRqI4lxuXAw

Ellerby, M. (2013a). How compassion may help me. *Psychosis, 6*(3), 266–270.

Ellerby, M. (2013b). Schizophrenia, Maslow's hierarchy and compassion-focused therapy. *Schizophrenia Bulletin, 42*(3), 531–533.

Ellerby, M. (2014a). Resisting voices through finding our own compassionate voice. *Schizophrenia Bulletin, 43*(2), 230–232.

Ellerby, M. (2014b). Schizophrenia, losers and compassion-focused therapy. *Psychosis: Psychological, Social and Integrative Approaches, 6*(4), 359–362.

Engaging with Voices. (2019). *Engaging with Voices.* [Video playlist]. www.youtube.com/playlist?list=PLOP1SbuZkEPwWlsOdfnRr5ZDDgiTN6FE5

Gilbert, P. (2009). Introducing compassion-focused therapy. *Advances in Psychiatric Treatment, 15*(3), 199–208.

Heriot-Maitland, C. (2020). *Social influences on dissociative processes in psychosis.* Unpublished PhD. King's College London. https://kclpure.kcl.ac.uk/portal/files/130519645/2020_Heriot_Maitland_Charles_1276898_ethesis.pdf

Heriot-Maitland, C. & Russell, G. (2018). Compassion-focused therapy for relating to voices. In C. Cupitt (Ed.), *CBT for psychosis: Process-orientated therapies and the third wave* (pp.98–113). Routledge.

Heriot-Maitland, C., McCarthy-Jones, S., Longden, E. & Gilbert, P. (2019). Compassion focused approaches to working with distressing voices. *Frontiers in Psychology*, 10:152. doi: 10.3389/fpsyg.2019.00152

Jung, C.G. (1917/2014). On the psychology of the unconscious. In C.G. Jung, *Collected works of C.G. Jung, volume 7: Two essays in analytical psychology* (2nd ed.) (pp.3–120). Princeton University Press.

Kennedy, A. & Ellerby, M. (2016). A compassion-focused approach to working with someone diagnosed with schizophrenia. *Journal of Clinical Psychology, 72*(2), 123–131.

Mayhew, S.L. & Gilbert, P. (2008). Compassionate mind training with people who hear malevolent voices: A case series report. *Clinical Psychology & Psychotherapy, 15*(2), 113–138.

Varese, F., Smeets, F., Drukker, M., Lieverse, R., Lataster, T., Viechtbauer, W., Read, J., van Os, J. & Bentall, R.P. (2012). Childhood adversities increase the risk of psychosis: A meta-analysis of patient-control, prospective- and cross-sectional cohort studies. *Schizophrenia Bulletin, 38*(4), 661–671.

30 Working with voices using the narrative genogram

Lykourgos Karatzaferis

The narrative genogram is a 'tool' that is used to work with families, as a way of showing how relationships between members of the family are formed through time. The basic guideline, when conducting the genogram, is to ask the person to choose an important relationship in their life (e.g. the one with their mother or father) and think of some stages (e.g. moments, experiences, time periods) of this relationship that they consider to be important 'milestones' in the development of the relationship. Then, they are asked to make some drawings (using symbols and such like) that will represent the person's sense and feelings regarding each 'milestone', culminating in the final drawing, which shows how the person imagines the relationship in the future.

In this chapter, I present the use of the narrative genogram with people who are experiencing distress in the relationship with their voices. A narrative genogram, when used with voice hearers' relationship to their voices or other non-shared experiences, can create a very helpful depiction of the relationship dynamics between them. Our experience with the narrative genogram involves the basic principles of the Hearing Voices Movement (HVM) being applied together with the dialogical self theory (DST). For example, one of the core values of the HVM states that it may be possible for voice hearers to learn to relate to their voices as a social network, and for some this may even turn into relating to them like a 'family'. In this way, it is like a system with which the person interacts. The relationships with the voices may be dynamic and change over time; there can be conflicts, negotiations, exchanges and debates. There may be more prominent and dominant or quieter and less dominant voices, which usually have specific names, their own stories, and so on. Such an understanding is very similar to the view of DST, which views the self as a society, with oppositions, conflicts, negotiations, cooperation and coalition between positions (Hermans, 2002).

We also know that people who get along with their voices, as opposed to those who do not, are more likely to cope with the experience of hearing voices. The use of the narrative genogram can thus be helpful for voice hearers who want to change their relationship with their voices, which may in turn also lead to positive relationship changes with other people.

This chapter reflects on practical experiences with the narrative genogram in relation to voice hearers' relationships with their voices and other non-shared experiences as they emerged during my collaboration with the Athenian Hearing Voices Network self-help group. As a co-founder of the Athenian Hearing Voices Network, I have worked with many people (voice hearers, professionals, family and so on) over time, facilitating workshops, presentations and seminars. In this way, we worked on the narrative genogram in order to propose a way of dialogical engagement with voices that could prove beneficial.

A voice is rarely just a voice

The Hearing Voices Movement (HVM) recognises that people hear voices in a wide range of circumstances. For some, it is an unremarkable feature of everyday experience; for others, it is a part of religious and spiritual devotion, an aspect of bereavement, or a source of intense creativity. A voice is rarely 'just a voice'; as personal as it might seem, it comprises cultural, political and sociological traits that we could explore (Woods, 2015). It is recognised that voice hearing has meaning, and therefore hearing voices cannot be regarded as a useless, meaningless symptom, regardless of its severity. The HVM does not focus on voices as being a sign of illness but as an experience that is rich in meaning, which, if properly deciphered, can yield important information (Corstens et al., 2014). So, before reading any further, let's consider the following:

> *Learning point 1*
> - Have you ever considered that hearing voices is a common human experience, which could be meaningful and understandable in the context of life events?
> - You may have found yourself hearing difficult or troubling voices, but could you imagine this relationship with voices changing over time?
> - Did you know that for many voice hearers understanding and accepting the voices has proved to be more beneficial for recovery, compared with continued suppression and avoidance?
> - Did you know that there are people who hear voices who have a more balanced, harmonious relationship with their voices than voice hearers who are troubled by distressing voices?

The voices may represent a part of the person that wishes to be heard. Many voices are experienced as aggressive and malicious; yet even an angry person needs to have an opportunity to express their anger and let off steam. It is important to note that often it is the case that anger hides other emotions. Many angry people might suppress other emotions, as they may not have felt that they have had an opportunity to express how they actually feel. The HVM recognises that some voices can come across like 'normal' people or be related to in that way. That is, voices may have feelings, motives, failings, capacities and opinions. Voices may use strategies that are not based on just thinking about things or rationalising them. Instead, they might react when they are upset. In that sense, a process of understanding and accepting one's voices may be more helpful for recovery than continued suppression and avoidance (Corstens et al., 2014).

The collaborative origins of the HVM, coupled with the contemporary developments in service user/survivor-led research, mean that the HVM approach necessitates the full participation of experts-by-experience at all stages. For voice hearers, this principle can be summed up by the phrase 'Nothing about us without us', which opens various perspectives for collaborative work at all levels: in recovery, research, therapy, peer support, and more (Corstens et al., 2014).

This emphasis on the partnership between voice hearers and professionals marks an important shift away from most existing approaches, which rarely shed light on the views of those who have actually experienced the mental health difficulties (Baker, 1989).

Seeking for meaning in dialogues

Human beings often search for meaning. Meaning may emerge from an interactive exchange between two or more people that takes place in an interpersonal space. Both the listener and the speaker produce the meaning of an expression, because a response is required for words to have meaning (Seikulla & Trimble, 2006). Thus, human behaviour can only be understood by navigating our way through a complex network of social, cultural, historical and political contexts.

Important theorists like Nietzsche, Bruner and Vygotsky have argued convincingly that there is a constant interaction between internal and external dialogues (Lysaker et al., 2001). Our narratives, our point of view of ourselves and the world are shaped by our resources (internal stimuli) and social expectations (external stimuli), thus maintaining a dialogue between the self and the environment (Lysaker et al., 2001).

We all grow in dialogue and being open to dialogue means being open to learning. Learning is a process where the individual recognises that their state of mind does not hinge on any particular identity but on the relationship between various different sub-selves that together make up the person (Bateson, 1972).

Human life and consciousness are dialogical (Bakhtin, 1984); we observe, think, question, make meaning and so on as part of an uninterrupted dialogue in which we are fully involved throughout our lives. As people, we are surrounded by discourses that pervade the whole structure of human life.

> *Learning point 2*
> - Voices are not meaningless.
> - Seeking for meaning could prove a wonderful collaborative work between the voice hearer and a professional.
> - Knowledge doesn't emerge in empty space. Learning from your experience is a process of dialogue and exchange.

Listening to the experts

Before reading any further, I invite you to reflect on the following:

> *Learning point 3*
> - Have you ever considered yourself to be an expert-by-experience?
> - Who else do you need to include in your dialogue about your voices, and what would their reactions be to what is happening? How can another person collaborate to make this a better way of working?
> - Sometimes we cannot simply get away from a person we do not like. But we could possibly change our relationship with him/her. Would you like to dream of a different relationship with your voices? If yes, what steps should be taken?

When psychological experiences or problems are perceived as barriers to the fulfilment of our dreams, it will likely lead to seeing these experiences as a deficit. In contrast, perceiving psychological problems or experiences as 'messengers' for being in touch with our needs and emotions opens up new ways into exploring future dreams. Many professionals are trained to detect and, ideally, eliminate so-called symptoms, as these are considered unhelpful deficits. In this way, the potential of simply being present and approaching an experience such as hearing voices with curiosity about what the voices need and what their message might be is excluded. It might also be helpful to hypothesise about a helpful function that phenomena that are experienced as problems (as voices often are) might have in the person's life (Lang & Markou, 2017).

Peter Lang and Elspeth McAdam (1997) introduced the Systemic Appreciative Approach, offering an important paradigm for learning, dialogue and acceptance. Their techniques provide a way to open a dialogue so that a path for appreciation can emerge. It is not their techniques or their ideas that make their work unique, but mainly their ethos and values. For Lang (Lang & Markou, 2017), the 'heart' of their approach is the ethical stance of a 'not-knowing position' – the belief that people are experts in their own lives.

Speaking about 'a Systemic way of thinking' means taking into account the richness of the system, the coherence of the system, the idea that it is eco-systemic. (Lang & Markou, 2017, p.10)

When we don't place our expertise first but we really listen to what people say, we prioritise their narratives and their truth and regard them as experts on their own experience. Bateson (1972) suggested that we should look at the whole richness of the stories in the system of people that we are talking about. Following his example, Lang poses the following questions: 'Who else do we need to include? What would their reactions be to what is happening? How can they collaborate to make this a better way of working?' (Lang & Markou, 2017, p.10). Having such questions in mind when working with voices can lead to a better observation of what is happening and what kind of changes occur. Similar to voice hearing, any part or member of the system that is ignored might return to haunt you later.

Lang used the narrative genogram as the main tool when working with families. It reflects the progress of relationships – both 'intrasystemic' ones among members of the family and relationships with the external environment.

First of all, the members of the family are invited to choose a specific moment of the past and to depict the relational patterns that they experienced at that time. Following this, the members reflect on how their relationships have progressed (from the past) until now.

When using the narrative genogram, we are interested in what stories the family members tell about their relationships and how they usually deal with any crisis in the family relationships in a functional way. Through the use of the schemata of the traditional genogram, the distance and the closeness among people over the years, as well as the conflicts, identifications, infusions, differentiations, losses, reparations, repetitions and so on are depicted. It is important to offer family members the possibility to comprehend that relationships are not static. They are sometimes repeated from generation to generation, or up to a certain point. Relationships do not necessarily progress in a way that is acceptable for all family members, but in time these relationships can change according to the desires and dreams of the family members (Gotsis, 2017).

Learning while playing – experience of the narrative genogram with voice hearers

The following structure was formulated in collaboration with the Athenian Hearing Voices Network self-help group, which has a 10-year history and, crucially, has adopted the principle of participation of voice hearers at all levels of action. Apart from 'spreading the word' about the normalisation of hearing voices, in line with HVM principles, the Athenian Hearing Voices Network runs internal and external activities, contributing to the empowerment of everyone included. One of these activities is the formation of the self-help group, which consists of people who hear voices or have other unusual/non-shared experiences. Their weekly meetings provide peer social support and a sense of belonging that does not constitute therapy or treatment. The number of participants varies each time, as some might take a break or leave the group, while others may join.

So, when I came up with the idea of facilitating a workshop using the narrative genogram in relation to voices, I addressed the group by sending a brief description, in plain language, of the concept of such a workshop. As the whole idea should be adapted to the needs of the members of the group, we worked together and co-constructed a plan that included the adaptation of the narrative genogram for voices, and developed a list of the possible questions to be asked, as well as some basic ground rules. The main intention was to highlight the key concept, which is that 'It is of cardinal importance for human beings to give meaning to their lives', while inviting people to share (or not share!) and creating space for all voices.

There are six steps that we identified in our process of using the narrative genogram with voice hearers and voices, which are briefly described below.

1. Definition: 'Which voice do we want to focus on together?'

This phase is used to clarify the area of work to be considered. Therefore, the voice hearer could be asked to recollect memories regarding their relationship with their voices from two important dates in the past and one in the present. These would then be referred to as 'stages'. They could be regarded as important 'milestones' in their relationship with their voices. It also seemed to be helpful for the voice hearer to concentrate on and work with only one voice at a time.

2. Discovering: 'How did the relationship evolve and what was helpful during this process?'

This is about reflecting on voice hearers' abilities to relate in a dynamic way to their voices. Moreover, we try to find what works beneficially in relating in a helpful way to the voices. This phase is about rediscovering and remembering the successes, strengths and periods of excellence in dialoguing with the voices.

3. Drawing: 'How would you draw on paper the relationship's milestones?'

One could use colours of any kind to depict the various voices and the relationships to them. In general, relationships can be presented in any creative way that one may think of. Symbols that can be used for the voices and the relationships can include natural phenomena, lyrics and so on. For each stage/milestone, a (nick-) name can be given. Pluymaekers & Nève-Hanquet (2008) state that the obligation to represent the information graphically (i.e. on an A3 sheet of paper or on a chalkboard) encourages the participants to be spontaneous, with each participant drawing whatever comes to their mind at that moment. Some choose colours and drawings, others choose text, or underlining, arrows and so on. And so, a complete story emerges…

4. Dreaming: 'Could you dream of yourself and your relationship with the voice in the future?'

The narrative genogram facilitator encourages the participant to choose a point in the future (e.g. 10 years ahead) and talk about how they dream their relationships evolving. Dreaming uses past achievements and successes that are identified in the discovery phase to imagine new possibilities and a preferred future. It allows people to identify their dreams, having discovered 'what is best'. They have the chance to project their dream into their wishes, hopes and aspirations for the future. This process is not fixed in advance and, therefore, a voice hearer might dream of patterns that increase closeness or distance, or those that reflect the breakage or reparation of the relationships.

5. Design: 'What steps have you made to fulfil your dream?'

Following this, voice hearers are invited to talk about their future as if it is happening now: for example, 'Imagine we are at a point 10 years from now and your dream has already come true. We meet again at this specific time and you are telling me in detail what exactly you have done to achieve it.' The discussion is conducted as if the future has already happened. *Design* brings together the stories from *Discovery* with the imagination and creativity from the *Dream*. It is called bringing the 'best of what is' together with 'what might be', to create 'what should be – the ideal'. In the final stage, the voice hearer designs the steps that would help them in the relationships with their voices according to the way that they imagined the relationships during the previous stage.

6. Delivery: 'What would be your first step tonight as commitment to fulfilling your dream?'

At this stage, we are interested in the clear expression of the first action to be undertaken. The basic question encourages the voice hearer to undertake simple actions (e.g. 'Take care of myself') that will help us to see how they are achieving their dream. It also strengthens the participant´s commitment to the previous steps.

The structure above could be used either for peer-to-peer work or in a group. It is important to mention that, during the whole process, the voices might get actively involved, consulting the voice hearer or providing ideas. When using it as part of a workshop for voice hearers, it could provide even more fruitful exchanges. Participants could be invited to briefly present whatever they want and new ways of engaging may possibly appear. Questions may lead to new directions in our discussion. Below are some useful questions that could shape the process:

- 'Reflecting over the process of design, what feelings and ideas arose for you?'
- 'What difficulties did you meet?'
- 'As you observe your drawings, what do you discover? How was your experience?'

It is important to highlight the steps made at each stage and to highlight the abilities of the person while their relationship with their voices evolves. This provides a direct reference to the work of Elspeth McAdam (McAdam & Mirza, 2009), which is known as ability-spotting: that is, skills that have never been recognised and valued before become part of a person's identity and their new resources for the future. McAdam and Mirza (2009) use 'back-lighting' as a technique that could also be applied: looking back on the story of the relationship and shedding light on the strengths and resources. This includes describing the obstacles that we have encountered on the way and how we overcame these obstacles. Furthermore, instead of seeing them as obstacles, they become landmarks of achievement and celebration along the road.

Paul's drawing – an anonymised example

Paul chose one of his voices, a male voice, that he had heard at the age of 25. He recalls this as his first milestone. He calls this voice 'the grim reaper', since it caused him great pain. It was very hard for Paul to listen to this voice, as it caused a lot of disturbance. It is one of the most difficult voices that Paul has ever had. In the beginning, the voice was positive but it quickly changed to being negative. Paul does not know why it changed to a negative voice. This was the voice he drew. At the age of 31, Paul had taken out some sticks to fight it ('do battle'). He managed to face the voice and threaten it, using these sticks. In this way, Paul treated the voice as it had treated him. Sometimes Paul regrets doing this, but it had been called for. And now, at 40, Paul feels himself to have come to be in a bizarre relationship where he threatens the voice with sounds and words! Choosing strong sounds, small verses and lyrics, Paul tries to draw the voice with sound and word symbols. In fact, Paul had heard a song and dedicated it to the voice. Paul threatens the male voice that if he does something to him, the song will not be dedicated to him anymore. The voice does then behave itself. That is how Paul threatens the voice. He feels that their relationship has gone to a weird place. Sometimes, when Paul tells the voice to leave him alone, he stops. Sometimes Paul tells him, 'Aren't you bored?'

Today, Paul can say: 'I am an ally with this voice in the world of voices,' as he has taken a small step by dedicating a song to the voice.

Conclusion

The narrative genogram encourages voice hearers to retrace the history of their relationship with their voices, from a present viewpoint. At the very least, it facilitates an opportunity for the voice hearer to say something about that history that stresses the emotional and metaphorical aspect of the voices, rather than just their genealogical aspect. The difficulty is, therefore, not simply the act of being able to write out how a person's relationship with voices evolves over time, but rather the emotional and metaphorical confrontation with this history, which will shed light on strengths and potentials that are inherent in this experience.

As we have learnt from the exercises, the main objectives of a narrative genogram can be summarised as follows:

> *Learning point 4*
> - Take a look at the dynamic character of a person's current relationship with their voices.
> - Focus on the way in which we continually change and reconstruct our relationships
> - Acknowledge the fact that the depiction of the process opens up not only the possibility to reflect on them, but also to redefine relationships.

The narrative genogram reveals information that is interesting, because it tells us something about the history of the voices and the way that those voices evolved over time. The graphical representation and the associated remarks suggest analogies and metaphors whose depth of meaning will be the basis for the healing process of creating a potentially more constructive dialogue with the voices (Pluymaekers & & Neve-Hanquet, 2008).

Working with the narrative genogram can therefore be potentially beneficial for the recovery journey for voice hearers, as it offers a means to understanding and accepting their experience. The depiction of one's relationship with one's voices through a *genogram* (visual stimuli), combined with the *narration* of the story (oral stimuli), provides a considerable amount of information and enriches the experience. Questions arising from the perspective of a 'not-knowing curiosity' may stimulate inner reflection and links between the voices and other life experiences or relationships.

The use of a narrative genogram should only be conducted as part of a genuine collaboration with voice hearers at all levels, as this is of the utmost importance both for their recovery journeys and also in affording us new insights in research settings. We have to look deeper and listen more carefully to what people with lived experience have to say.

Acknowledgements

With respect and appreciation to Artemis Kolomvrezou, Danae Kokorikou, Peter Bullimore and all the members of the Athenian Hearing Voices Network self-help group for their invaluable support.

References

Baker, P. (1989). *Hearing voices.* Manchester Hearing Voices Network.

Bakhtin, M. (1984). *Problems of Dostoyevsky's poetics.* (C. Emerson Ed.). University of Minnesota Press.

Bateson, G. (1972). *Steps to an ecology of mind: Collected essays in anthropology, psychiatry, evolution, and epistemology.* University of Chicago Press.

Corstens. D., Longden, E., McCarthy-Jones, S., Waddingham, R., & Thomas, N. (2014). Emerging perspectives from the Hearing Voices Movement: Implications for research and practice. *Schizophrenia Bulletin, 40,* 285–294.

Gotsis, I. (2017). Training with Peter Lang (Part 2): Transferring and implementing in the Organization against Drugs (O.KA.NA) during the years 2013–2016. *Metalogos, 30.*

Hermans, H. (2002). The dialogical self as a society of mind: Introduction. *Theory & Psychology, 12*(2), 147–160.

Lang, P. & Markou, S. (2017). Interviewing Peter Lang. In S. Markou (Ed.), A tribute to Peter Lang. *Metalogos, 30.*

Lang, P. & McAdam, E. (1997). Narrative-ating: Future dreams in present living jotting on an honouring theme. *Human Systems: The journal of systemic consultation and management, 8*(1), 3–12.

Lysaker, P.H., Lysaker, J.T. & Lysaker, J.T. (2001). Schizophrenia and the collapse of the dialogical self: Recovery, narrative and psychotherapy. *Psychotherapy, 38*(3), 252–261.

McAdam, E. & Mirza K.A.H. (2009). Drugs, hopes and dreams: Appreciative inquiry with marginalized young people using drugs and alcohol. *Journal of Family Therapy 31,* 175–193.

Pluymaekers, J. & Nève-Hanquet, C. (2008). Training of family therapists and the landscape genogram: A tool for personal development and supervision human systems. *The Journal of Therapy, Consultation & Training, 19*(3), 212–221.

Seikkula, J. & Trimble, D. (2006). Healing elements of therapeutic conversation: Dialogue as an embodiment of love. *Family Process, 44*(4), 461–475.

Woods, A. (2015) Voices, identity and meaning-making. *The Lancet, 386*(10011), 2386–2387.

31   Mindfulness and hearing voices
Rufus May and Elisabeth Svanholmer

Mindfulness is increasingly used in mental health settings as a gentler approach to managing challenging experiences and relationships. Mindfulness is about learning how to sit with sensations and one's reaction to them with non-judgemental awareness. Through mindfulness exercises, we can learn to be more aware of where we put our attention and how we can have more choice about this.

We see it as complementing the accepting approach to hearing voices as developed and particularly encouraged by the Hearing Voices Movement since its beginning in 1987 (Romme & Escher, 1993). We have now been active members of this movement for many years. However, we recommend using mindfulness with discernment and in a way that is flexible and tailored to each person who uses it.

For the purpose of this chapter, we asked people to contact us and share their personal experiences of hearing voices and using mindfulness. We have found both from using mindfulness in hearing voices groups and workshops and in the responses to us on the internet that it is important to for mindfulness to be used creatively and tailored to the individual (as opposed to a manualised approach). One person talked about the benefits of mindful smoking – they felt that the commonly cited exercise of 'eating a raisin mindfully' was not helpful. Another person described how they had found their own kind of mindfulness by taking simple pleasure from 'a damn good cup of coffee or the smell of fresh cut grass'.

We have included anonymised personal accounts (unless otherwise described) later in the chapter to illustrate the different experiences people have had with using mindfulness. (The accounts are shortened for this chapter. You can find the full accounts at openmindedonline.com)

Research evidence

There is a danger in being too reliant on evidence from academic research to inform decisions about whether something is useful or not in practice. The so-called evidence-based approach can encourage working in a rigid way and shuts down the creative potential of working individually, tailoring your approach and technique to each person or group.

There has been relatively little research specifically looking at hearing voices and mindfulness. Strauss and colleagues (2015) conducted a review of 15 studies, with a total of 479 participants, looking at the evidence for mindfulness being accessible, engaging and helpful for people who hear voices. They concluded that the results were encouraging and that more research was needed. Stephanie and colleagues (2018) carried out research with 63 people who heard voices and found that mindful relating to voices was associated with less voice-related distress, less avoidance and less internal struggle with the voice-hearing experience. Dudley and colleagues (2018) surveyed 128 voice hearers and found that developing mindful attitudes towards voices and greater self-compassion were associated with less voice-related distress.

There have been more studies looking at mindfulness and psychosis, which will likely have included people who hear voices (as this is often considered to be a psychotic experience), even if they did not specifically focus in on the nature of their experience. In this larger category of psychosis, there have been several studies showing how mindfulness group courses can improve general clinical functioning and an improvement in mindfulness skills (Chadwick et al., 2009; Langer et al., 2012; Bardy-Linder et al., 2013; van der Valk et al., 2013).

In a qualitative study of a mindfulness group, Abba and colleagues (2008) reported that participants learned to recognise and let go of 'self-defeating thoughts' about difficult voices and difficult thoughts, and that this led to an increased sense of empowerment and acceptance of themselves and their experiences.

Chadwick (Chadwick et al., 2016) suggested that guided mindfulness exercises can be more accessible to people hearing distressing voices or experiencing paranoia if the guidance is more frequent. We imagine this can reduce the chance of being distracted by voices' expressions. Chadwick suggested a normalising approach to voice hearing that will help the person learn to be more accepting of their experiences. Hearing voices groups can be helpful in promoting this accepting attitude (Romme & Escher, 1993, 2000).

Introduction to mindfulness

Mindful approaches aim to bring us back to our senses – to what is happening in the here and now. Mindfulness is rooted in Buddhist meditative practices and has been developed in Western contexts to help people manage things like stress and pain to improve their mental and physical performance.

In pain management, mindful body scans are used to help people both be more accepting of their pain and be aware of the parts of the body that are not in pain. Pain is thought to be intensified by people's resistance to it. Thoughts such as 'Why is this happening to me?' or 'I hate this pain' can increase the experience of the actual physical pain. Mindfulness exercises can help people become aware of the pain as it is, without adding to it by fighting it, and help them feel they have more agency in how to respond to and look after the pain.

In the Hearing Voices Movement, there is a similar ethos that, if we can encourage the voice hearer and their social network to be more accepting of the voices, the experience of hearing voices can become more manageable.

As well as learning to adopt an accepting attitude, there is a range of mindfulness exercises that people who hear voices might find helpful. Exercises can help people feel more grounded and more in touch with things happening both around them and within them.

Our values are that everybody has wisdom about their own experience and their own bodies, so if you try the exercises in this chapter, please listen to your own wisdom on how you experience them. An exercise that is useful to one person might be another person's nightmare. Some people find one exercise that works for them and stick with it and other people use a range of exercises and develop them over time to fit their need.

Mindfulness principles

When the concept of mindfulness was developed for use in Western contexts, it moved away from being a spiritual practice with a strong philosophy and ethos. Today, mindfulness is often described as a tool and it can be used in a targeted way to manage unwanted experiences. However, some people advocate using mindfulness exercises as more than a way to calm ourselves, the argument being that it can also help us build up and sustain particular mental and emotional skills that can help us in all parts of life.

Jon Kabat Zinn (2001), a mindfulness teacher, was one of the first people to make mindfulness more mainstream. He emphasises the importance of these mindful attitudes:

- acceptance – accepting what is present rather than suppressing it or wishing it was not there
- non-judging – observing objects and events without evaluating them
- patience – we stay with the present moment and don't rush towards the next exciting event
- beginner's mind – seeing things with an open mind and noticing their unique qualities
- letting go – developing the ability to switch attention and let go of one object of concentration and focus on another
- being with – as opposed to trying to fix, control or achieve
- non-striving – letting go of constantly striving for better moments
- non-attachment – relating to things with kindness but not clinging onto them, and recognising that everything changes.

> ### *Learning point 1: Reflecting on mindful attitudes*
> Think about which of the attitudes above you have some positive experience with and which attitudes you find challenging.

Ways to practise mindfulness with the body

The most well-known way to practise mindfulness is by using breathing exercises or breathing meditation. Again, we want to emphasise that different exercises and strategies suit different people. In relation to breathing exercises, some people find them calming or grounding. Others can find breathing exercises put them in touch with feelings that are too uncomfortable for them to focus on, such as a tightening in the chest or a panicky feeling. If so, it may be better to find another mindfulness activity to use.

Other commonly used practices are body scans and Yoga Nidra. These are guided meditations that encourage people to focus on different parts of their body and slowly scan across the whole body. They can help people relax and may also strengthen the ability to be more fully present while staying flexible and able to let go.

> ### *Learning point 2: Mindful breathing exercise*
> Find a comfortable place to sit. Notice how your body feels. Notice how your shoulders feel and how the ground feels beneath your feet. Focus about 25% of your attention on your breathing. Try not to force the breath; notice it coming and going.
>
> Time yourself for three to five minutes, or as long as you feel comfortable with.
>
> If it is the first time you have tried this, we recommend keeping the exercise brief as it is more about noticing what it is like for you than managing to do it for a certain amount of time.
>
> You could try these other options:
>
> - Put one hand over your heart area and the other hand over your belly and notice how your body moves as you breathe in and out.
> - Count your in-breaths and out-breaths up to 10. In your mind, say 'Breathing in one, breathing out one, breathing in two, breathing out two', and so on, up to 10. When you get to 10, you count from one again. If you get distracted at any point, go back to the last number you remember being at.

Mindful movement is another way to practice mindfulness using the body. For some people with a lot of thoughts or energy, it can be uncomfortable to sit and focus on the breathing. Mindful movement can be more accessible and grounding than physically inactive practices.

There is a practice called 'Ten mindful movements', guided by Thich Nhat Hanh, which can be found on YouTube.[1]

People have variously described tai chi, chi gong, yoga and pilates as well as other more Western intense exercise regimes like spinning, circuit training and boxercise as being helpful and grounding.

> *Learning point 3: Movement*
>
> Go for a 15–30-minute walk or try some of the movement exercises at openmindedonline.com. Take time to notice – and maybe write down – how you feel before, during and after the exercise.

This is Louisa's experience (anonymised):

> I have tried breathing exercises, but I get too anxious. Yoga is like a breathing exercise but you're moving around and engaging a lot of your body so it's easier for me to concentrate. Also running while singing has become a very good mindful exercise for me. I don't know if this counts, but when my voices are getting too difficult, I remind myself that they are just voices, they cannot hurt me or force me to do anything.

Mindfulness using our senses, the environment and different activities

Mindful activities that use our senses can help us ground ourselves and shift our attention. Some people find that their mind gets a chance to calm down when it is regularly applied to mindful activity.

It can be helpful to spend time each day doing one thing mindfully. Mindful activity means trying to focus our attention wholeheartedly on the thing we have chosen to do.

First, decide what to do. Then focus fully on it. Every time you get distracted, bring your attention back to what you are doing. You will probably need to do this a lot of times. If you keep getting distracted by something, give it some attention, as it may be important. Or pencil in a time to address the distracting issue later, and return to your mindful activity.

There are many ordinary, everyday activities that can be done mindfully, such as washing up, dog-walking, cooking, cleaning, gardening and exercise. Other activities could be colouring in and crafts like knitting, woodwork, felting or embroidery.

---

1. www.youtube.com/watch?v=4mz-dJFkmrk

> ***Learning point 4: Mindfully noticing your environment***
>
> Try using an exercise called '5, 4, 3, 2, 1'. Take the time to notice five things you can see, five things you can hear and five things you can feel. Then do the same thing with four things, then three, then two and finally one. When you've finished, reflect on how you found this.
>
> - Was it difficult, annoying, fun, calming or something else? How much was your experience influenced by the environment you were in? Might it be different if you tried it in a different place?

Mindfulness and hearing voices

When people practise mindfulness, they may feel restless. People can become more aware of their emotions, uncomfortable sensations in their bodies or how active their mind is.

The same is true with hearing voices – the voices might become clearer or they might seem to become more talkative or aggravated. This may be because some voices find it threatening when the person practises mindfulness. The voices may feel jealous and try to distract the person from their mindfulness exercise.

Some people have found it helpful to include their voices in the exercise. For example, you could explain the exercises to the voices and tell them they are welcome to join in. Also, if you are comfortable with this, you can invite the voices to choose which exercise they would like you to practise. The aim here is to share choices with the voice, but only do activities that you are comfortable with. You can also dedicate soothing exercises to voices that are obviously upset, such as crying voices or voices urging self-harm. This involves telling a voice you are dedicating the exercise to him, her or it before carrying out the soothing exercise. Many people have reported that crying voices calmed down when they dedicated a breathing exercise or a face massage to them.

This is Ander's experience (Anders Vo Shakow is an active member of the Danish Hearing Voices Network):

> It wasn't actually my idea to start using mindfulness. I was in my mid-20s, had been given a diagnosis of paranoid schizophrenia and was living in a 24-hour supported institution. I was hearing three voices and the voices wanted me to become a Buddhist monk as a punishment.
>
> At the time I had a support worker who practised Buddhism and she knew about the voices I was hearing and what they were saying. But she didn't want to impose any Buddhist practices or teachings on me because she didn't know if it was something I really wanted.
>
> I was in a pretty desperate place and I decided I was willing to accept the punishment the voices were suggesting because I was hoping the voices would take a step back or be less distressing. I started looking into

Buddhism myself and I eventually approached my support worker about it. She suggested some books I could read, and she taught me a couple of meditation exercises. There was only one of the exercises that I kept using. It was a pretty simple breathing meditation where you focus on the sensation at the top of your nasal passages. I had to practise a lot before I felt able to use the exercise when I felt anxious.

I practised the exercise with my support worker sitting with me while she guided me verbally. I needed somebody there to keep an eye out because it was very scary for me to close my eyes. A lot of my paranoia was about people coming to kidnap and torture me, so I was always on high alert. Having somebody there helped me practise the breathing exercise.

I found that I could use the meditation to deal with my anxiety, which would be at its worst in the evening when I was supposed to go to sleep. Nothing had really helped me. I was on a lot of medication and still I couldn't get to sleep because I was so scared of people coming to get me. The beliefs and the voices would feed into each other and they had a lot of power over me. Sleeping meant I couldn't keep watch and protect myself and this would make me so scared I would have something like panic attacks, with palpitations, struggling to breathe and sweating.

When I was overwhelmed by fear, it was hard to do the breathing exercise, so it was important for me that I kept practising. It made it easier to access when I had the panic attacks. What I found was that, by being able to control my breathing and ground myself through my breathing, I didn't get drawn into the panic. This also meant my physical responses would change. I wouldn't get all the weird sensations that happened when I was hyperventilating. When I was able to control my breath, then my body and my heart would calm down and I started being able to get to sleep by meditating.

And then there was a point where I stopped seeing the meditation as part of a punishment or a task I had to complete. It was probably sometime after I started working more directly with the voices and was able to link them to my life story. So my understanding of the voices changed. I stopped getting so drawn into this different universe and I could see my experiences as linked to painful stuff I had been through in my life. It was a slow process. There was a long time where I still felt uncertain about what to believe and the anxiety only went away very slowly. I did a lot of work with my anxiety and through all that I found the breathing meditation useful to help me calm myself.

I don't think people can expect mindfulness techniques to directly affect the voices or make them go away. Maybe it's more likely that mindfulness can help you cope with anxiety caused by the voices. But learning to be in control of your body and its responses might help you feel you have more power and more choice, which could help in dealing with voices. The ability to accept what you hear without getting drawn in and being able to shift your focus can make you feel more in control and give you confidence and skills you can use in other situations with voices and in life.

> *Learning point 5: Thinking about your motivation*
>
> If you hear voices and want to try mindfulness, it might be helpful to explore what you hope to achieve. Maybe you hope to get a break from the voices? To feel less afraid or emotional? To focus on tasks and not be distracted by the voices? Do you hope to get better at managing stress? Or it might be something completely different.
>
> Having a clear idea about your hopes for practising mindfulness might help you decide whether an exercise works for you or not.

Mindfulness in groups and with other people

For some people, mindfulness is easier to practise in a group. We have found that people often value doing a grounding exercise at the beginning or end of a hearing voices group meeting, or when the group has been talking about something that has evoked strong feelings. In the Bradford hearing voices group, we sometimes do an exercise called 'do-in', where you gently tap different parts of the body (see openmindedonline.com).

Mindfulness used in clinical settings has been criticised for neglecting the social causes of distress. If it's used as a mental 'band aid' or a panacea, it can mean we miss other possibilities that practising mindfulness can bring to our lives, such as helping us in our relationships with others. Thich Nhat Hanh, a Buddhist monk and mindfulness teacher, has emphasised that mindfulness is a way of life that promotes more peaceful relationships in the wider world as well as between individuals. Hanh (2001) has been part of an engaged mindfulness movement that has sought to work in war-affected areas such as Vietnam, where he is from. He suggests finding ways to be with people who are suffering is an important mindfulness practice that awakens us to social and psychological realities.

> *Learning point 6: Using mindfulness with other people*
>
> Try to think of situations where you might be able to use mindfulness with other people. Do you attend meetings where it might be nice to do an exercise together – at the beginning or the end or as a way to take a break? Do you spend time with someone who talks a lot or is very quiet – could you use mindfulness to sit with them, however they are? Do you spend time with children – could you play with them in a mindful way – perhaps by being aware of your senses? If a friend is in distress, could you use a calming exercise for yourself to help you be with them in their distress?

Problems with ways mindfulness can be used

In my (Rufus) clinical experience and in both of our experience organising training and peer support spaces for people who hear voices, we have come across people who hear voices who have been put off by the prescriptive way they have been introduced to mindfulness exercises. That's why we say it is important to listen to your own wisdom about what feels manageable at any one time when trying out new exercises.

If mindfulness is practised obsessively and too intensively, it can be destabilising for some people. What seems to prevent this destabilisation is having other people to share experiences of practising mindfulness with and not overdoing it. Some people have run into problems when they have done an intensive retreat without building up to it more gradually with a regular mindfulness practice.

Another difficulty can be that practising mindfulness may sensitise us. We become more aware of our bodies and our senses when we use mindful exercises, which means we can acquire a heightened sensitivity. For some people, this is a wonderful thing, because they become more aware of pleasurable sensations and the beauty of the world around them. In a more spiritual context, people might call this transcendence, and some teachers see this as something to pursue.

However, some people find this heightened sensitivity overwhelming and may need support to manage it. They may decide it isn't something they are interested in continuing to develop. A heightened sensitivity has its pros and cons and, depending on your social and environmental context as well as your life history, it might not be what you want.

> *Learning point 7: Taking a person-centred approach to mindfulness*
> - Are there parts of practising mindfulness that you feel concerned about?
> - Have you heard stories from other people that have put you off or have you had your own experiences of trying mindfulness and not liking it?
> - We have a website www.openmindedonline.com where we have 26 different mindfulness exercises we have called Mindful Minutes. Try some of the different exercises and notice how you find them.
> - Can you see a way of changing an exercise so that it works better for you?
> - Are there things you already do that you could adapt and make into a mindful activity?

Using a trauma-sensitive approach

Because research has shown that a high number of people who hear voices have experienced trauma, we think it important to take a trauma-sensitive approach when using mindfulness with voice hearing.

Trauma-informed approaches recognise that mindfulness, yoga and other awareness practices can open people up to trauma memories (Treleaven, 2018).

Practitioners of trauma-informed approaches emphasise the importance of avoiding exercises that may trigger high levels of discomfort. They advocate tailoring exercises to the individual and being guided by the person's intuitive sense of what feels safer and more grounded.

If a mindfulness exercise does seem to initiate high levels of stress, it is wise to avoid this particular practice, or, if the person prefers, try it again at a later date.

Supporting people to develop a sense of their own authority and choice can be useful. Mindfulness can be used to help do this. In her book *8 Keys to Safe Trauma Recovery*, Babette Rothschild (2010) talks about helping people develop a 'mindfulness gauge' for decision-making. People are encouraged to check in with their felt sense when making decisions. Rothschild encourages people to start with simple choices, like whether to have tea or coffee, an apple or an orange, and learn to listen to how the body responds at the thought of each choice.

This is Jake's experience (anonymised):

> I find mindfulness practice impossible to do. However, I find the principles very important. It seems very useful in order to survive being overwhelmed to be able to step back from what your own mind is doing.
>
> I find practitioners of mindfulness are rather over-zealous and not trauma sensitive.
>
> For me, guided practices don't feel safe, but I can see it might be safer than being alone for other people. I tend to find one thought or image that I can return my attention to, and these tend to be linked to spirituality.
>
> Mostly I cannot cope with being aware of my breath, and ground myself by thinking of my toes, elbows, heels or something like that. I think mental health practitioners don't understand that bodies can be deeply terrifying and sources of harm, because it is literally unthinkable to them that forms of abuse can cause such intimate damage and that this damage can be so different for different people.
>
> What I took from the things that work for me is that mindfulness and spirituality go hand in hand, so for me secular mindfulness is missing something. For me, finding meaning in suffering is spiritual, so secular mindfulness teaching feels very flat and lacking in richness.
>
> I think for mindfulness to work better we need a better understanding of trauma. Safe ways of doing it and how to stop safely need to be established first. Flexibility is needed.
>
> At the moment, I focus on breathing. Earlier in my life, I focused on an image of light, or of being at ease with pain rather than fighting it. At bad times I do tai chi rather than yoga, and walking or moving mindfulness rather than mindful sitting. I try being aware of washing up or chopping – being aware of the moment, but outside of me rather than inside. This is helpful and essentially a way of not spacing out, so it helps me find a way to be more present, not less.

Conclusion

Research looking at using mindfulness to help people with distressing or challenging voices suggests it may be helpful in a number of ways. This includes leading to less distress relating to voice hearing and greater levels of compassion for oneself. An accepting attitude is an important principle in mindfulness practice. This is also an important theme in the Hearing Voices Movement, which aims to promote accepting attitudes towards voice hearing in individuals and their support networks. In this chapter, we have shared principles and examples of a range of different ways one can practice mindfulness. We have shared a number of personal accounts of the different ways people who hear voices have used mindfulness to their benefit. We suggest people adopt a person-centred approach to using mindfulness. This means trying out different exercises and styles of mindfulness and listening to one's own wisdom on what feels comfortable to practise and develop. We think it is supportive to practise mindfulness with others and have spaces to reflect on how it is useful or how it may also be unhelpful. With such support networks, we think mindfulness practices offer different ways that can help people who hear voices ground themselves and tune into their own intuitive sense of how to best respond to inner and outer experiences.

Acknowledgements

Thanks to everyone who contacted us via social media and provided personal accounts. And thanks to our Hearing Voices Movement colleague Anders Vo Shakow for sharing his experiences.

References

Abba, N., Chadwick, P. & Stevenson, C. (2008). Responding mindfully to distressing psychosis: A grounded theory analysis. *Psychotherapy Research 18*(1), 77–87.

Bardy-Linder, S., Ortega, D., Rexhaj, S., Maire, A., Bonsack, C. & Favrod, J. (2013). Mindfulness training in group to cope with persistent psychotic symptoms. *Annales Medico-Psychologiques 171*(2), 72–76.

Chadwick, P., Hughes, S., Russell, D., Russell, I. & Dagnan, D. (2009). Mindfulness groups for distressing voices and paranoia: A replication and randomized feasibility trial. *Behavioural and Cognitive Psychotherapy, 37*(4), 403–412.

Chadwick, P., Strauss, C., Jones, A.-M., Kingdon, D., Ellett, E., Dannahy, L. & Hayward, M. (2016). Group mindfulness-based intervention for distressing voices: A pragmatic randomised controlled trial. *Schizophrenia Research, 175*(1-3), 168–173.

Dudley, J., Eames, C., Mulligan, J. & Fischer, N. (2018). Mindfulness of voices, self-compassion, and secure attachment in relation to the experience of hearing voices. *British Journal of Clinical Psychology, 57,* 1–17.

Hanh, T.N. (2001). *Anger: Buddhist wisdom for cooling the flames.* Random House.

Kabat Zinn, J. (2001). *Full catastrophe living: How to cope with pain and illness using mindfulness meditation.* Piatkus.

Langer, A.I., Cangas, A.J., Salcedo, E. & Fuentes, B. (2012). Applying mindfulness therapy in a group of psychotic individuals: A controlled study. *Behavioural and Cognitive Psychotherapy 40*(1), 105–109.

Romme, M. & Escher, S. (1993). *Accepting voices*: Mind Publications.

Romme, M. & Escher, S. (2000). *Making sense of voices.* Mind Publications.

Rothschild, B. (2010). *8 keys to safe trauma recovery: Take-charge strategies to empower your healing.* W.W. Norton & Co.

Stephanie, L., Rossell, S.J, Lin T.W., Monique, S. & Thomas, N. (2018). Does mindfulness help people adapt to the experience of hearing voices? *Psychiatry Research, 270,* 329–334.

Strauss, C., Thomas, N. & Hayward, M. (2015). Can we respond mindfully to distressing voices? A systematic review of evidence for engagement, acceptability, effectiveness and mechanisms for change for mindfulness-based interventions for people distressed by hearing voices. *Frontiers in Psychology, 6,* 1–12.

Treleaven, D. (2018). *Trauma-sensitive mindfulness: Practices for safe and transformative healing.* W.W. Norton & Co.

Van der Valk, R., van de Waerdt, S., Meijer, C.J., van den Hout, I. & de Haan, L. (2013). Feasibility of mindfulness-based therapy in patients recovering from a first psychotic episode: A pilot study. *Early Intervention in Psychiatry, 7*(1), 64–70.

Part three

Creative approaches to working with voices

32 Creative ways to engage with voices
Rufus May and Elisabeth Svanholmer

The Hearing Voices Movement (HVM) has been arguing for an accepting approach to hearing voices since 1987. The HVM is made up of networks of self-help groups for voice hearers as well as mental health practitioners, researchers and volunteers who support this approach. Research carried out by Romme and Escher from the late 1980s onwards (Romme & Escher, 2000) found that many people lived harmoniously with their voices. Romme and Escher suggested that, rather than trying to get rid of voices, the aim should be to help people live with their voices.

This involved changing the relationship with voices from one that is antagonistic to one that is more equal and mutually respectful. Romme and Escher's research suggested that voice hearers didn't have to be stuck in a distressing relationship with voices. They found that people who hear voices could change the power relationship with their voices by building their confidence and assertiveness, learning negotiating skills, finding an accepting community and accessing support to make sense of their voices in relation to their lives in ways their community respected. In the book *Living with Voices: 50 stories of recovery* (Romme et al., 2009), many of the contributors describe how they found ways to achieve this so they no longer lived in fear of their voices.

Mainstream research has not yet caught up with this change in the direction of what the aim of helping people should be. For example, as yet there is no measure that looks at the quality of people's relationship with their voices. Rather, rating scales tend to look at the presence or absence of voice hearing as a measure of mental wellness.

Several therapeutic approaches have been developed that seek to help people change the relationship with their voices, many of which are covered in other chapters in this book. This chapter will focus on using the Talking with Voices approach (Chapter 19) and exploring creative ways to engage with voices as part of that approach.

Getting to know voices better

Our values are that everyone has expertise and wisdom about their voices and there is no single best way to see or understand voices. When we engage with people who hear voices and the voices they hear, we emphasise being open-minded, curious, respectful and non-judgemental.

More often than not, at the core of the distress people experience when hearing voices are problematic ways of relating, and the relationship between the person and the voices they hear is shaped by the person's life experiences (Heriot-Maitland et al., 2019). Ways of relating are learned through relationships, and modelling equal and non-judgemental ways of relating can be an essential part of supporting people to find ways to live with their voices. Our attitudes and values might be just as important – if not more – than the model of understanding or therapeutic technique we use.

It is easy to make assumptions about voices as we are exposed to stereotypical stories about voice hearing through the media and popular culture. But, in reality, we never know what a voice is like, what its history is or why it is saying and doing the things it does until we have listened to the person hearing voices and the voice itself.

In a culture where listening to voices is still seen as possibly damaging and dangerous, it can feel daunting to spend time being deeply curious about a voice. This is especially so if the voice and its behaviour seem to be the cause of great distress to the person hearing it and the only relief they can get is by pushing the voice away and distracting or numbing themselves.

> *Learning point 1*
>
> The way the media and people around us talk about hearing voices can have a big impact on how we feel about ourselves if we start hearing voices. If we only know of stories about people being 'crazy' or 'ill', it can be very scary to experience voices and it's easy to lose confidence in oneself. We can internalise the stigma and judgements that we hear from other people. An antidote to this can be finding stories where people live well with voices or even use them as inspiration, support or something to learn from.
> - Can you think of any stories about voice hearing that gives a positive view of voices? You could research historical accounts of people whose voices have been an inspiration or useful (e.g. Gandhi, Joan of Arc, Swedenborg, Hildegard of Bingen, Jung, and many more).

Getting to know voices better is about gathering information: about the person, their life, the voice and the relationship between them. It can be helpful to see the relationship between the person and the voice as like living with a family member and there being no way of moving out or avoiding them. The more information we have about this family member, the better we can support the person to find ways to live in the same house as them.

> *Learning point 2*
>
> Here are some examples of questions that can help to build a better picture of the voice and its individual traits and personality.
>
> - Does it sound male or female?
> - Does he/she/it have a name? If not, would you or they like to give the voice a name?
> - How old does the voice sound? Has it got older as you have got older or has it stayed the same age?
> - What kind of things does the voice say?
> - What is important to the voice (e.g. performance, safety, power, control)?
> - How does the voice relate to other voices you hear (if this is relevant)?

> *Learning point 3*
>
> We can ask questions about the relationship between the voice and the person's life.
>
> - Does the voice sound like or remind you of any person you have known?
> - How long have you been hearing the voice?
> - What was happening in the period just before you started hearing this voice?
> - What is your relationship with the voice like?
> - Are there significant life experiences the voice might be linked to?

Creative ways to get to know voices better

We live in a very visual world and something that is difficult about voices is that no one else can hear or sense them like the voice hearer does. It can feel very lonely, and it can be difficult for other people to understand or empathise with what the person is going through.

Finding different ways to represent the voices can help the hearer see the relationship between themselves and the voice differently. It can also make it easier to talk about the voices with others and make it easier to engage in a dialogue with the voices (Craig et al., 2016).

Drawing

If people feel comfortable with drawing or painting, you can work with them to create images that represent the voices. The images can be abstract; they can use colours, textures, patterns or words – anything that captures some of the characteristics of a voice for the hearer.

This can also be done using a paint programme on a phone, tablet or computer. Rachel Waddingham, a trainer, advocate and campaigner with lived experience, has made a film about living with voices, *Short Thought #2: Get to know your voices*.[1] In it, she suggests drawing circles for each voice and filling the circle with colours, patterns, doodles or textures that represent the voices. This can be a way of checking in with the voices regularly and keeping a record of how they are at different times.

Collages

Creating collages can feel less intimidating than drawing. Find some old magazines, tear or cut out pictures, colours, words and anything else you can find that represent the voice for you and glue them to a piece of paper or card. Or you can invite the voices to choose the images or words that they think represent them.

Puppets

Make finger puppets with masking tape and cardboard or by cutting off tips of old garden gloves or similar. Or you can use a wooden spoon to make a puppet core – the bowl forms the face.

Once you've created a core for the puppet you can decorate it with wool for hair and draw a face on it and wind fabric or tissue paper around it to depict the kinds of clothes the voice might wear.

Learning point 4

Try drawing your voices, making finger puppets or making collages to represent your voice or voices. If you don't hear voices, you could do it for parts of yourself.

If you don't feel comfortable doing this, maybe think about or talk with someone you trust about why it feels difficult to do.

- How do your voices feel about being represented?

You may be able to involve your voices in making decisions about how best to represent them. You can try asking your voices for ideas and suggestions about how you can represent them. Or, when using different media, collage, drawing, craft and so on, you could ask for their input – for example, what colours to use in drawings or which images to choose for collages.

---

1. See www.behindthelabel.co.uk/short-thought-2/

Mapping out voices in space

Map out voices using the space you are in. Mapping out voices can be a good way to generate a conversation about the different voices, their role in your life and the relationship between you and the voice, or between different voices if you hear several voices.

You can do it with chairs (or pillows and stools), or you can do it using objects to represent yourself and the voices. If you have limited space, you can draw the relationships on a piece of paper or use small objects on a table or the floor.

Figure 32.1: Mapping the voices

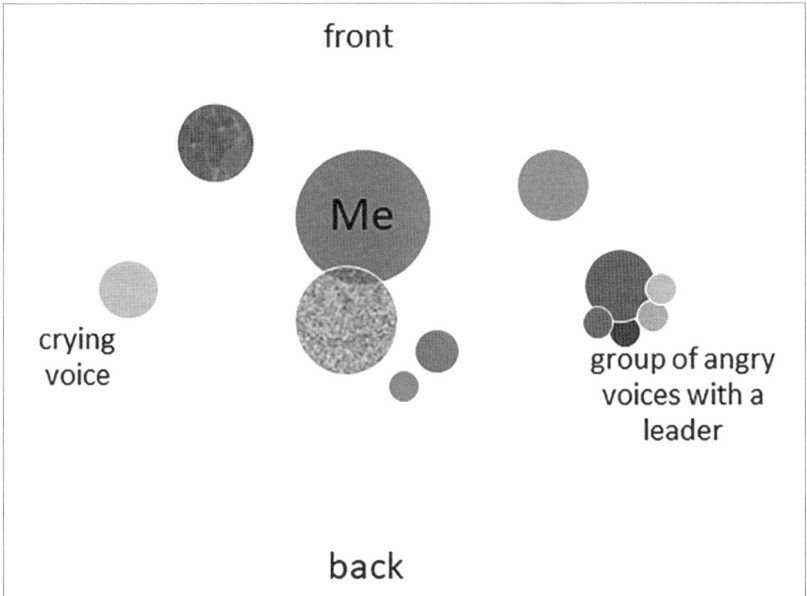

Choose a chair or an object to represent yourself and place it in the room. Then decide where each voice should be positioned in relation to yourself (see Figure 32.1). Are they in front or behind? Are they far away or close by, or even inside you? Are they protecting something – an emotion, a secret or part of the person? Are they facing away from you or towards you? Are they positioned higher or lower than you?

If you are using objects, try to find a broad selection of objects that somehow remind you of the voice it represents. Or ask the voices if they have an opinion on the object that should represent them.

Your map is likely to change over time. If it's not on paper, you could take photos of each map and use them as reference points to see how the relationship patterns change over time.

Sculpting

This use of sculpting has been adapted from family therapy by Ron Coleman and Karen Taylor (who have been very influential in the HVM). Sculpting voices is where a group of people help the person represent their voice-hearing experience.

The voice hearer asks them to stand in a particular place that symbolises the relationship they have with the voice. They can then act in a similar way to how the voices act, using posture and/or words. The hearer can ask someone else to represent them, standing in the middle of the role-play. Someone can take the role of facilitator and freeze the role-play at a particular point and imagine with the voice hearer how they might relate to their voices differently and encourage them to try them out or watch someone else try them out.

Talking with voices

The Talking with Voices technique (Corstens et al., 2012) has also been influenced by the Voice Dialogue approach (see Chapter 19), which was developed by psychologists Hal and Sidra Stone (Stone & Stone, 1993) to help couples relate better to each other. They describe it as a self-development tool rather than therapy.

So, originally, the Voice Dialogue approach was not aimed at people who hear voices, despite its title, but to explore different parts of people's personality. Voice Dialogue theory suggests we all have different sub-personalities or parts of self (selves) and that it can be helpful to get to know these different parts better.

The aim of the Voice Dialogue approach is to increase the person's awareness of their inner parts and support them to better manage and negotiate between different selves and their different needs. One way to get to know our different parts better is for somebody else to interview them one at a time. This is done by asking the voice hearer to identify a part they want to get to know better and then change chairs to sit where they feel that part to be in the room. Then the facilitator (as the interviewer is usually referred to in Voice Dialogue practice) of this Voice Dialogue process conducts an interview with the part. (The process is described in more detail in Chapter 19.)

Let's say it's the voice hearer's ambitious part. The facilitator can ask this part questions about its relationship to the person and what it wants for them. The facilitator does not try to change the part/self/sub-personality. Instead, they take a more curious and neutral stance, exploring the role of the part, its history and its opinions. Questions might include: 'How are you?', 'What is your job?', 'What do you want for the person?', 'What would their life be like if you were not there?', 'Do you have any advice for the person?' The ambitious part may say it wants the person to get up earlier and create more of a routine and believe in themself more.

Then, when the conversation is complete, the voice hearer moves back to their original chair and, with the facilitator, reflects on the views of the ambitious part and whether they want to take on board some of its advice.

The interview is conducted in a non-judgemental and respectful way towards the part of the person. When the interview is finished, the part is thanked for their contribution.

It's important to take a balanced approach to negotiating with the parts. You don't want to give one part too much power, but you need to be careful not to deny a part because it can then go into opposition to the rest of the self. Voice Dialogue recommends a middle way where parts are listened to and negotiated with but not blindly obeyed. This is called 'honouring the different parts of the self'. So, using the example above, the person may find it helpful to listen to the ambitious part but also create space for a self-caring part that doesn't want to push them so hard and allows them to rest and recuperate.

You can read more about this in the Stones' book, *Embracing Our Selves* (1993).

> ### Learning point 5
>
> It can be interesting to think about personality as made up of a group of selves.
>
> - Have you noticed that you behave differently at different times and in different situations?
> - Think of three strong characteristics in your personality. For example, are you competitive, or very helpful, or very good at problem-solving? Are you good at organising, being creative or doing things to a high standard? Are you laid back, confident, diplomatic and good at keeping others happy?
>
> As you reflect on your different parts, consider what might be each part's strengths and weaknesses.
>
> - Can you think of times when a part of you has made decisions that you later have regretted? Despite this, can you see how that part of you was trying to help you?

Interviewing the voices

The Voice Dialogue interviewing style can also be used to help voice hearers better understand their voices. For example, the facilitator can ask the hearer to move to a different chair (or cushion or part of the room) and report what the voice is saying from there. They can ask the voice similar questions to those asked in Voice Dialogue, as suggested above. So, questions might include: 'How are you?', 'What is your job?', 'What do you want for the person?', 'What would their life be like if you were not there?', 'Do you have any advice for the person?'

When the hearer is comfortable to be interviewed and answers directly as the voice, or lets it speak through them, we call this *direct* interviewing. An example of direct interviewing would be to ask a voice, 'How are you?' and the person would then say exactly what the voice tells them: for example, 'I am not happy because Christmas is coming.'

But some hearers feel more comfortable if the voice is interviewed *indirectly*. This involves asking the hearer to ask their voice questions themselves and report indirectly (in the third person) what the voice is saying. An example of *indirect* interviewing might be: 'Can you ask your voice how he is?' and the person responding: 'He says he is not happy because Christmas is coming.'

Like Voice Dialogue, the interviewer is not trying to change the voice; rather, they are interested to explore what is important to the voice, what its intentions are and how it perceives things. New information may emerge from the interview that can help the hearer understand their voice in a different way.

For example, a voice that tends to talk a lot when the person is trying to sleep may explain in an interview that it feels anxious at night and would like a bedtime story to help it relax.

Voices that sound like abusers will sometimes share that they are not the abuser but a younger part of the person that was around and took some of the abuse.

The aim of a facilitator talking with another person's voice is to help the hearer find new ways to relate to their voice and find time to regularly talk with their voice themselves. We have several films that demonstrate talking with voices, which are available online.[2]

Talking with voices as self-help

Some people are comfortable talking with voices on their own, but others can find it very overwhelming and scary. They may need support to find ways to make it feel safer to talk with voices themselves.

Making conversations with the voices part of their routine can be helpful for some people and it can be helpful for the voices too. Routine can be about both time and space as well as about having certain activities planned before and/or after talking with the voices.

It might be important to have designated space where the hearer can talk with voices. It could be in the morning, in bed, or bed may be the worst place. Maybe it works well to talk with voices while going for a walk. The hearer will need to work it out with the voices, through trial and error.

Planning a regular time to engage with the voices can be useful. It could be a certain time each day or certain times during the week, when the hearer will give the voice quality time and the voice will have the experience of being listened to and taken seriously. If the person is worried about getting drawn in by the voices, they can set a timer to remind them and the voices that the allotted time has come to an end.

It is important to support the hearer to find a balance between listening and talking to voices and engaging with the rest of their lives.

If voices are particularly aggressive or critical, it may be helpful to learn about non-violent communication (see below).

Writing down what the voices are saying can be one way to show the voice that they are being listened to. Writing can also be used to dialogue with a voice. The hearer can write out both what they are saying and what the voice is saying (perhaps using different coloured pens to signify who is speaking). This is also called 'journalling with voices'.

---

2. At www.openmindedonline.com

> **Learning point 6**
>
> Trying to engage with voices can be daunting. If you would like to try this approach, you can watch the videos on www.openmindedonline.com and notice how you feel about talking with voices. You can consider these questions:
>
> - What is your motivation for talking with your voices? Do you hope to achieve something in particular – for example, negotiate times when they give you a break, feel less scared of them, get space to do activities you enjoy without the voices interrupting you?
> - What would give you more confidence to try talking with your voices?
> - Is it something you feel ready to try or do you need more support or safety to try it?
> - How might someone provide that support or sense of safety?

Talking with voices with other people present

We attended a meeting about Talking with Voices in 2018 at Reading University, where Matt Ball, a mental health practitioner with lived experience who lives in Australia, showed us how it can be supportive to have more than one person engage with a voice. It helps break down the hearer's sense of isolation and it can also be a way to bring talking with voices into the community and out of the specialised, professionalised and pathologised bubble where it usually happens. Safety, consent and respect is still essential and bringing in other people may mean spending some time talking about values and taking an accepting approach to voices.

One of the important values in a group Talking with Voices session is that everyone is equal, including the voices. At the beginning of a session, everyone shares how they are feeling and whether they have any concerns or anything in particular they are interested in finding out or understanding better. We make sure that the voice knows what is going on and if it is interested in being asked questions by everyone present.

The facilitator usually starts by engaging with the voice and then can take a break to let everyone reflect on what they have heard. This is when there can be space for the other people present to ask the person or the voice questions. It is important that their questions come from a personal perspective and that they don't take an inquisitorial, objective stance.

Tips for talking with voices that seem critical or destructive

We have found non-violent communication useful for dialoguing with aggressive-seeming voices (Rosenberg, 1999). Non-violent communication assumes that all communication is fundamentally trying to express legitimate feelings and needs.

If we can help a voice express its deeper intentions, it may seem less threatening, and if we can help the voice to feel heard and understood, it is likely to calm down.

There are lists of feelings and needs you can find online.[3] Using the lists, you can ask a voice to choose the feelings and/or needs that it can relate to.

Here are some examples of questions you can ask critical-seeming voices to learn more about why they say the things they say (these are adapted from Sarah Peyton's book *Your Resonant Self* (2017):

- Are you disappointed and do you long for a sense of achievement and belonging?
- Do you feel sceptical of people and long for relationships you can trust and have faith in?
- Do you feel hopeless and tired of trying and not getting acknowledgement?
- Do you feel annoyed that your attempts to help me survive have not been acknowledged?
- Are you tired and exhausted and would you like me to take more responsibility for how I truly feel?
- Does self-harm help you get a break from fearful and angry feelings you experience?
- Do you feel livid and furious and would you like to destroy people to acknowledge the amount of loss you have experienced?
- Are there times when you want me to kill myself because you long for peace? Could we together look at other ways to get your need for peace met?

It is important to emphasise that asking questions that try to be empathic to a voice does not mean agreeing with it. Marshall Rosenberg (1999), in his book *Nonviolent Communication: A language of life*, shares how to empathise with people who are expressing painful feelings aggressively. We recommend reading this book if you want to dialogue with voices that seem angry. Just like people, voices can use blaming and defamatory language when they are feeling unsafe. For example, a voice that calls someone an idiot for falling over may actually be feeling anxious and wanting the person to take more care of themselves.

We think that, if the hearer understands what is driving the voice to be critical or urge destructive behaviour, it can make the voice less frightening and help the hearer find ways forward and so calm the voice down. For example, an aggressive and intimidating voice may deep down want the person to become more assertive and expressive about what they want and need, and this can emerge from a dialogue with the voice.

---

3. We recommend www.cnvc.org/training/resource/feelings-inventory and www.cnvc.org/training/resource/needs-inventory

Learning point 7

Even voices experienced as critical or destructive may have started out having a protective role. The voice may start out in a similar way to a teacher or parent who criticises a child because they want them to become better at something and see them achieve, or a parent who shouts angrily at a child out of fear because they were about to run across the road or reach up for a boiling saucepan. The parent might be feeling scared and act out of love for the child, but they express themselves very aggressively.

- Write down how a critical voice that you hear (or critical thoughts you experience) might be trying to help or protect you.

Conclusion

Historically, hearing voices has been something to try to get rid of, or at best ignore and endure. However, many people in the Hearing Voices Movement have found it helpful to change the relationship with their voices through assertiveness, creativity and empathic communication.

In this chapter, we have looked at some of the ways people can do this. This includes different ways of representing the voices and getting to know the characteristics of each voice through using creative arts approaches such as collage, puppet making and role-play. Speaking directly with a voice can also be helpful and there are different ways to facilitate this. The aim is to help the person be less afraid and feel that they have more choices in how they respond to their voice-hearing experience.

References

Corstens, D., Longden, E. & May, R. (2012). Talking with voices: Exploring what is expressed by the voices people hear. *Psychosis: Psychological, social and integrative approaches*, 4, 95–104.

Craig, T., Ward, T. & Rus-Calafell, M. (2016). AVATAR therapy for refractory auditory hallucinations. In B. Pradhan, N. Pinninti & S. Rathod (Eds.), *Brief interventions for psychosis: A clinical compendium* (pp.41–54). Springer International Publishing.

Heriot-Maitland, C., McCarthy-Jones, S., Longden, E. & Gilbert, P. (2019). Compassion-focused approaches to working with distressing voices. *Frontiers in Psychology*. https://doi.org/10.3389/fpsyg.2019.00152

Peyton, S. (2017). *Your resonant self: Guided meditations and exercises to increase your brain's capacity for healing*. W.W. Norton & Company.

Romme, M. & Escher, S. (2000). *Making sense of voices: A guide for professionals who work with voice hearers*. Mind Publications.

Romme, M., Escher, S., Dillon, J., Corstens, D. & Morris, M. (2009). *Living with voices: 50 stories of recovery*. PCCS Books.

Rosenberg, M. (1999). *Nonviolent communication: A language of life*. Puddledancer Press.

Stone, H. & Stone, S. (1993). *Embracing our selves: The voice dialogue training manual*. Nataraj Publishing.

33 Dramatherapy for people who hear voices
Louise Combes

In this chapter I explore how dramatherapy helps when the voices people hear and are distressed by are beyond language: perhaps they are not yet intelligible or too difficult to be discussed. I will include some exercises I used with someone using NHS Early Intervention in Psychosis (EIP) services, which she found helpful and might help people in a similar position.

What is dramatherapy?

The drama of dramatherapy is not acting; rather, it's self-expression, and it starts without words. The developmental model of dramatherapy is widely practised in the UK (Jennings, 1990, 1994, 2011), and begins with whatever creative expression is most comfortable for the client. **E**mbodied movement, creative **p**rojection onto objects and **r**ole exploration (sometimes abbreviated to EPR) are all entry points, as I will explain. They allow expression of the client's outer world (their social environment) and inner world (their internal mix of voices, feelings and state of mind), without the need for explanation or fear of judgement.

Dramatherapy is person centred. Working within metaphors means that clients choose what to share and what to keep private. They can explore meaning in a way that is relevant to them. Some use this process to externalise issues freely, without feeling self-conscious and without having to share verbally. The therapist values the client's process through witnessing and discussing only what the client chooses to share.

Dramatherapy is one of the arts therapies used in the NHS, along with art and music. Dramatherapists must be trained to Master's standard and be registered with the Health and Care Professions Council. Rather than just using dialogue between client and therapist, arts therapists use the object of creative expression as a third presence in the therapy session. This may be developed by the therapist as directed by the client; it may be created solely by the client, or it can be co-produced with others in a group. This element is a metaphor often containing healing information from our subconscious.

Why drama?

A theatre can safely contain any story. However brutal and destructive the story, theatrical conventions boundary it and protect the witnesses. Theatre is useful to explore the unspeakable. Anyone who saw Gareth Malone's TV choir programme *Our School by the Tower* (Rumney, 2019) will understand how theatre can give permission to safely engage with dangerous material. In this programme, children living near Grenfell Tower in London devised a silent theatrical piece depicting the moment they realised that the tower was on fire and that their friends might be inside. Their teachers worry that the drama is too powerful for the community to witness, just a year after the disaster. In fact, it proves to be a safe way for everyone to acknowledge this terrible shared experience. Tears are shed. The audience is appreciative of the cathartic experience.

Casson's book *Drama, Psychotherapy and Psychosis* (2004) details how theatre has, from its beginnings, been 'a psycho-spiritual forum where sanity and madness are explored' (p.51). He references many examples of theatre that portray non-shared realities, including Shakespeare's Hamlet, who sees the ghost of his dead father, and Aeschylus' Orestes, who is tormented by the Furies, who sing:

> Over our victim
> We sing this song, maddening the brain,
> Carrying away the sense, destroying the mind. (Cited in Casson, 2004, p.51)

Drama involves every kind of human communication that uses human movement, gesture and sound. Just like newborn babies, when we use drama we don't need words to express ourselves and be understood. It enables us to articulate pre-verbal, unspoken emotions and unspeakable thoughts, however light or dark. It occupies the full range of experience. In drama, we work with what we bring. However random and seemingly irrelevant, this playful approach connects us rapidly to our true selves. It brings a new perspective on who we are.

Drama has long functioned as a psycho-social education tool to help people whose experiences and expressions of traumatic distress lead to mental health interventions. Van der Kolk, for example, the well-known international trauma expert, included a chapter titled 'Finding your voice: Communal rhythms and theater' in his important work *The Body Keeps the Score* (2014). Since then, other neuroscientists have identified emotional disconnect as a common problem for people who have been given diagnoses of schizophrenia (Torregrossa et al., 2019) and identified embodiment of feelings as a key component for their recovery (Thirioux et al., 2020). Most recently, Nelson and colleagues (2020, p.2) have argued for more inter-relational approaches in Early Intervention in Psychosis (EIP) services so that clients can experience 'being with' others and explore mood in a more distanced, gentle way than is possible through the current model of cognitive behavioural therapy offered in many services after a psychotic episode.

Drama in therapy can give us sufficient distance from distressing feelings, events or experiences to explore them safely. Landy (1993, p.149) calls this 'aesthetic distance' – a place and moment where creative, playful freedom is possible. Casson (2004, p.120) developed this concept specifically for people experiencing psychosis. He beautifully describes how some people are easily engulfed by emotions and lose their sense of self (they are 'under-distanced'). Others are isolated and, although they may talk easily about emotions, they are split off from feeling them ('over-distanced'). Casson demonstrates how dramatherapy supports the client to find a balanced 'middle distance' (2004, p.122) where healthy relationships between self and other are possible.

Drama in other therapies, what is the difference?

Many therapies are relational. The use of physical space to gain new perspective on the differences between ourselves and others was developed by Moreno and is used in many approaches, including systemic (family) therapy and psychodrama (Marineau, 1989; Compernolle, 1981).

Psychodrama and dramatherapy use theatrical conventions to protect the client. Both divide the therapy room into two realms of the client's experience. The audience space becomes the physical 'real' world. The stage space represents the world that the client wants to explore. However, while psychodrama focuses on re-enactment of real experiences, dramatherapy is useful when people are too confused or uncomfortable to talk directly. In dramatherapy, we work metaphorically, rather than literally.

As an example, in Chapter 19 of this book, Lafferty and Allison explain using chairs in Voice Dialogue for voice hearers. In dramatherapy, I use chairs as a way to unravel a bundle of voices early in a voice hearer's experience. With the action kept separate in a clearly marked area that represents a theatrical stage, it is possible for the client to externalise their internal world safely. I facilitate; the client directs from the audience. Different cloths and objects placed on each chair capture the quality of each voice and help differentiate between them: the powerful, the cruel and the kind. We can go further and use this stage space to understand how the voices interact. With each voice represented by a different piece of material, we can externalise the territory taken by them in the client's head, in the same way that people attending an open-air concert might lay out picnic blankets to mark their seating area as their territory. Filling the stage with colour in this way helps us to understand where the power lies between the voices. So the stage space is used to better understand and control the voices, as directed by the client. The space is a place where clients' hopes can become real, without the limitations of reality. With the greater distance from the problem, clients can work with anything they wish to bring, in a gentle metaphorical way.

Such exercises help people to unpack what is in their heads; to externalise without words. Indeed, a large part of the work is about the client exercising their autonomy to choose what is shared and what is kept private, unarticulated and contained.

Dramatherapy in early intervention services

Since 1999, the NHS has provided an EIP specialist service in the UK. Following a first episode, EIP teams visit the person regularly, with the aim to 'improve short- and long-term outcomes by reducing the duration of untreated psychosis (DUP), protecting social support networks, involving families in care, and providing prompt and intensive pharmacological and psychological treatment' (Neale & Kinnair, 2017). This is based on an initiative from Australia (McGorry & Jackson, 1999), which found that people who engage with services soon after a first episode of experiences that meet the diagnostic criteria for psychosis are less likely to go on to develop enduring mental health problems (NHS England, 2016).

Aspire, the Leeds EIP service, noticed that 15–20% of their clients weren't benefiting from talking therapies. Some were disengaging from the service altogether; some felt that they had failed at talking therapies. Others were not talking at all, which made it difficult for the service to know how to help. Aspire applied to Comic Relief for funding to trial dramatherapy for this group.

With little research evidence available, we created a new approach based on Casson's and others' evidence-based practice (Emunah, 1985, 1994; Landy, 1993; Landy & Butler, 2011; Read Johnson, 2012; Lahad & Dent-Brown, 2012; Röhricht, 2006; Romme & Escher, 1993). Over a three-year period, this was honed to include only what clients fed back as being useful (NICE, 2019). This led to the adoption of a set of principles, listed below.

The model is designed for all service users, not specifically voice hearers. Romme and Escher's (1993) understanding of what they term the 'startling phase' and Romme and colleagues' publication of voice hearers' testimonies (2009) support our observation that many voice hearers choose to withhold information about their experience for a variety of reasons.

The therapy principles are as follows:

- *The client is in control* – the client controls the frequency of individual sessions, who attends (family/staff) and what role everyone takes in the session, and decides if and when they feel ready to progress to the group.
- *The client is the expert* – the client chooses the activity and decides on the speed, pace and length of activity.
- *The client has freedom* – the client chooses when to watch and when to take part, the physical or metaphorical space they need and whether to share or contain their experience.
- *'No' is a positive choice* – this is a way to keep activities safe and relevant. Even when a client finds it hard to say 'No', they can show 'No' by sitting in the audience space.
- *The work is future-focused* – activities focus on enjoying the dream without the burden of thinking through the practical steps involved in making it a reality.

Dramatherapy aims to support clients to work out what they want for their future by staying positive and light-hearted. It can be fun. Once they have developed a relationship of trust with the therapist, people may choose to use dramatherapy to express unarticulated experiences and challenge their frightening voices. With better understanding and a language for their voices, they may then find it easier to progress to talking therapies.

How dramatherapy has helped

I asked Zakki (the name is a pseudonym), who is open about her voice hearing and had recently completed a dramatherapy group, to identify examples of exercises that might be useful for other voice hearers. She suggested three to demonstrate the three different elements of the EPR model. I've slightly adapted them so they can also be used by people on their own at home, as learning points.

Zakki attended six sessions of individual dramatherapy. After four sessions, she decided to attend group dramatherapy and used the remaining individual sessions to prepare for this. The group included seven other people within the service and ran for one and a half hours every week for 12 weeks.

Role exercise

This is an exercise for people at the start of dramatherapy. It was developed by Robert Landy (Landy & Butler, 2011, p.148). Landy has spent many years identifying the roles in theatre that make stories possible. He has researched how role-taking supports healing. He believes that inhabiting a narrow range of roles makes us unwell. In the exercise, we use Landy's original categories with a refined set of 58 key roles, which include fictional (Vampire, Zombie) and real (Mother, Helper). The client is given a deck of role cards portraying each of the 58 roles and sorts them into four categories: what I am; what I am not; what I am not sure about; and what I'd like to be. They are then invited to use the cards to map out the roles according to how much time they spend inhabiting each (more time = core roles; less time = fleeting roles) and consider for themselves what they might change in the future. This can be done on their own or with me.

Zakki said that doing this exercise enabled her for the first time to experience distance from her voices: 'I think I created a character. I feel I viewed myself as a second person and the character was myself. It was very important. To identify, recognise and play that role at the right time, that really helped me and really solved a lot of situational problems that I had been through in my past… That killer instinct, killer role was a brilliant one that I discovered within myself, that I was denying… then I accepted it and I know that every role has its own prioritised time. If it is not required, you can keep it down, tuck it inside your sleeve or have it somewhere in there. That killer was really a very powerful tool. I think equally important was accepting it and not denying it all the time there was denial there, like a ripple inside, a ripple in the emotional dimension.'

Zakki realised that, once she had identified the voices, they could be controlled: 'I think it was the beginning point of something like self-analysing…

when I recognise these roles within myself, I am getting a different point of view of myself, like a second person, myself, watching myself, and I could shift roles. I got that killer instinct.'

This helped Zakki reach a point where she could assert herself over the voices. She used the 'killer' role to guard an imagined 'pot', 'the container of emotions'. She began to see that she had choices about how to engage with the voices. 'So when the voices are on and on and on, the killer role can shut them up straight away.'

> *Learning point 1*
>
> You can use Landy's original list in his book or find lists online by searching 'Landy Role Profiles'. As a first step, I suggest considering:
>
> - What roles do you take? What roles do the voices take?
> - Which would you like more of? Which would you like less of?
> - What kind of a container would work for you? Which voice would be your guard?

Zakki found group work brought benefits – new ideas resulted from being with others, as well as new stimuli and new coping strategies.

Embodiment exercise

Everyone has had experience of EPR by the time they enter the group, but they need a transition to reconnect with the group each week. This relaxation, followed by a silent check-in, enables us to re-engage.

On arrival, each person takes the space they need to stretch out on the floor. Deep breaths taken while lying on the floor are very grounding. So I ask people to empty themselves of air. Then I ask them to take deep breaths, consciously, filling ourselves right to our edges, focusing on fingers, toes, nose, mouth, and remembering where we end and the world starts. Remembering how 'to be' in our bodies is the ideal way to start embodying our feelings.

We emerge from this without talking. This next exercise is based on Emunah's Partner Mirror (1994, p.151). Standing in a circle, the group follows my request to 'copy me'. Everyone mirrors my actions, like a reflection. I slowly explore my understanding of what it is to be 'open' and 'closed', as a reminder that both are accepted. Then I silently pass the leadership role to the next person. The group now copies their expression of 'open' and 'closed' until this person passes it on. If someone doesn't want the role, they pass it on with cupped hands to the next person, until we have gone, silently, around the whole circle. Then we repeat it, this time sharing just a gesture with the group, which everybody mirrors back.

> ### Learning point 2
>
> Try this with someone you trust. After the breathing relaxation, ask them to mirror your physical exploration of the words 'open' and 'closed' for one minute. Then swap and you mirror them for one minute. Next repeat the exercise, but this time share and mirror any actions that have surfaced for each of you.
>
> - What do you notice when you mirror the actions that have surfaced for your partner?
>
> It is important to remain silent, move slowly and stay focused on your partner. It should be so synchronised that anyone watching would not be able to tell who is leading or following.

Zakki said of this exercise: 'There are so many thousands of emotions that are not represented in language. Now I realise that I can identify them without words. If I identify the emotions at this point, non-verbally, they may not progress to voices and certainly they don't get strong.'

Zakki noticed how copying other group members' movements helped her to shift her own feelings of depression because they helped her move in a way that she would not have thought of. 'When I get voice attacks out of nowhere and I'm feeling depressed, and someone gives you a chunk of their emotions through action – a new emotion flowing from somewhere – you know what to do with it, because now you know how to operate the emotion. You get their movement and it takes you to a new place you have never experienced before. Over time, this helps you become more fluid.'

Zakki found this useful because: 'It heightens your awareness of how much we live in a world that operates through non-verbal cues. My voices used to be triggered by other people. The stress I used to feel coping with voices and trying to go about daily life is much less now I realise that everyone I meet, or just pass in the street, is following these non-verbal cues; they do not need me to engage with them verbally. As long as I look presentable and follow the logic of how people co-exist, there is no need to deal with the voices or explain them. They are contained inside.

'I now have boundaries and I am not triggered by other people. I can just stand in a queue in the supermarket. I have a new perspective on this. I experience other people differently. The new perspective is I don't have to explain and talk. We can do so much without a single word. There is telepathy and I can rely on not crashing into people; we communicate subconsciously and it's not a danger. This is a new freedom. I don't have to tell. The world is going on without me talking. There are in-built rules and language. There is so much non-verbal communication. That's how the traffic works, driving cars, it's how we work at the supermarket or walking in the street.

'If I look presentable, I realise I don't have to reply. I feel much more relaxed about being silent. I have been given permission to go about my daily business without reaching for any words. I realise the infinite power of "No" that cannot be argued with. I can use this anytime I choose.'

Projection exercise

This exercise helps members consider what they have gained from the process towards the end of the dramatherapy group. It invites the possibility of continuing individual progress after the group has ended.

Using a bridge as a metaphor for future change (Casson, personal communication), we review pictures of different types of bridges. Every person chooses an image that best captures their own group journey. Group members then privately reflect what it is like to stand in the middle of their chosen bridge, looking forward to a new life after the group and backward to this, more familiar world.

Working together on the floor, we create a shared montage to represent our group experience, capturing the comfortable space we have created together, using material and objects to express this without words. I mark out a metaphorical 'bridge' with yarn reaching across to another part of the room. Group members are invited to decorate this second area with symbols of our individual future hopes. I invite each group member to bring at least one symbol of their dreams for the future to this new shared space.

People are encouraged to spend time exploring. They are free to stay in one area or venture across the bridge. As the exercise progresses, some group members will cross the bridge and others will stay on one side, adding more symbols. Some people experiment by moving to and from the two places, over the bridge.

Zakki said: 'The bridge brought future hope. We were playing like little children, picking something that was safe, travelling across the bridge, but on an emotional level I felt like I was making a resolution for my future. Crossing the bridge was like, "I can do anything." It was a spatialised adventure. It played the game emotionally. When I got home, I was able to challenge negative thoughts verbally and make improvements. I have taken on so many things. Building up a resolution that means, "Okay, sometime in the future I will cross the bridge and get things done." It's empowering. It is conscious. I can do it six months from now.'

Learning point 3

Find some images of bridges by searching online. Choose the one you are first drawn to.

- What do you notice about the bridge? How sturdy is it? Which side are you starting on? What do you notice on the other side? Where are you most comfortable on the bridge? Why? Where would you like to go next? What attracts you to this place?

Note down your thoughts. After a week, return to your notes and the picture and do the exercise again.

- How are the voices reacting to you doing this? How do you feel about staying at your starting point? If that was where you felt most comfortable last week, do you feel any different now?

Conclusion

In my chapter, I've tried to show how dramatherapy may be useful when working with people who are distressed by hearing voices for the first time or struggling to verbalise their experience of hearing voices. It might provide a form of pre-therapy as a route into engaging with talking therapies, or simply help the voice hearer gain new perspectives on issues that keep recurring.

Hopefully, the reader will come away with the knowledge that:

1. Role work can help contain and name voices, so that we can take a more powerful role in our relationship with them.
2. Embodiment helps us better understand and trust silent interactions in daily life. We do not have to talk in order to negotiate situations.
3. Projection can help us find hope and visualise dreams beyond what is currently considered possible.
4. Group dramatherapy is a useful space to learn from others.

Overall, I believe that using the three elements of dramatherapy – **e**mbodied movement, creative **p**rojection and **r**ole exploration – enables us to access unconscious information that helps us understand better what makes us feel good now and what we might want more of in the future. This knowledge may then become a bridge or springboard to our taking action to achieve it.

References

Casson, J. (2004). *Drama, psychotherapy and psychosis: Dramatherapy and psychodrama with people who hear voices*. Routledge.

Compernolle, T. (1981). J.L. Moreno: An unrecognised pioneer of family therapy. *Family Process 20*, 331–335.

Emunah, R (1985). Drama therapy and adolescent resistance. *The Arts in Psychotherapy, 12*(2), 71–79.

Emunah, R. (1994). *Acting for real drama therapy: Process, technique and performance*. Bruner Routledge.

Jennings, S. (1990). *Dramatherapy with families, groups and individuals*. Jessica Kingsley.

Jennings, S. (1994). *The handbook of dramatherapy*. Routledge.

Jennings, S. (2011). Assessment through embodiment-projection-role (EPR). In D. Read Johnson,

S. Pendzik, & S. Snow (Eds.), *Assessment in dramatherapy* (pp.177–196). Charles C. Thomas Publishing.

Lahad, M. & Dent-Brown, K. (2012). Six piece story making revisited: The seven levels of assessment and the clinical assessment. In: D. Read Johnson, S. Pendzik & S. Snow (Eds.), *Assessment in dramatherapy* (pp.121–147). Charles C. Thomas Publishing.

Landy, R. (1993). *Persona and performance: The meaning of role in drama therapy and everyday life.* Jessica Kingsley.

Landy, R. & Butler, J. (2011). Assessment through role theory. In D. Read Johnson, S. Pendzik & S. Snow (Eds.), *Assessment in dramatherapy* (pp.148–176). Charles C. Thomas Publishing.

Marineau, R.F. (1989). *Moreno, 1889–1974: Father of psychodrama, sociometry and group psychotherapy.* Routledge.

McGorry, P.D. & Jackson, H.J. (1999). *The recognition and management of early psychosis: A preventative approach.* Cambridge University Press.

Neale, A. & Kinnair, D. (2017). Early Intervention in Psychosis services. *British Journal of General Practice, 67*(661), 370–371.

Nelson, B., Torregrossa, L., Thompson, A., Sass, L. A., Park, S., Hartmann, J.A., McGorry, P.D. & Alvarez-Jimenez, A. (2020). Improving treatments for psychotic disorders: Beyond cognitive behaviour therapy for psychosis. *Psychosis, 13*(1), 78–84.

NHS England (2016). *Implementing the Early Intervention in Psychosis access and waiting times standard: Guidance.* NHS England/National Collaborating Centre for Mental/National Institute for Health and Care Excellence.

NICE (2019). *Dramatherapy in Early Intervention in Psychosis: Guidance.* NICE. www.nice.org.uk/sharedlearning/dramatherapy-in-early-intervention-in-psychosis

Read Johnson, D. (2012). Diagnostic role playing test. In D. Read Johnson, S. Pendzik & S. Snow (Eds.), *Assessment in dramatherapy* (pp.61–90). Charles C. Thomas Publishing.

Röhricht, F. (2006). Effect of body-oriented psychological therapy of negative symptoms in chronic schizophrenia. *Psychological Medicine, 36*(5), 669–678.

Romme, M. & Escher, S. (1993). *Accepting voices.* Mind Publications.

Romme, M., Escher, S., Dillon, J., Corstens, D. & Morris, M. (2009). *Living with voices: 50 stories of recovery.* PCCS Books.

Rumney, B. (Dir.). (2019, March 11/18). *The choir: Our school by the tower.* BBC Two.

Thirioux, B., Harika-Germaneau, G., Langbour, N. & Jaafari, N. (2020, February 6). The relation between empathy and insight in psychiatric disorders: Phenomenological, etiological, and neurofunctional mechanisms. *Frontiers in Psychiatry.* https://doi.org/10.3389/fpsyt.2019.00966

Torregrossa, L.J., Snodgress, M.A., Hong, S.J., Nichols, H.S., Glerean, E., Nummenmaa, L. & Park, S. (2019). Anomalous bodily maps of emotions in schizophrenia. *Schizophrenia Bulletin, 45*(5), 1060–1067.

Van der Kolk, B. (2014). *The body keeps the score.* Penguin Books.

34 Dance movement psychotherapy and voice hearing: looking outward and inward

Mary Coaten

My experience in dance movement psychotherapy (DMP) and voice hearing has been primarily in NHS acute adult inpatient settings in the UK. For the past decade I have run DMP groups on wards, and people attending have often experienced voice hearing. As a dance movement psychotherapist, I do not specifically focus on the voice hearing but simply receive and respond to whatever the person brings to the session. They may decide not to bring the voices as a focus. My work involves taking an embodied approach to working with distress, in whatever form, and this chapter briefly describes the nature of that process, and invites the reader to engage in the experience through the learning points.

In recent years, embodied approaches to dealing with severe mental distress have attracted much interest (Fuchs & Schlimme, 2009; Brauninger, 2014; Bryl, 2018, Biondo et al., 2021). The potential relevance of embodied approaches to voice hearing should not be surprising if one considers that voices very regularly appear to be connected to unexpressed emotions (see, for example, Chapter 18 on experience focused counselling, and many other chapters in this book). At the same time, there is a real lack in current mainstream mental health service provision in offering ways for people who are distressed by their voices to express their emotions, let alone physical ways. However, emotions are generally experienced primarily in the body. So it makes sense that the body would be used as a tool to express them, too. DMP is one such embodied approach and concerns the 'moving body' (Jeong et al., 2005; Koch, 2011; Meekums, 2002). Dance movement psychotherapists learn to tune in or attune to the person in and through their body movement in dance. They are interested in how people express their emotions creatively through dance and movement, thus embodying their emotions, thereby providing another means for expression other than the verbal, and one that looks both inward and outward at the same time.

In this chapter I am not including direct examples of how people's voices may have changed as a result of DMP. My aim is to explain DMP and its relevance as an emotion-expressing tool. From my work and research, it is clear that progress in reducing distress in the voice-hearing experience can be made even if one does not work directly with the voices, by working with thus far unexpressed emotions. When unexpressed emotions that are connected to voices are expressed, the voice-hearing experience may also become less distressing or intense.

What is dance movement psychotherapy?

DMP in the UK is governed by its professional organisation, the Association for Dance Movement Psychotherapy (ADMP) UK. Founded in 1982, its current definition of DMP states:

> DMP recognises body movement as an implicit instrument of communication and expression. It is a relational process in which client(s) and therapist engage creatively using body movement and dance, as well as verbal and non-verbal reflection.[1]

DMP provides embodied interventions that link with the individual's lived experience in the context of the social system they live in. It is also concerned with how they experience living in their body and their relationship to it; how they think about themselves and their relationships, as well as emotional responses that may be hard to put into words. At the heart of this is the fundamental belief in the inter-relationship between psyche, soma (the body) and spirit. It is used for a range of neurological, psychological, relationship and social problems, and also for people who wish to develop their creative potential.

The experience of DMP can be understood as engaging the body and the senses. It is a way to sense our connections with the outer world. Through moving, the individual is creating something that holds meaning. The dance can be seen as a product of our own creativity. Moving together, we experience not only our own dance but also that of the other, joined with us in the dance. This is important if we consider that an erosion of trust in others may come from previous traumatic experiences. Being more present as a sensing being through the very process of dancing can strengthen our sense of self. Dancing demands awareness in terms of selecting moves and creating improvisations; it produces a sense of freedom and joy through movement. The shaping of feelings through movement also provides a way of experiencing distressing feelings at a safe distance. This opens up the possibility for a creative reflection on the feelings, fantasies and emotions brought up during the DMP process. Additionally, being part of a group promotes social cohesion and a collective body response. The created dance thus becomes a bridge rather than a barrier between each other.

DMP can be offered in both group and individual sessions and is based on the premise that body and mind interact, so that a change in one will influence the other and have an effect on overall body-mind functioning (Berrol, 1992; Stanton-Jones, 1992). Central to this approach are four key concepts: body action, symbolism,

---

1. www.admp.org.uk

therapeutic movement relationship and rhythmic group activity (Chaiklin & Schmais, 1979). The creation of a therapeutic movement relationship is at the heart of all DMP practice, which essentially is about seeing and being seen by the 'other'. In the past decade, several studies have explored the use of DMP in severe mental distress, with varying outcomes, but all have demonstrated the benefits of using body-oriented therapies (Martin et al., 2016; Priebe et al., 2016; Savill et al., 2017; Bryl, 2018).

Often people attending a DMP group will have experienced some kind of trauma, whether past or recent, and they may be presenting with distressing experiences, such as voice hearing and psychosis, PTSD and so forth. The link between trauma, psychosis and negative content of voice hearing has, for example, been highlighted by Read et al., (2014). The experience of trauma, especially childhood trauma, may have led to an erosion of trust in others (Ratcliffe, 2017). I have become increasingly interested in this erosion of trust in others caused by trauma and how that is expressed through movement and dance.

The erosion of trust may have an impact on how we view the world and can be exacerbated by further stressful events. These traumatic events may manifest in a variety of ways: for example, through hyperarousal, hypervigilance, non-shared auditory and visual realities and unusual beliefs. It may also manifest in somatic or body-based disturbances, with a disruption in where we place ourselves in space and time. It is important to emphasise that the presence of trauma is only one aspect of voice hearing; not everyone who hears voices will necessarily identify any traumatic experiences in their history.

The phenomenon of voice hearing can be viewed in different ways (Cooke, 2014). One view is that hearing voices places something outside oneself that feels too difficult to hold within oneself. This may be a consequence of traumatic experiences in one's life. Understanding what the voice is saying and understanding the content in terms of what is or has been happening in one's life can be translated into the dance process. Furthermore, through connecting with others non-verbally and creatively using music, movement and dance, the person may, in fact, feel able to express emotions and experiences that they would otherwise still experience as too difficult to acknowledge or express verbally or fully consciously. Movement metaphors are central to this process (Meekums, 2002, pp.19–20). A movement metaphor is a symbol of something felt or thought and reflected in either a movement or a posture and can be seen as a form of non-verbal communication. For example, a person may adopt a sunken posture when describing anxieties that they feel overwhelmed by. Movement metaphor is also embedded in the English language; we talk, for example, about 'going out on a limb', 'elbow room', 'jumping out of one's skin', 'falling to pieces', and so forth. These may be represented in movement or in posture and can become a means to facilitate therapeutic change through movement and verbal and non-verbal processing.

A session in practice

My doctoral research (Coaten, 2020) in the acute adult inpatient mental health setting included an evaluation of working through movement and creating dance and the importance of symbol and metaphor in communication within these interactions. Kalsched (2013), a Jungian analyst, talks about the importance of the symbol offering a connection between what one feels internally and the expression of it externally. A typical session on the ward takes place on a weekly basis for one hour. The room is located on the ward. During the session, there is no direct invitation to dance. I set up a speaker and use my mobile phone and Spotify to provide the music. I place art materials around the rooms, and provide props such as cloths, scarves and different textured materials. Props act as a bridge between participants. They allow participants to communicate and connect when it may be too difficult to use words. A piece of cloth can be held at each end by two people. They can move it in response to the music, and others can dance beneath it. The art material can allow participants to create a visual image that may arise from the dance or act as a focus to express how they may be feeling. I initially choose music with a strong beat, which helps to give a sense of togetherness. Heavy metal music, hip-hop, rap, Bhangra and Bollywood are all very popular. As the group proceeds, participants ask for different types of music and I am able to provide this. I often use music from around the world. Sometimes there may be someone attending from a specific country, and they request music from that country. This can provide a strong personal sense of connection between the person and the music, which is also important.

Learning point 1

Choose a particular music with a strong rhythm – for example, heavy metal, rap or Bhangra. Try different types of rhythm – strong, slow, fast. Move in relation to this rhythm. Notice if there are any changes between various rhythms.

- What do you feel?
- Are you able to express yourself?
- If so, notice in what ways you feel more connected.

During the session, individuals dance alone and collectively, and sing and draw. As I move, I respond to the individuals in the group. I may 'mirror' movement, which gives the person the sense of being seen and valued. If a group forms, we may move collectively, sharing the movements in rhythmic activity. This shared rhythm creates a sense of cohesiveness, connection and community. I keep an eye out for opportunities to dance – a form of 'creative alertness' or sense of attunement to the individual and the group. I create a space that people can enter into and respond in whatever way they choose, and I in turn respond to this. At the end of the session, I place some chairs in a circle and there is an opportunity for participants to reflect and share anything arising for them during the session.

What follows are some examples from my doctoral research. The names and all other information in these stories has been anonymised.

Alan and Daniel

Alan enters the room. He is a young man, in his early 20s, who has become distressed, although no one is quite sure why. His movements are very stiff; he has no torso movement and his eyes dart from side to side, giving the impression of suspicion, or of a private detective or spy casing the joint.

What is striking about his movement is that it is very limited and guarded. Alan begins to dance with me. He begins to make little movements, but still with no movement in the torso. The movements are, however, comfortable – small, twisting, cautious, but perfectly rhythmic and interactional. We dance to Dragon Magic, his favourite band. I note the symbolism in this name as I am aware that Alan is having difficulties with his father. I reflect inwardly on the archetypal image of George and the dragon. At one point, Alan dramatically lifts his arm up and then plunges it down, in a strong descending movement, as if, I think, he is slaying the dragon. We mirror each other's movements. We are dancing together, creating a dance. He has little facial expression. Then, suddenly, we are side by side and he is rolling his arms around, turning, moving in complete synchronicity with me. This movement seems to come out of nowhere, like a sudden burst of perfect synchrony. Previously, it had felt as if he had not noticed me, but this seems to indicate that he had completely taken everything in and was waiting, watching for that moment.

When these moments happen, I am amazed at the aliveness and connection that did not seem to be there before. The change in the state is dramatic, and it makes me ponder about the conditions and factors that allow this to take place. Under what conditions does a person move from seemingly complete de-animation to one of complete animation? Even under the influence of powerful antipsychotic medication, which can slow the body down, the person is still able to respond to the dance and, in fact, seems to be drawn to the aliveness in the DMP group. Maiese (2016) asserts that it is the re-inhabiting of the body, through the DMP process, that leads to change. There is a building up of the 'who we are', culminating in a stronger sense of self.

> ### *Learning point 2*
>
> Have you ever had the experience of dancing in a group or with another person where a powerful and palpable sense of synchrony and connection has come through the dance and the pulse and rhythm of the music? Choose a piece of music that you feel connected to and simply dance to it, by yourself or with other/s.
>
> - Do you notice a sense of aliveness, a change in your energy, a connection to self/other?

Alan and I continue, tumbling arms up into the air, moving side by side. Then he sits down and stays sitting, quietly. Then, suddenly, Daniel enters the room and

Alan immediately 'springs to life'. This contrasts with the quieter energy before. There is much more energy. They begin to dance with such explosive energy. They cross hands and begin to spin around and around together, faster and faster, controlled but almost spinning out of control. It looks very funny, the two men having great fun. Daniel is in his 30s and Alan in his early 20s. They come to a halt and Alan stumbles back, laughing, having clearly enjoyed it. He has 'come to life'. They then begin to engage in shadow boxing, again with great energy and hilarity. This then evolves into bouncing off each other's chests. They connect in a very powerful way. There is an intense connection between the two. I watch as this happens, mesmerised; it reminds me of two sumo wrestlers.

Daniel then asks for very loud heavy metal music and does an intensely strong movement backwards and forwards, backwards and forwards while playing air guitar (colloquially known as 'head-banging'). Arching his back, he sings very loudly and we all try to join in to varying degrees, although he seems to be completely on his own with this movement.

> ### Learning point 3
>
> The importance of movement, dance and free improvisation are all at the heart of this chapter. Consider your own relationship to these aspects in your own life. Try tuning in to your 'self' as you move – your sensations, thoughts, images, emotions and feelings. Put on some music that you like, either at home or in another place of your choosing, and simply let your body respond to it in any way you like. There is no right or wrong way to move.
>
> - What comes up for you?
> - What changes do you notice?
> - What sensations (outside) and feelings (inside) are you noticing?

Radu

Radu joins for the last two sessions of the study. He is aged 20 and comes from an Eastern European country. His movements are very slow, guarded, bounded and neutral. He is wide-eyed, taking in his surroundings through his eyes with almost no movement in his body. I put on folkloric music from his country. It is fast, lively, intricate. On hearing it, he leaps into action, his body flying across the floor as if he has taken off – quick, nimble, sprightly. I join him, taking his hand, and fly alongside him in a line formation. We move quickly across the floor. He is completely animated and full of vitality. He laughs; he comes to life.

When the music stops, he sits down and puts this movement and feeling into an image. He draws a very detailed picture with a very vibrant yellow thunderbolt that comes down to strike the earth at the point of a deep, blue pool of water. It is like a map of his world. There is also a large egg, a cosmic egg symbol.

> *Learning point 4 – the importance of symbol and metaphor*
>
> While moving freely in a space, notice whether any particular symbols or images arise for you. Try moving with them, or make a drawing of these images and then improvise in response to the drawing. You could perhaps try some 'free association' writing: put the pen on the paper and just allow a stream of consciousness to emerge.
>
> - What are the themes that are emerging for you?
> - What are you noticing about how you like to move?
> - What is the process revealing to you about yourself?

Conclusion

I have given a brief outline here of DMP as a therapeutic intervention in the context of my experience as a dance movement psychotherapist working with people who hear voices in the acute adult inpatient setting. I have looked at the impact of trauma and the ensuing erosion of trust on the individual and on their relationships with others. I have also described how DMP can strengthen the person's sense of self in relation to others through the pulse and rhythm of music and dance, of which expression of symbol and metaphor is an essential part. The practice examples also show how, under the influence of the music and dance, there is a sense of vitality, of 'coming back to life', and of playfulness and joy. These practice examples underline the importance of expressing oneself either through the dance, through symbol and metaphor or via visual imagery that may also come out of the dance. Creating images allows the individual to express their distress in a way that feels possible and safe for them, which they can explore either by themselves and/or in conjunction with the dance movement psychotherapist.

> *Learning point 5*
>
> Read this chapter again and allow an image to emerge out of your reading. Spontaneously, without judging the image, or images if a whole series comes into your mind, note if it is possible to see new connections. Are images or symbols emerging that speak to you in a new way? Perhaps to the dancer inside you?

References

Berrol, C. (1992). The neurophysiologic basis of the mind-body connection in dance/movement therapy. *American Journal of Dance Therapy, 14*(1), 19–29.

Biondo, J., Gerber, N., Bradt, J., Du, W. & Goodill, S. (2021). Single-session dance/movement therapy for thought and behavioral dysfunction associated with schizophrenia: A mixed-methods feasibility study. *Journal of Nervous & Mental Disease, 209*(2), 114–122.

Brauninger, I. (2014). Specific dance movement therapy interventions – which are successful? An intervention and correlation study. *The Arts in Psychotherapy, 41*(5), 445–457.

Bryl, K. (2018). The role of dance/movement therapy in the treatment of negative syndrome and psychosocial functioning of patients with schizophrenia: Result from a pilot study mixed methods intervention study with explanatory intent. *Schizophrenia Bulletin, 44*(s1), s315–s316.

Chaiklin, S. & Schmais, C. (1979). The Chace approach. In P.L. Bernstein (Ed.), *Eight theoretical approaches in dance-movement therapy* (pp.51–70). Kendall/Hunt Publishers.

Coaten, M. (2020). Dance movement psychotherapy in acute adult psychiatry: A mixed methods study. Unpublished thesis. Durham University. http://etheses.dur.ac.uk/13548/

Cooke, A. (Ed.). (2014) *Understanding psychosis and schizophrenia*. British Psychological Society.

Fuchs T. & Schlimme J. (2009). Embodiment and psychopathology: A phenomenological perspective. *Current Opinion in Psychiatry, 22*(6), 570–576.

Jeong, Y., Hong, S.-C., Lee,. M.S., Parek, M.-C., Kim, Y.-K. & Suh, C.-M. (2005). Dance movement therapy improves emotional responses and modulates neurohormones in adolescents with mild depression. *International Journal of Neuroscience, 115*(12): 1711–1720.

Kalsched, D. (2013). *Trauma and the soul: A psycho-spiritual approach to human development and its interruption*. Routledge.

Koch, S. (2011). Basic body rhythms: From individual to interpersonal movement feedback. In W. Tschacher & C. Bergomi (Eds.), *The implications of embodiment: Cognition and communication* pp.151–171. Imprint Academic.

Maiese, M. (2016). *Embodied selves and divided minds*. Oxford University Press.

Martin, L.A.L., Koch, S.C., Hirjak, D. & Fuchs, T. (2016). Overcoming disembodiment: The effect of movement therapy on negative symptoms in schizophrenia – A multicentre randomized controlled trial. *Frontiers in Psychology, 7*, 483. doi: 10.3389/fpsyg.2016.00483

Meekums, B. (2002). *Dance movement therapy*. Sage.

Priebe, S., Savill, M., Wykds, T., Bentall, R.P., Reininghaus, U., Lauber, C., Bremner, S., Eldridge, S. & Röhricht, F. (2016). Effectiveness of group body psychotherapy for negative symptoms of schizophrenia: Multicentre randomised controlled trial. *British Journal of Psychiatry, 209*(1), 54–61.

Ratcliffe, M. (2017). Selfhood, schizophrenia, and the interpersonal regulation of experience. In C. Durt, T. Fuchs & C. Tewes (Eds.), *Embodiment, enaction, and culture: Investigating the constitution of the shared world* (pp.149–171). MIT Press.

Read, J., Fosse, R., Moskowitz, A. & Perry B. (2014). The traumagenic neurodevelopmental model of psychosis revisited. *Neuropsychiatry, 4*(1), 65–79.

Savill, M., Orfanos, S., Bentall, R., Reininghaus, U., Wykes, T. & Priebe, S. (2017). The impact of gender on treatment effectiveness of body psychotherapy for negative symptoms of schizophrenia: A secondary analysis of the NESS trial data. *Psychiatry Research, 247*, 73–78.

Stanton-Jones, K. (1992). *An introduction to dance movement therapy in psychiatry*. Routledge.

35 Awesome metalcore therapy: using heavy metal music in therapeutic work with voices

Kate Quinn and Daniel Baines

Current research on working with people who hear voices who are identified as having an 'at-risk mental state' emphasises the use of cognitive behavioural approaches (e.g. van der Gaag et al., 2019). However, it is also suggested that pluralistic, integrated approaches and tailoring therapy to individual need may be helpful (Cooper & McLeod, 2007). This chapter was co-written by Kate Quinn, a psychologist and therapist, with one of her clients, Danny, who gave his written informed consent. It is a case description of how metalcore music and lyrics were integrated into a programme of therapy with a young man who was hearing distressing voices, because these were of specific interest to and had resonance for him, and fortunately also for Kate, the therapist. This is not a music therapy case study, although there is some evidence that therapy using music can be useful for people who hear voices (Geretsegger et al., 2017). Rather, it is intended as an example of how therapy can be adapted in an idiosyncratic and creative manner to best suit the needs of and better engage the voice hearer.

Metalcore is a subgenre of heavy metal music that combines influences of extreme metal and punk. It originated in the 1990s but came into prominence in the 2000s and remains popular to date. There is some limited evidence that people with emotional vulnerabilities may be attracted to listening to heavy or extreme music (Baker & Bor, 2008), and various researchers have proposed mechanisms for why people may find it helpful for managing their wellbeing, including that it helps with the processing of anger (Sharman & Dingle, 2015).

In this chapter, Kate will describe her work with Danny, a 19-year-old man with a history of voice hearing and difficulties managing emotions, who was referred for psychological work to an NHS early intervention service. Kate has been working in early intervention services for several years, predominantly with young people who hear voices, using Voice Dialogue and cognitive approaches.

We initially attempted to work together using CBT but, when this wasn't successful, we agreed to try an adapted and integrated approach, using our shared interest in metal music and in particular Danny's strong identification with metalcore as a source of help to him in coping with life events and for emotional regulation.

> ### Learning point 1
> - Many voice hearers have existing coping strategies based on their experiences and interests. What resources do you (or your client) have that may already be helpful and could be built on?

The main body of this chapter comprises selected extracts from the narrative letter that Danny and Kate co-produced at the end of therapy. At the end of the chapter, there is a link to the playlist and the speech quoted in the letter. There are two aspects to the extracts: Danny's history in his own words and how this relates to his connection with music, and the therapeutic strategies we adopted, written mainly from Kate's perspective.

> ### Learning point 2
> Voice hearers may find it helpful to write their own narrative of their life experiences and what they find useful for managing their difficulties (with voices or more widely).
>
> - How could you (or your client) do this creatively?
> - What kinds of media (drawing, poetry, collage, music and so forth) might work for you?

The awesome metalcore therapy letter

Part 1: Extracts from Danny's life history pertaining to voice hearing (written by Danny)

When I was 12 years old, I moved out to live with my dad. I didn't see my mum or sister for six months – I was fuming with the world for quite a long time. This reflected in my behaviour at school. I got less bothered about moving schools all the time, though. I remember going on holiday and listening a lot to 'Sempiternal' by Bring Me The Horizon (BMTH). I was in a weird place (mentally) but it kind of grounded me, and I realised how important music was to me. I started hearing the odd laugh or scream from like a demon and it felt like my head was in hell.

Song: 'Can You Feel My Heart' – Bring Me The Horizon

When I was 14 my friend killed himself and I found him. Neck Deep was one of his favourite bands.

Song: 'Smooth Seas Don't Make Good Sailors' – Neck Deep

I started hearing his voice, it was a comfort thing and helped a bit, but in some ways it made it harder, 'cos I used to see him. I couldn't accept that he was dead. Sometimes I feel he isn't real or that I can't remember him properly anymore. I still hear his voice sometimes.

Things carried on in terms of my low mood and voices for a while, and I started hearing more voices, some of which were nastier than my friend's voice. At this time, I came into [psychiatric] services. Later, another friend tried to kill himself. He survived, but it brought a lot of the stuff back and things were difficult for a bit.

Song: 'Don't Pray for Me' – Asking Alexandria

Part 2: Therapeutic strategies (written by Kate with parts in bold italics written by Danny)

'What brings me back round when my head goes off....'

Given that we had used music and lyrics as a way to describe things that had happened in your life, we wondered whether this would also be useful as a way of thinking about things that might be helpful for managing some of the struggles that you are facing. You particularly identified that [the band] Architects have been a specific source of helpful ideas. You said that in particular you started really listening to the album 'Holy Hell' and reading into what the lyrics meant for you. We've picked a couple of examples from their music.

'I think Architects are part of the reason now why I'm still alive.'

Song: 'Holy Hell' – Architects

One of the issues that we have talked about a lot is that you sometimes have big emotional responses to things that happen in your life, or, as you put it, 'the littlest thing can start the biggest problems', and that this can tip you 'over the edge'. This sense of being up and down all the time can be really difficult to manage, especially when you are in the middle of experiencing a lot of difficult feelings.

Song: 'Doomsday' – Architects

We talked about how you use the idea from this song that everything leads to a 'bigger picture', so it is good to hold this in mind when you are experiencing difficult emotions, as these often pass in a short time. Instead, it is important to think about the bigger picture and what you are aiming for long-term. This can be the same with voices. They are experiences that can represent difficult feelings, but we can relate to them differently if we keep in mind the bigger picture. You said that now your voices are more like a 'background noise'.

Song: 'All Love is Lost' – Architects

You identified this song as being particularly important, because it reminded you about all of the people who have low mood at times, including ones that are famous! Or, as you put it, '***He's a rock star so if that's what he feels like…***' We talked about how highs and lows of mood can be part of the human experience and knowing that other people are also going through difficulties can make you feel less alone.

One of the best things that you came across was this speech that Sam Carter (vocalist in Architects) made at a concert. It's kind of long, but worth it!

> I had a conversation today and a lady asked me, 'When you lay in bed what do you think about? What do you worry about?' I paused 'cos that's a fucking hard question to answer. But what I said was: 'In a world that we live in right now, when every day you wake up, and you look at your phone or your laptop, you read a newspaper, you are filled with the worst kind of shit you could possibly read. You are filled with negativity from the moment you open your fucking phone.' And I said to her, I said: 'I'm scared of people giving up, I'm scared of people losing that fire in their fucking heart, because you are born an empathetic human, you are born someone who cares about your brother or sister. It is society that pushes that out of you. It is society that pushes hate upon you.' So what I'm saying to you right now is that it's okay to feel scared in this world that we live on. What is not okay is to feel alone, because you are not alone, you are not alone in your empathetic state of mind. You are not alone in how much you care, you are not alone in how much fire is in your fucking stomach. If you want to make a difference, you fucking can, and I'm telling you this, we who live every day, we are lucky to see every day. But when you see something that is wrong, whether it's sexism, homophobia, racism, or just outright hate towards anyone, don't be a fucking sheep. Stand up, and stand up for what is fucking right. Don't be the person that goes home wishing they did something, be the person that goes home proud that you stood up for somebody and you showed them love, and you showed them compassion, because love will always fight over hate, and it will always fucking win. (Architects, 2018)

We talked about how you found this speech to be really powerful and that it highlights a lot of things that you connect with – *'He's a smart guy!'* We discussed that it's kind of about continuing to fight for things that are important to you. It is important to keep this in mind when moving forwards. I was telling you about one idea in psychology, where it can be helpful to have a 'compassionate ideal' (e.g. Gilbert, 2015). This involves keeping your imagined 'ideal person' in mind when you think about how you respond to yourself or your voices, especially if you criticise yourself. We wondered if Sam was kind of similar to how you would want this person to be. We also noticed how positive this speech was compared with some of the ideas that you may have if you are experiencing low mood, and that this was similar to the responses we generated when we practised challenging negative thoughts with more balanced, compassionate ones.

As we came to the end of our time together, we talked about how things are now, and the ways that you have learned to cope with things. I think we both realised that things might never be 'perfect'. However, you said that you now *'move past shit in my own way'*, and a lot of this is about being able to clear your head by re-focusing or re-directing your attention. As you might expect, music can be a big part of that, but you also said that it helps you to watch or listen to something you are familiar with, that this fills your head with things that you know you like. In particular, where this is an 'opposite' action to how you are feeling (so, happy stuff when you feel sad), this can work sometimes. You mentioned watching happy films as an example. You also said that you still use the playlists[1] that you made in the beginning that described different emotions. As part of this, it seemed apt to have a playlist that goes with this letter with all the songs in it that you mentioned. ☺

'I am okay to me, wouldn't say that I'm not okay.'

> *Learning point 3*
>
> As well as, or instead of, written or visual narratives, voice hearers may find music or sound-based material that has personal meaning to them helpful. What would you include on your own playlist of music or sounds?

Reflections on the work from client and therapist

At the start, Danny couldn't really discuss his feelings in therapy, despite there being a positive alliance between us. The use of playlists allowed us to consider things less directly through this shared medium. Danny felt that, at least in the first instance, it was important that Kate would also listen to the music in between the sessions to facilitate the discussion in the session and because this felt less exposing than listening together, which may have conveyed feelings of vulnerability more directly. In this way, it was possible to create some distance from his feelings of vulnerability. The discussion of lyrics and the themes in them allowed us to talk through how this related to certain of his life experiences.

For example, the first playlist Danny produced contained many references to feeling abandoned, and this made it possible for us to have a discussion about the changes in some family relationships in his life. This was the start of the process of mapping Danny's life events onto the music, which enabled him to tell his story in a way that he couldn't before. Once he started to tell his story through the music, Danny found it easier to talk about other aspects of his life in his own words. Danny also used the playlists to help him manage difficult emotions, which we then built on to create strategies that could help him to manage his difficult feelings generally. Legitimising this strategy and the importance of the meaning of the music validated what Danny was already doing and meant we did not need to 'start from scratch'. In addition, it was motivating for Danny, as it meant the between-session work was interesting and he was therefore more likely to do it.

The use of Sam Carter's speech and lyrics was important as Danny identified him as a strong role model, particularly as Sam has been public about his own adverse

---

1. You can listen to the playlist of songs in Danny's awesome metalcore therapy letter and watch a video of Sam Carter's speech at heavymetaltherapy.co.uk/awesomemetalcore

experiences. Kate could then integrate therapy ideas such as thought-challenging by basing this on other things that Danny felt he could relate to. This is important as Danny found structured, traditional CBT quite challenging because it reminded him of difficult educational experiences, but he could use some of the CBT ideas once they were adapted (by, for example, using a lyric as a positive self-statement).

Danny also identified strongly with the wider metalcore community and felt that they shared his core values, which fostered a sense of belonging. He regularly attended live metalcore concerts and was active on online social media metalcore sites and said that the shared expression of emotion at live concerts, both with the artists and with the audience, was an important source of social support for him. He spoke about talking with other people at concerts about their interpretations and understanding of particular lyrics or songs and telling people stuff that he would not usually be able to speak about, even with close friends. Kate gained a sense that this was a community helping each other and that this was another important aspect of the metalcore scene for him.

> *Learning point 4*
>
> Identification with role models, individuals and communities may be helpful for voice hearers in terms of development of social supports and coping strategies. This doesn't have to be metal music related ☺.
>
> - Which people would you identify for yourself or the person you are supporting, and what is it about them that you/they admire?

The work emerged from the principles of Voice Dialogue and the theory that people have a range of 'Selves' or aspects of self that represent different parts of their personality. This theory has been adapted for working with voices, which may be similar, for example, to pushed-away parts of self in this model (Corstens et al., 2011; see Chapter 19 in this book). Metalcore, and heavy metal music more generally, often expresses themes that may 'tap into' pushed-away selves, such as parts that are angry. There are also frequent references in metalcore lyrics to experiences like hearing voices. In these cases, the voices often express angry feelings, and Danny said that listening to music that specifically mentioned voices had a calming effect on his mental state. We therefore used the music to work with three aspects of self: the angry part, as represented by the voices; the sad part, as identified in a number of the lyric themes, and the aware ego – the part that is able to take a step back and pay attention to all the other selves. Kate did not attempt direct dialogue work or talking with the voices, partly as Danny did not feel he could directly dialogue with his voices. Also, Voice Dialogue ideas are very compatible with compassion-focused therapy, and Kate was able to integrate the use of the compassionate ideal as the development of a compassionate aspect of self (Gilbert, 2015) into the work, using Sam Carter's speech as a basis.

> *Learning point 5*
>
> Voices and aspects of self may like different kinds of music or different activities. Some people find it helpful to 'honour' these parts by engaging with the preferences of voices/parts in a positive way.
>
> - What activities do you think that your voices/the voices of the person that you are supporting would enjoy?

That Danny and Kate shared an interest in metalcore was a happy coincidence and something that Danny felt was important, as he was scared he might otherwise be judged. He had had some negative reactions to his musical preferences, so it was important for him to feel that Kate had some background knowledge and genuinely liked the music. However, there may not always be the luxury of a therapist and their client having a shared interest. This should not preclude the possibility of including the client's interests in therapy anyway. It may be possible to adapt therapy to include the interests and existing coping skills of voice hearers, with some research and creative thinking on the part of the therapist.

In terms of outcome, Danny is now discharged from psychiatric services and is managing well with the coping strategies he has in place. His voices are still present but only as background experiences that he can choose to engage with or not. He has good insight into where they come from and what helps him cope with them. He continues to be a keen member of the metalcore scene and likes to share his experiences and ways of overcoming difficulties with other metal fans in order to help others.

Music references

Architects. (2016). 'All love is lost'. From *All our gods have abandoned us*. Epitaph Records.

Architects. (2018). 'Doomsday'. From *Holy hell*. Epitaph Records.

Architects. (2018). 'Holy Hell'. From *Holy hell*. Epitaph Records.

Asking Alexandria. (2013). 'Don't pray for me'. From *Death to destiny*. Sumerian Records.

Bring Me The Horizon. (2013). 'Can you feel my heart?' From *Sempiternal*. RCA Records.

Neck Deep. (2015). 'Smooth seas don't make good sailors'. From *Life's not out to get you*. Hopeless Records.

References

Architects. (2018). *The Devil is Near & Sam Carter Speech (Live, Alexandra Palace, London 2018).* https://youtu.be/qxElulzTVaU

Baker, F. & Bor, W. (2008). Can music preference indicate mental health status in young people? *Australasian Psychiatry, 16*(4), 284–288.

Cooper, M. & McLeod, J. (2007). A pluralistic framework for counselling and psychotherapy: Implications for research. *Counselling and Psychotherapy Research, 7*(3), 135–143.

Corstens, D., May, R. & Longden, E. (2011). Talking with voices. In M. Romme & S. Escher (Eds.), *Psychosis as a personal crisis: An experience-based approach* (pp.166–178). Routledge.

Geretsegger, M., Mössler, K.A., Bieleninik, Ł., Chen, X.J., Heldal, T.O. & Gold, C. (2017). Music therapy for people with schizophrenia and schizophrenia-like disorders. *Cochrane Database of Systematic Reviews, 29*(5), CD004025

Gilbert, P. (2015). Self-disgust, self-hatred, and compassion-focused therapy. In P. Powell, P. Overton, J. Simpson (Eds.), *The revolting self: Perspectives on the psychological, social, and clinical implications of self-directed disgust* (pp.223–242). Karnac Books.

Sharman. L. & Dingle, G.A. (2015). Extreme metal music and anger processing. *Frontiers in Human Neuroscience, 9*, 272.

Van der Gaag, M., van den Berg, D. & Ising, H. (2019). CBT in the prevention of psychosis and other severe mental disorders in patients with an at-risk mental state: A review and proposed next steps. *Schizophrenia Research*, 203, 88–93.

36 A safe space: sound therapy and hearing voices

Jane Ford

Recent interdisciplinary research aimed at furthering our understanding of the experience of people who hear voices has demonstrated that this phenomenon is widespread and most people who hear voices are not distressed by them. Only a minority may end up seeking additional mental health support for these experiences, and some of these may be given a diagnosis of psychosis (Corstens et al., 2014; Johns et al., 2014; Wilkinson & Alderson-Day, 2016). For those voice hearers who are given a diagnosis of psychosis, there often may not be much choice of therapeutic interventions beyond medication, which is of course problematic. In either situation (where voice hearers have been given diagnoses and where they have not been diagnosed), it is now widely accepted that an emphasis on acceptance of the voices and their integration into that person's life, rather than trying to eliminate them, should be the focus.

This chapter will consider the role that sound therapy can play in achieving this objective by describing work at Cygnet Victoria House in Darlington and One One Eight and The Recovery House in York. These were all privately run, secure residential inpatient settings for adults with short- and long-term mental health issues. As a result of the work that I and a colleague, Dianne Jackson-Roberts, carried out, we have achieved the only evidence that is currently available, as far as we know, for the significant benefits of sound therapy for people experiencing voice hearing. The feedback that we received from people who took part in these sessions was extremely positive and most felt that sound therapy helped significantly in enabling them to live with the (often) distressing effects of hearing voices. Dianne and I, as well as the staff, also noticed a reduction in symptoms of stress, improved concentration, a reduction in tendency to self-harm and, in one case, the ability to move from full-time care to semi-independent living.

Sound therapy

It is important first to clarify what sound therapy is, because it differs from music therapy in the following ways:

- First of all, it is cross-cultural and not rooted in the Western musical tradition. The instruments used include Himalayan bowls, frame drums, gongs and tuning forks, which produce sounds to which the Western ear is generally unaccustomed.

- The sonic landscape created by these instruments assists in inducing an altered state of consciousness (ASC)[1] in the listener, which is similar to that employed by shamans in indigenous cultures (Winkelman, 2000; Boyce-Tillman, 2000). This is a key aspect of sound therapy, but an essential difference is that a shaman creates the ASC for *himself*, in order to travel to other realms for the purpose of bringing about healing for an individual or community, whereas the sound therapist will provide sounds designed to bring about an ASC for the *client*.

- Ancient shamans may have used hallucinogenic drugs to enhance their powers. Modern sound therapists are highly trained professionals working in hospitals, care homes, hospices and many other environments where their skills are making a real difference to people's lives, without the use of drugs.

- One further essential difference between the disciplines lies in the fact that sound therapy tends not to use recognisable melodies, or, indeed, any melody at all. As a result, each sonic experience is unique and tailored to the needs of the individual at the time.

- Finally, whereas music therapy is a participatory practice, the sound therapist usually has sole responsibility for providing the sounds. That said, when the therapist is working with a voice hearer, they encourage them to actively participate, and this involvement can form an integral part of the recovery process.

Sound therapy and voice hearers

The willingness to embrace complementary practices into mainstream healthcare is a welcome development and offers an exciting opportunity for sound therapy to demonstrate how instrumental it can be in the recovery process of voice hearers. Recent literature has highlighted the need for a reappraisal of how people who hear voices are viewed (McCarthy-Jones 2012; Romme et al., 2009), with the emphasis on the integration of the voices into the individual's life rather than efforts to eliminate them. With this in mind, several aspects of sound therapy practice suggest that it might be a highly appropriate therapeutic intervention for voice hearers:

---

1. ASC refers to any state of consciousness that is *different* for that individual and is usually measured by brain wave activity. Examples are the dreaming state, daydreaming, the meditative state and achieving the runner's 'high'. See Ludwig (1966) for a detailed examination of this phenomenon.

- Somewhat paradoxically, most sound therapists are not privy to any diagnostic information relating to individuals in hospitals or other community care centres. Although this may seem unhelpful, it has the effect of ensuring that the therapist remains neutral. In this sense, a basic phenomenological requirement, that of suspending preconceived notions as far as possible, is met.
- Sound therapists are trained to 'meet the energy'. That is to say, they will relate to the individual 'on that person's terms' and respond with appropriate sounds for that person on that day. This is one of the four conditions for successful holistic healing, according to Stanley Krippner (1992, p. 365).
- The use of sounds such as repetitive drumming to bring about an ASC is a vital aspect of the therapeutic process, allowing for a suspension of the client's ordinary consciousness. This affords the possibility that, during the session, the voices may not seem as intrusive, thereby creating the potential for healing.
- There is the additional benefit of distraction. Even if no long-term improvements can be achieved, there is at the very least the advantage of short-term distraction from the voices.
- Voice hearers with an accompanying diagnosis of psychosis can feel isolated and unable to communicate with clinicians for a variety of reasons (such as not feeling heard by professionals; feeling distracted by the voices, and so forth). They may feel themselves to be 'different' or set aside from the rest of the population, and prefer to inhabit their own world, even when the voices are harsh, critical and frightening. Sound therapy 'speaks' a language that could also be considered 'different' or outside the bounds of 'normal' clinical practice, and so is often welcomed by people in this situation. Some of the strange sounds that can be elicited from a singing bowl by, for example, over-toning with the voice may not seem at all strange to someone whose waking consciousness is already permeated with unusual sonic experiences.

Sound therapy in practice

Having provided a necessarily brief summary of the background to sound therapy, I want to consider some examples of how this works in practice. I would like to offer some reflections on work carried out at Cygnet Victoria House, Darlington from 2015 to 2017 and One One Eight and The Recovery House, York during a similar period by my colleague Dianne Jackson-Roberts. I should point out that this was not part of a research programme; these observations are retrospective accounts of treatment sessions.

Cygnet Victoria House[2] is a mental health hospital managing people with severe and enduring mental health needs. In some cases, the extent of these needs means that they may continue to require long-term support. One One Eight and The

---

2. www.cygnethealth.co.uk

Recovery House are run by Amitola,[3] which offers care and support services to adults with enduring and complex mental health issues and (or) learning disabilities.

Before any client work can commence, it is important that the sound therapist has a picture of what is going on for the person at that point in time – not in a clinical sense but, rather, how do they view the world? How do they view their place in it? What is important to them? These are the kinds of questions that are not perhaps specifically asked but which a sound therapist will address through casual enquiry or intuition in order to assess how best to proceed. The ability to 'speak the language' of the client is vital and this is particularly true of people who are hospital inpatients and may have serious mental health issues, making ordinary communication a more complex task at times.

> ### Learning point 1
> By considering the situation holistically it is often possible to gain clues about the underlying causes of the problem. You could, for example, ask:
> - How do you view the world and your place in it?
> - What is special or 'sacred' to you?

One resident at Victoria House, for example (all practice examples have been anonymised in terms of location, gender and background), had an extremely advanced knowledge of the chakra system,[4] and wanted to explain his symptoms using that as his basis. The fact that he and I were able to discuss his health and wellbeing in this way was very helpful in establishing an environment in which he felt supported, safe and free to express his thoughts.

In his case, we found that playing a Himalayan singing bowl and chanting were highly beneficial. He reported that repetitive chanting of a Sanskrit mantra (*om gum ganapatayei namaha*) helped him relax and gave him some temporary respite from the voices. Likewise, he said the sound of the singing bowl took him 'somewhere else', and meant that, for the duration of the session, he had some relief from the all-consuming sound of the voices. As the sessions continued, he decided he would like to use the chants and learn to play the bowl himself so that he could gain some control over his situation. This development is consistent with the recommendations of the Hearing Voice Movement, which asserts that therapeutic approaches should be directed towards acceptance and empowerment of the voice hearer (Romme et al., 2009).

After several months of weekly sessions, this man was able to contextualise his experience and reported that he no longer felt controlled and compelled to act on the sometimes violent orders he received from his voices. He expressed visible relief once he was able to accept that, although the voices were a very real part of his life, he could exercise choice over whether or not to obey them.

---

3. www.amitola-communities.co.uk

4. This is based on Ayurvedic medicine, which recognises seven main energy centres in the body

> *Learning point 2*
>
> Being 'held' in a safe space is very important for healing:
>
> - Would you feel able to accept your voices if you were 'held' in this way?
> - Try saying a mantra or affirmation, such as 'I am safe and protected' (this will only work if you use it as a means to increasingly assert your ability to look after your personal safety and protection), for 10 minutes each day and see if this makes a difference to the sound of the voices.

Another resident at Victoria House who also heard voices reported feeling calmer after regular tuning-fork treatments. I worked with a pair of tuning forks, C4 and G4 – 256Hz and 384Hz respectively – which I placed at either side of his head, and activated at regular intervals for approximately 15 minutes, creating a sonic 'cradle'. During this process, the resident repeated phrases such as: 'I am good and worthy', 'I own my feelings' and 'I will do what is right for me'. This patient had chronic low self-esteem, but used the opportunity of being 'held' by the sound of the tuning forks to express his inner conviction that he could overcome his feelings of unworthiness, which he felt the voices were keeping him ensnared in. For this brief period, he was able to articulate feelings of strength, in stark contrast to his habitual demonstrations of powerlessness. It is possible that the combination of the two tuning forks created a form of binaural beat, a phenomenon that has been shown to be highly relaxing in a number of different situations (Alipor et al., 2014; Isik et al., 2017).

However, this is one example of a therapeutic intervention that requires further investigation, because research suggests that, for the establishment of a binaural beat, the difference between the two frequencies cannot be greater than 40Hz, and the difference between 384Hz and 256Hz is 128Hz.

> *Learning point 3*
>
> Often, it is trauma from the past that keeps us locked in a troubled present.
>
> - Would you feel different now if the past were no longer difficult to accept? Do your voices remind you of past events?
> - How do you think the future might look if, in the present, you were able to experience more joy, for example, with the help of sound created by fork treatments, and separate from difficult feelings related to the past?

Mantra and tuning fork treatments can focus in on the voices but can also bring a general sense of empowerment.[5]

The frame drum[6] was, I found, one of the most valuable tools with which to work. It is a universally popular instrument, and I used it in a variety of ways:

- to provide a meditation by playing a regular beat over a sustained period of time. This had a calming effect on residents, but several also reported that they felt able to see things more clearly or had a revised perspective on their problems following the drumming.
- to encourage group participation where residents each had a drum and, while playing the instrument, were invited to express their thoughts, desires, fears and so forth. The drumming appeared to act as a kind of 'safety net' that made it safe for them to make statements that might otherwise have remained unsaid. This is an important form of empowerment.
- to create a sonic landscape in which past fears or traumas might be released. Often, voice hearing is linked to incidents from many years ago that are locked in the mind of the individual, sometimes on a conscious level, but often on an unconscious level. Drumming, particularly when incorporating voices as well, can evoke memories. If this happens in a 'safe space', the person can bring some meaningful reflection to that memory and begin to reframe their experience.

Learning point 4

Using a drum can be a rich means of self-expression:

- Try playing a steady rhythm and asking your voices to join in.
- Use your drum to play whatever you feel you want to 'say' – there is no right or wrong way of drumming.
- Play your drum whenever you feel upset, angry, lost or sad and see how uplifting this can be.

At One One Eight in York, similar work has been taking place with some highly significant results. One woman who had been hearing voices for many years attended fortnightly sessions where Dianne chanted the Sanskrit mantra *Sa Ta Na Ma*. This is traditionally held to be a transformation mantra, and it is reputed to be effective in breaking old, established patterns of behaviour. The resident responded very well to this mantra and was encouraged to join in, and eventually was able to chant it herself for around 20 minutes daily. Her initial response was that, when

---

5. Further advice can be obtained from the Therapeutic Sound Association at www.therapeuticsoundassociation.com
6. This is a hand-held drum played with a padded beater.

listening to the mantra, she felt it was keeping her heart beating and was a kind of 'life support'. Gradually, she assumed responsibility for her mantra practice, using it whenever she felt vulnerable and challenged by the voices. This woman reported that regular mantra practice was very beneficial and, having been almost immobile as a result of self-inflicted injuries, she is now living semi-independently.

Another woman who was being supported by Amitola had been hearing a loud, aggressive voice for many years, which she considered to be the devil. The voice threatened to harm her or her family members and seemed most prominent when she was feeling low and vulnerable. Dianne treated her with tuning forks, mantra and solfeggio pipes, all of which contributed towards bringing tremendous peace to this deeply troubled soul. The woman reported feeling 'uplifted, empowered and wonderful', both during the treatment sessions and for sustained periods of time afterwards. After some months of regular sessions, she reported that the previously loud voice 'in the front of her head' was now only 'a quiet whisper somewhere at the back of her head'.

During the treatment sessions, both women also received sounds from Himalayan bowls, and positive results were reported, similar to those reported by the people with whom I had been working at Victoria House.

It is striking that, in both cases, these women had been abused/attacked and traumatised when very young. When a 'safe space' was created with sound, the women felt courageous enough to take control of their situation and became sufficiently empowered to 'own' their experience and begin to exercise some choice about the impact of the voices on their lives.

Final remarks

It has to be recognised that most people who hear voices and are hospitalised will undoubtedly also be receiving medication. Therefore, until further research is conducted, it is impossible to state with any certainty the extent to which the sound therapy was the decisive factor in improving the health of these people. Importantly, however, if we look at the first-person reports from the people receiving the therapy, the feedback seems to suggest that the sound was the pivotal aspect of the treatment. This phenomenological evidence cannot yet explain why or how it is that sound therapy aids recovery in the way that it does. More work needs to be done to elucidate the connection between the ASC – a fundamental aspect of sound therapy – and the responses from the people who have benefited from this practice.

For interested researchers, there is tremendous scope in this largely unexplored arena, given the considerable potential for real, tangible help towards managing the devastating effects when a person has not yet found a way of being less distressed by their experience of hearing voices. Neurological testing might help ascertain what happens in the brain when sound is being used, or a qualitative piece of research could examine and collate the statements provided by voice hearers following sound therapy.

I would like to thank Dianne Jackson-Roberts for her valuable contribution, and also Cygnet Victoria House, Darlington, and Amitola, which operates One One Eight and The Recovery House in York.

Further reading

Aldridge, D. (2004). *Spirituality, healing and medicine: Return to the silence.* Jessica Kingsley Publishers.

Aldridge, D. & Fächner, J. (Eds.) (2006). *Music and altered states: Consciousness, transcendence, therapy and addictions.* Jessica Kingsley Publishers.

Barrett, F.S., Johnson, M.W. & Griffiths, R.R. (2015). Validation of the revised Mystical Experience Questionnaire in experimental sessions with psilocybin. *Journal of Psychopharmacology, 29*(11),. 1182–1190.

Becker, J. (2004). *Deep listeners: Music, emotion and trancing.* Indiana University Press.

Clarke, D. & Clarke, E. (Eds.) (2011). *Music and consciousness: Pphilosophical, psychological and cultural perspectives.* Oxford University Press.

Clarke, I. (Ed.) (2010). *Psychosis and spirituality: Consolidating the new paradigm* (2nd ed.). John Wiley.

Eliade, M. (2004). *Shamanism* (2nd ed.). Princeton/Bollingen.

Farhall, J., Greenwood, K.M. & Jackson, H.J. (2007). Coping with hallucinated voices in schizophrenia: A review of self-initiated strategies and therapeutic interventions. *Clinical Psychological Review, 27*(4), 476–493.

Gioia, T. (2006). *Healing songs.* Duke University Press.

Glicksohn, J. (1993). Altered sensory environments, altered states of consciousness and altered-state cognition. *The Journal of Mind and Behaviour, 14*(1), 1–12.

Griffiths, R., Johnson, M.W., Richards, W.A., Richards, B.D., Jesse, R., MacLean, K.A., Barrett, F.S., Cosimano, M.P. & Klinedinst, M.A. (2017). Psilocybin-occasioned mystical type experience in combination with meditation and other spiritual practices produces enduring positive changes in psychological functioning and in trait measures of prosocial attitudes and behaviours. *Journal of Psychopharmacology, 32*(1), 49–69.

Kerri, M. & Hunt, H. (2013). Creativity, schizotypicality and mystical experience: An empirical study. *Creativity Research Journal, 25*(3), 266–279.

Krippner, S. & Welch, P. (1992). *Spiritual dimensions of healing.* Irvington Publishers.

McCarthy-Jones, S., Krueger, J., Larøi, F., Broome, M. & Fernyhough, C. (2013, April 9). Stop, look, listen: The need for philosophical phenomenological perspectives on auditory verbal hallucinations. *Frontiers in Human Neuroscience.* https://doi.org/10.3389/fnhum.2013.00127

Peters, E. (2010). Are delusions on a continuum? The case of religious and delusional beliefs. In I. Clarke (Ed.). *Psychosis and spirituality* (pp.127–138). Wiley & Sons.

Snell, T.L. & Simmonds, J.G. (2015). Mystical experiences in nature. *Archive for the Psychology of Religion, 37*(2), 169–184.

Thomas, N., Hayward, M., Peters, E., van der Gag,g M., Bentall, R.P., Jenner, J., Strauss, C., Somner, I.E., Johns, L.C., Varese, F., Garcia-Montes, J.M., Waters, F., Dodgson, G. & McCarthy-Jones, S. (2014). Therapies for auditory hallucinations (voices): Current status and key directions for future research. *Schizophrenia Bulletin, 40*(s4), s202–212.

Ward, C.A. (Ed.) (1989). *Altered states of consciousness and mental health: A cross cultural perspective.* Sage.

References

Alipoor, A., Oraki, M. & Sabet, M.Y. (2014). Efficiency of brainwave entrainment by binaural beats in reducing anxiety. *Journal of Kermanshah University of Medical Sciences, 18*(1), 19–26.

Boyce-Tillman, J. (2000). *Constructing musical healing.* Jessica Kingsley Publishers.

Corstens, D., Longden, E. McCarthy-Jones, S., Waddingham, R. & Thomas, N. (2014). Emerging perspectives from the hearing voices movement: Implications for research and practice. *Schizophrenia Bulletin 40*(4), s285–s294.

Isik, B.K., Esen, A., Buyukerkman, B., Kilinc, A. & Menziletoglu, D. (2017). Effectiveness of binaural beats in reducing preoperative dental anxiety. *British Journal of Oral and Maxillofacial Surger, 55*(6), 571–574.

Johns, L.C, Kompus, K., Connell, M., Humpston, C., Lincoln, T.M., Longden, E., Preti, A., Alderson-Day, B., Badcock, J.C., Cella, M., Fernyhough, C., McCarthy-Jones, S., Peters, E., Raballo, A., Scott, S., Siddi, S., Somner, I.E. & Larøi, F. (2014). Auditory verbal hallucinations in persons with and without a need for care. *Schizophrenia Bulletin, 40*(4), s255–s264.

Krippner, S. (1992). Medicine and the inner realities. In B.J. Horrigan (Ed.). Voices of integrative medicine (pp.360–370). Elsevier Science.

Ludwig, A.M. (1966). Altered states of consciousness. *Archives of General Psychiatry, 15*(3), 225–234.

McCarthy-Jones, S. (2012). *Hearing voices – The histories, causes and meanings of auditory verbal hallucinations.* Cambridge University Press.

Romme, M., Escher, S., Dillon, J., Corstens, D. & Morris, M. (2009). *Living with voices: 50 stories of recovery.* PCCS Books.

Wilkinson, S. & Alderson-Day, B. (2016). Voices and thoughts in psychosis: An introduction. *The Review of Philosophy and Psychology, 7*(3), 529–540.

Winkelman, M. (2000). *Shamanism: The neural ecology of consciousness and healing.* Bergin and Garvey.

37 How writing memoirs and poetry may help voice hearers

Isla Parker

Many people hearing voices who enter mental health services are given a diagnosis of 'schizophrenia' or 'psychosis'. The Hearing Voices Movement, which views voices as an understandable reaction to trauma, argues that there is a lack of scientific validity for the concept of 'schizophrenia' itself. As Woods (2013, p.265) notes, 'voice hearers sometimes share not just a common experience of hearing voices but also a (frequently negative) experience of mental health services'. For these reasons, voice hearers often reject psychiatric labels, such as that of 'the schizophrenic' (Woods, 2013, p.265), as stigmatising and unhelpful (see Coleman, 2004, pp.55–56; Longden, 2009, p.143). The clinical view of schizophrenia is that people often lack a sense of self and the insight to provide a coherent, reflective account of their experiences. In recent years, this viewpoint has been challenged; the narratologists Roe and Davidson, for example, argue that people with schizophrenia can be agents of their own lives, capable of constructing their own stories. However, they recognise that people with schizophrenia can 'face a struggle with accepting and incorporating their illness as only one dimension of an expanded sense of self' (Roe & Davidson, 2005, p.91).

In recent years, some voice hearers have been able 'to speak out' about the experience of hearing voices, although some face stigma when disclosing this.[1] Voice hearers often describe their journey to come to terms with the challenges presented by psychosis in terms of the traumatic impact of some kind of a breakdown and their struggle to reframe their sense of identity as they continue to live with voices and unusual experiences. In this chapter, I will explore how voice-hearer authors bear witness to trauma and distress through their accounts of living with voices by discussing Tracy Harris's use of music and metaphor in her account of having schizoaffective disorder, and Emily Knoll's use of the memoir

---

1. There has been an increase in the number of memoirs of voice hearing that have been published in the last 15 years. The emergence in the 1980s of the Hearing Voices Movement encouraged voice hearers to challenge stigma by writing their stories so that they could share with others their recovery journeys. For a list of published memoirs, see Hornstein, 2011.

to explore her relationship with her voices, before discussing a poem by a voice hearer who I will call Simon (a pseudonym). I will relate my close reading of these texts to the theoretical literature that challenges views about schizophrenia being non-narrative.

Telling a story: exploring voice hearers' different modes of autobiography

The Music of Madness (2001) is Tracy Harris's first book, which she wrote 20 years ago. In it, she describes the voices she hears as being a very uncomfortable intrusion on her inner mental world. The voice is 'a loud coarse voice, like an aged operatic soprano reaching for a note well beyond her range' (Harris, 2001, p.60). She gives it a name – the Soprano. It distracts her, a professional flautist, from her flute practice, as she feels 'terrified'. The anthropologist Els van Dongen observes how 'it is assumed that schizophrenic people live outside reality… [and] that the psychotic world is irrational'. But, as van Dongen notes, 'the mad world has its own universe of discourse, its own conception of reality and criteria of rationality, perhaps different from the non-psychotic world' (Van Dongen, 2010, p.214). Harris fittingly draws on the musical world that she is knowledgeable about to describe how alone she feels with her tormenting voice. 'This ungodly voice is giving a contorted, private concert, just for me', she writes (Harris, 2001, p.61).

The power balance is clearly weighted in favour of the voice. Harris initially feels powerless to challenge it; she can only wait for the 'screaming' to finish, when 'the angry voice has mercifully concluded its performance' (Harris, 2001, p.61). Harris could be said to be experiencing what the Romme and Escher identify as 'the startling phase' in voice hearing (Romme & Escher, 1993), when the voice hearer feels confused and overwhelmed by the voice she hears. The voice quickly colonises many of the spaces that have hitherto been private to Harris. Interestingly, she maps her relationship to this voice spatially. She describes it as 'an unexpected guest, living with me in my house and callously commenting on all aspects of my life, my opinions, my love' (Harris, 2001, p.62). Harris then gives us specific details of how the voice inhabits different spaces: it 'shares my bed and the very intimate dream that should be left to me alone' and 'is there even during my bath' (Harris, 2001, p.62).

> ### *Learning point 1*
> Now that you have read Tracy Harris's account of hearing voices, think about how voice hearing is a spatialised experience.
>
> - Could you think of an example when your voices tried to 'colonise' your space?
> - Do you try to assert a boundary with your voice/s in these spaces? Does this change the voices that you hear?

Despite the distress that Harris feels at the invasion of her private space, she continues to separate herself from the Soprano's voice. Sometimes Harris refers to what she experiences as 'a brain disorder' (Harris, 2001, p.51). But her lengthy description of the Soprano's voice shows that this is an experience that has personal meaning for her. My 'brain chose something that I loved deeply and warped it into something ugly and disorientating' (Harris, 2001, p.62). This description conveys to the reader how traumatic this experience is for her. Trauma is a very complex term. In essence what I mean by it is that a psychotic episode may be very distressing for the individual, and they may feel unable to articulate their feelings or return to key memories associated with that episode, such as feeling persecuted by a voice. As Roe and Davidson note, the types of explanations people with schizophrenia give for unusual experiences 'are often viewed as delusional ideas that are attributable to the illness, serving simply as one of its more characteristic symptoms' (2005, p.91). But Harris is keen to approach her experiences from what Roe and Davidson describe as 'a narrative perspective', as demonstrated by her active search for musical language to define the voice. She speaks of the Soprano's voice 'with words that I love, such as aria and concert, in order to smooth the edges of her viciousness' (Harris, 2001, p.63). Harris describes a person-centred recovery. She makes it clear that her focus is regaining her musical career. Harris chooses to narrate her story in a narrative that is rich in musical imagery.

By 'narrative perspective', I mean that the voice hearer may be able to construct their own story. I take 'narrative' here to mean the discourse that conveys a certain meaning or story (Ryan, 2010, p.24). But the voice hearer's world, as voice-hearer authors describe, itself creates disruptions and disjunctions that ultimately threaten to undermine their agency as an author, and each is concerned that they present their own story in a way that doesn't make them seem too destabilised to tell it.

Narrative and self have traditionally been denied by psychiatry to those it diagnoses with schizophrenic illness because of the prevailing belief that people with schizophrenia lack insight into their condition. But, as Roe and Davidson point out, 'Were this true, it certainly would then be a challenge with schizophrenia to describe how the illness has affected their lives and sense of self, since they would be unaware of such changes' (Roe & Davidson, 2005, p.90). In recent years, researchers have argued that voice hearers may have the insight to provide a coherent account of their experiences. Lysaker and colleagues (2003), for example, suggest that the narratives of people with a diagnosis of schizophrenia frequently lack coherence, as these people have difficulty locating the self as the agent-protagonist in the teller's story. Therefore, people with a diagnosis of schizophrenia benefit from the development of greater flexibility in their narratives. Lysaker and colleagues (2003) argue that this gives these individuals a sense of owning their stories as the protagonists of their own stories.

Arts and written expression as a tool of personal recovery

In recent years, researchers have begun to argue that narrative plays an important role in recovery from schizophrenia. According to van Dongen, the stories of people with mental health issues 'put culture at work and become "the weapons of the weak" in order to control what usually remains beyond their control' (van Dongen, 2010, p.207). That is, language and storytelling give power to people who are stigmatised and often lack the resources to have influence and authority. The narratologist Clive Baldwin recommends that we pay attention to these fragmented stories of people diagnosed with mental illness 'in all their complexity, collecting them in different times and settings so that we can learn to understand how they contribute to the development and maintenance of the self' (Baldwin, 2005, p.1027).

> *Learning point 2*
>
> Do you feel that you have a lost a sense of your self? Would you like to write your own story or a poem about your voice-hearing experiences? One way to start to write a story is by mind-mapping. Try creating a 'spider diagram' when planning and organising your story, either using pen and paper or software such as XMind, which is free.[2] To prepare for writing the story, think about the following points:
>
> - Do your voice/s have any defining characteristics? For example, are they male/female, a certain age, positive or negative?
> - Would you like to create a visual representation of your voice? You could draw the voice, or take photos of images that remind you of the voice.
> - How often do you hear the voice/s? Do you hear them at a particular time of day?
> - What triggers hearing the voice/s?
> - Write about the time when you first started to hear voices. What was going on for you?
> - Would you say that you have a relationship with your voice/s?

Emily Knoll's book, *Emily's Voices: A memoir* (2018), is a semi-fictional account of voice hearing that is based on a composite of several voice hearers. The book provides a moving account of a young woman's experience of hearing voices. The book was self-published and launched at Blackwell's bookshop in Oxford in September 2018, at an event attended by researchers, mental health professionals and voice hearers. Several posts and reviews were published on Durham University's 'Hearing the Voice' blog[3] over the next two years. One reviewer was the psychologist Simon McCarthy-Jones (2018), who has published widely in the voice-hearing field.

---

2. https://www.xmind.net
3. www.dur.ac.uk/hearingthevoice/

Writing provided a useful filter for Emily to reflect on what it was like to receive various diagnoses, treatments and therapies when she was hearing voices. Voice hearing can be an intense, overwhelming experience, and writing helped Emily get a sense of distance from her voices. In *Emily's Voices: A memoir*, Emily describes how she must find a way of accepting that she hears voices or she can't be in the world. In the following extract, Emily is encouraged by her therapist, Daphne, to change her relationship with her voices.

> Daphne was keen for us to talk about the voices. 'The spiteful woman is part of you. She's the critical part,' she said.
> 'But she feels separate,' I shot back.
> 'Yes, I know it can seem like that. That's because the voice is outside your head.'
> 'So why does the voice sound like she's a woman?' I replied.
> Daphne said, 'That's what the voice-hearing experience is like. It's a paranoid voice that says nasty things to you. But you need to remember they're your voices. They are parts of you.'
> 'But I wouldn't tell myself these things,' I replied.
> 'Your unconscious mind would, and that's where the voices come from,' Daphne replied. (Knoll, 2018, p.128)

Emily struggles to recognise the voices as being parts of her 'self', particularly when they are saying frightening or distressing things to her. One of her coping strategies is to set a boundary with the voices: she tells them to 'Shut up and go away!' At other times she 'listened to my favourite music, and told myself that the voices were just another noise. This way the voices didn't intrude too much, and I could keep working' (Knoll, 2018, p.203). Emily is studying for a Master's degree, and it is important to her that she continues with her research.[4]

> ### Learning point 3
>
> In the extract above, Emily and her therapist are exploring Emily's voice.
>
> - Why may it help the voice hearer to describe the identity of their voice?
> - Do you think that it is a helpful strategy for the voice hearer to be encouraged to recognise the voice as being 'a part' of them? What may help the voice hearer to identify the things that the voice says as being their own fears or concerns?
> - For the voice hearer: Do you see your voice as a 'part' of you?

---

4. Emily Knoll is a pen name. Emily has an interest in geography, and recently assisted Assistant Professor Marijn Nieuwenhuis with a paper titled 'Towards a geography of voice hearing', published in the journal *Emotion, Space and Society* (Nieuwenhuis & Knoll, 2021).

Poetry as a helpful therapy for voice hearers

I will now move on to discuss how voice hearers use poetry to explore their voice hearing.

Research has shown that creating poetry can also be helpful as a therapy for schizophrenia, as the process releases emotions (Shafi, 2010, p.96). Furman (2003) has also argued that poetry can be used to help voice hearers manage their anxiety, cope with stress and express their emotions. Writing poetry may also help readers get an insight into a voice hearer's recovery story. Simon is in his 70s and enjoys writing poetry. Simon has heard voices since he was 20. During his working life, Simon was a labourer, digging trenches in roads to lay cables. I asked Simon to write a poem exploring his voices for this chapter. He wrote about an occasion when he felt persecuted by his voice.

Demonic electronic
Demonic electronic coursing through my brain,
The devil commanding me, 'am I insane?'
I look for the source of this onslaught
It does not follow
The logic that I have been taught.
I look in vain. There's nobody there.
But I hear it again. 'Kill yourself! Kill yourself!'
There's no relief.
It ransoms my soul, like a common thief.
Forty years on it has all died down.
These days I laugh
And say, 'You're only a clown.'

In this poem, Simon externalises the terror that his voice hearing causes him. He describes the experience as a high-voltage current running through his brain. During an interview about his voices, Simon told me that it felt to him as if he had metal spikes in his head, which he would try to pull out. The uncomfortable physical sensations of the voice are made more distressing by the content of the voice. The voice asks Simon, 'Am I insane?' He doubts his sanity, and this makes him afraid. He also experiences the voice externally but is unable to locate its source.

The voice is commanding Simon to kill himself. He says that there is 'no relief', which suggests that the voice continually torments him. Simon draws on his Christian upbringing when he interprets the voice in a religious way, and it feels to him as if this voice 'ransoms his soul, like a common thief', implying that he is powerless in his relationship with it. Forty years later, Simon is able to laugh at or with the voice and thinks of it as 'a clown'. He tells us that his terror has 'died down', and through the poem he is able to connect to his earlier suffering, his sense of fragmentation and his change to a positive sense of self where he is able to assert himself. He is now speaking to the voice, when he finishes by saying, 'You're only a clown.' Simon has found it therapeutic to write this poem.

> ### Learning point 4
> Simon finds it a therapeutic strategy to write a poem that explores his voices.
>
> - Do you think that writing a poem might help you to change the power balance with your voice, so that you feel more powerful than the voice?
> - Simon draws on his Christian upbringing when he interprets the voice in a religious way. Do you have religious or cultural beliefs that shape your understanding of your voices?

For the voice-hearer authors discussed above, presenting voice hearing in these ways allows them to make more sense of their experiences. They present them deliberately in a form that they can share with an audience that is unlikely to have heard voices. In each case, these accounts are insightful and highly reflective, due to the internal or external stigma that the writer experiences, particularly in the aftermath of a psychotic episode. The uniqueness of these accounts of voice hearing clearly shows that these voice-hearer authors have the agency to construct their own accounts of living with voices. Harris's, Emily's and Simon's difficulty in seeing the voice as part of themselves results in a continual battle with it. All of these authors have used memoir writing or poetry as an effective way to engage with sometimes traumatic memories of distressing voice-hearing experiences in ways that can vividly communicate the experience in a way that is accessible to a general audience.

References

Baldwin, C. (2005). Narrative, ethics and people with severe mental illness. *Australian and New Zealand Journal of Psychiatry, 39,* 1022–1029.

Coleman, R. (2004). *Recovery: An alien concept?* P&P Press.

Furman, R. (2003). Poetry therapy and existential practice. *The Arts in Psychotherapy, 30,* 195–200.

Harris, T.L. (2001). *The music of madness: Surviving schizoaffective disorder.* Writer's Club Press.

Hornstein, G. (2011). Biography of first-person narratives of madness: Personal accounts of madness written by survivors themselves (5th ed.) (p.1–25). www.gailhornstein.com/attachments/Bibliography_of_First_Person_Narratives_of_Madness_5th_edition.pdf

Knoll, E. (2018). *Emily's voices*: A memoir. Amazon (Kindle edition).

Longden, E. (2009). Eleanor Longden. In: M. Romme, S. Escher, J. Dillon, D. Corstens & M. Morris (Eds.), *Living with voices: 50 stories of recovery* (pp.142–146). PCCS Books.

Lysaker, P., Wickett, A., Wilke, N. & Lysaker, J. (2003). Narrative incoherence in schizophrenia: The absent agent-protagonist and the collapse of internal dialogue. *American Journal of Psychotherapy, 57,* 153–166.

McCarthy-Jones, S. (2018, February 2). Book review: Emily's Voices by Emily Knoll. [Blog]. *Freedom of Mind.* https://simonmccarthyjones.wordpress.com/2018/02/02/book-review-emilys-voices-by-emily-knoll

Nieuwenhuis, M. & Knoll, E. (2021). Towards a geography of voice-hearing. *Emotion, Space and Society, 40,* August, 100812.

Roe, D. & Davidson, L. (2005). Self and narrative in schizophrenia: Time to author a new story. *Medical Humanities, 31,* 89–94.

Romme, M. & Escher, S. (1993). *Accepting voices.* Mind Publications.

Ryan, M.-L. (2010). Toward a definition of narrative. In D. Herman (Ed.), *The Cambridge companion to narrative* (pp.22–38). Cambridge University Press.

Shafi, N. (2010). Poetry therapy and schizophrenia: clinical and neurological perspectives. *Journal of Poetry Therapy, 23,* 87–99.

Van Dongen, E. (2010). Walking stories: Narratives of mental patients as magic. *Anthropology and Medicine, 10*(2), 207–222.

Woods, A. (2013). The voice-hearer. *Journal of Mental Health, 22,* 263–270.

38 Finding an authentic voice: music therapy in multidisciplinary psychiatric support services

Stella Compton Dickinson

This chapter explores what happened when a man who was hearing voices and was distressed by them did not receive the right sort of support to enable him to lead a normal life and realise his full potential. I will call him George. This is not his real name. He has given me his consent to write his story in an anonymised way in the hope that it will help others in future.

I met George in a locked NHS hospital where he had no access to the community because the courts had sent him there for treatment after he had killed a man. At the time, he did not yet fully understand his own feelings, or how his negative formative experiences in life had eventually impacted on him as factors that led him to commit the offence.

It is important to say here that, although George did hear voices at the time of the offence, based on our understanding of research and contrary to an oft-held popular belief and highly publicised news stories, people who hear voices are no more likely to kill or harm anyone than those who do not. In fact, people with mental health problems and those who are distressed by their voice-hearing experience are much more likely to have been victims of severe trauma and more likely to suffer harm from others than the other way round (Pettitt et al., 2013). This was the case for George.

My aim is to illustrate how music therapy played a significant part in George's overall journey through the secure hospital system, where he had no freedom or access to the community. As part of his overall treatment, which included a choice of education subjects and psychology, the music therapy process helped him to understand his actions better and to relate better to other people, so that one day he could return to the wider community.

Voice hearing and the role of music therapy

It is frequently forgotten that people who have been diagnosed in the medical system with a serious mental illness and who have committed a violent offence have often themselves been the tragic victims of circumstances beyond their control, and sometimes they received no help.

Economic hardship, social exclusion and discrimination, which are more common in ethnically diverse populations, as well as neglect, physical and sexual abuse, social and emotional deprivation, domestic violence and substance misuse, are all factors that contribute to a person experiencing 'psychosis', which may include hearing voices (Hickling & Rodgers-Johnson, 1995).

Music therapy can therefore offer a way for people to openly express feelings and thoughts that are relevant to their voice-hearing experience. As voice hearing appears to be linked to unexpressed emotions and thoughts, discovering how to easily create one's own music with a trusted person/music therapist, along with reflective thinking and talking within the environment of safety and trust that develops in the musical therapeutic relationship, can offer a way to find expression for voice hearers. The 'therapeutic relationship' is all about mutual trust and can create a template for how to build future relationships. The feelings expressed without words may relate to difficult life events as well as the experience of voice hearing.

It is important to know that anyone using music therapy need not feel obliged to talk about things, and nor is any musical knowledge required. There is no such thing as a wrong note in improvised music therapy. The instruments made available in music therapy sessions can all be played without prior experience, and may be from many different cultures and countries. They may include, for example, djembe drums, rainmakers or ocean drums for sound effects, and tuned percussion instruments such as xylophones and glockenspiels. The music therapist will also have their own instrument with them, which may, for example, be a keyboard, flute or violin. Once an effective therapeutic rapport has been established, new and more effective relational strategies can develop that may later be replicated in relationships outside of the therapy room. Painful memories may be felt safely, becoming more bearable when an empathic response is received (Compton Dickinson & Jolliffe, 2021). Thus, a music therapy process can help with the gentle emergence of feelings and ideas as they are expressed within the music and without words, or in writing songs. In this way, difficult issues or confusing feelings may be processed so that they no longer risk being so overwhelming.

By creating music jointly with the client, the music therapist can support each individual to recognise and feel safe enough to think about and choose whether to share their experiences.

It can be long-term work to achieve a sense of mental integration between our thoughts and feelings after a trauma. Research by Tinnin (1990), Fachner (2009) and Blood and Zatore (2001) demonstrates how creating music together, when and if it is expertly tuned to the individual's mental health experience at the time, can affect our minds and our bodies positively. In this way, rapid trauma-based instinctual responses to fear, which may, for example, include an impulse to fight, flee from the situation or freeze (and can include feeling numbed-out, or 'out of body'), can gradually be better managed. This can be of importance as practice experience shows that the more feelings are pushed away, the more likely voices are to occur. This means, in turn, that the more a person is able to accept their fear, the less likely the voices are to occur.

The range of unconscious responses to fear may also include feelings of injustice and outrage, which may be triggering old memories that also resulted in strong feelings of rage. This may feel horrible and unhelpful for the person if they do not feel safe or are not able to deal with them in a non-violent manner. Importantly, music therapy can provide a safe space within which the person may feel safe enough to talk about or express these old memories more safely. In this process, the client should be supported by the music therapist to use ways of staying in the here and now, so that flashbacks (that is, being overwhelmed by old memories) do not occur. Therefore, the way the shared musical improvisations develop within the music therapy setting is carefully mediated by the music therapist's discreet input, tailoring it to each individual's needs, rather than it being an out-of-control, 'free for all' type of experience.

In this way, music therapy can provide a space within which the person can process difficult issues so that they do not feel so bad, and they can then understand themselves and their past actions better and feel more at peace. This usually involves reflecting on significant relationships with others. It can then become easier to relate to other people in everyday life.

When deeply held emotions become fully conscious to the person using music therapy, these may be openly expressed and actually heard in the 'feel' (the qualities) of the jointly created musical improvisation. Quite often the improvisations can be recorded and listened to together in the session. This musically creative process is mediated with an appropriate emotional balance. The music therapist may use various musical techniques to help, yet it will still feel like the individual's own music. This, because it is more personal and unique to the individual, is often of greater value than using known songs or riffs, although the latter might be a starting point and important to each person.

In order for the music therapist to engage well and appropriately in this process with their client, it is important that they understand the history and problems of the person with whom they are working. As with any other healthcare-approved therapeutic approach, the music therapist will have clinical supervision to ensure that all is going along safely and well.

Learning point 1

- Can you define the difference between recreational music-making and music therapy as a supportive process that can create inner and lasting changes in how people relate to themselves and to others?
- What do you think the barriers might be to a person who is distressed by their voice-hearing experience engaging in a jointly created musical improvisation with a music therapist?

Group cognitive analytic music therapy within a mental health service setting

The particular model of music therapy that has been developed to accommodate the restrictions of working in locked psychiatric hospital settings is called group cognitive analytic music therapy (G-CAMT) (Compton Dickinson & Hakvoort, 2017). It was developed in particular to meet the needs of people who hear voices and have felt distressed by them. It is also designed to help them to feel less isolated or withdrawn, and as a way for them to enjoy expressing a wide range of feelings. The purpose is to help them to understand themselves and others better, as well as explore new ways to relate to other people.

G-CAMT is unique in that it progresses through four stages. First, it is about the client developing 'musical mindfulness' by taking our time and simply observing an instrument, with no obligation to play unless we choose to do so. Group members may choose from a carefully selected range of instruments that anyone can make a sound on, regardless of whether they have any previous musical experience. It is important to both have one's own choice, and also to feel guided if needed.

We all learn from seeing what other people do, deciding whether we like it or not, perhaps waiting, learning how to listen intently, and finding and sharing new ways to make music together. By considering others and discovering how to find our own authentic voice in this way, we reflect on and value what each person brings to the group, without judgement.

Each person may then in turn move on to consider and perhaps be curious about the effect on their senses of the sound or the look or feel of an instrument. This is stage two, where we develop an emotional recognition of how the vibrations and sounds of an instrument feel, which may be different depending on who is playing it, and the mood of the music we create. We share, listen to and support each other as a group, rather than all doing things at the same time. If any one person decides to keep returning to a particular instrument, we call this their 'sound-print'. But we always keep in mind that the instruments stay in the room, and that we may want to share them with others during the session. Thus, we discover how to negotiate the sharing of musical resources when it feels like the person has found their own voice and self-expression through the particular qualities of an instrument. This is naturally different for each individual. For example, one person may like the African djembe drum and feel that they need to make a strong sound. Someone else may prefer a small instrument that makes gentle or scratchy sounds, depending on their mood that day. This process of choosing how to make their sound can heighten the person's awareness of their own uniqueness. Once all participants are content with their choices, they may feel ready to make some music together as a group. They can always change their mind and try something else as the session progresses.

Stage three involves the development of distress tolerance and the ability to discover new ways to manage potential conflict or difficult situations in everyday life. This occurs as the individual explores a greater range of musical expression and is helped to think about discord and dissonance as they occur naturally in the music and as a metaphor for how we relate to other people in life: for example, when people fall out with each other or discover how to make new friends.

Stage four is about attaining the ability to relate to others more effectively by discovering that endings (of formalised support or therapies) do not have to be traumatic or destructive. These are not like deaths, but can be the source of a new beginning if we can engage with having enjoyed the here-and-now experiences and forged some positive, happy memories of being together.

Naturally, the groupwork approach aims to be non-judgemental and provides an opportunity for the sharing of experiences and for peer support and acceptance. The process is contained and mediated by the music therapist, thereby reducing the sense of isolation and stigma that can so often occur for those who hear voices.

> *Learning point 2*
> - How do you think music therapy helps therapists and voice hearers feel safe, effective and respected?
> - Why do you think musical mindfulness may be helpful in the therapy?
> - If music therapy helps the voice hearer to manage potential conflict, how could they be supported so that this is a lasting change beyond the therapy setting? What might the role of music be in creating this lasting change? (Read on to find out.)

Practice example

This practice example is about a man for whom appropriate therapeutic services were not available for many years, and whose situation taught us many lessons about community care provision, which had failed him all those years ago. Since those days, greater care is taken towards helping people live a more normal life without being incarcerated. George had been given a diagnosis of paranoid schizophrenia. He had committed manslaughter and was sentenced to secure hospital treatment for an indefinite period, until he was deemed safe to be with other people again without hurting anyone. George had been desperate for help before he committed the offence. He had felt neglected and bereft.

George initially took part in individual cognitive analytic music therapy and, as he gained greater understanding of himself, he felt able to be with others and participate in G-CAMT. He had been labelled as untreatable and dangerous until he discovered music therapy. Like many people who are given a diagnosis of schizophrenia, George heard voices that talked about him in a nasty way. Some voice hearers may find it difficult to distance themselves from some seemingly negative things that the voices say or the suggestions or orders the voice gives, or they may mistake the voice for a real person.

I saw George once a week for individual, 50-minute sessions for several years. As the trust developed between us, we began to piece together his life story. George frequently expressed turmoil and confusion, and these feelings were reflected and could be heard in the musical improvisations that we created. As time went on, through our collaboration, George became more able to organise his thoughts and then to share his past experiences with me. He began to understand the events that led to his sense of downfall from what had been a promising career.

Following a particularly loud musical improvisation in which we both used drums, he disclosed how he had been violently abused by a man in his own family when he was a child. This abuse, he explained, always occurred unexpectedly, the result of which, we recognised together, was that George could not deal with surprises. Indeed, at that time, I too felt the same about 'surprises' in how he expressed this violence in his music and in his sharing of this shocking description of the beatings that he had received. He had been able to express those beatings in his loud drumming. As a child, he had done nothing to provoke the beatings. He had been minding his own business. Yet George had had high aspirations and had felt very special in his mother's eyes. He described that, just as he had started to gain recognition in his career, his mother developed a progressive disease and could no longer recognise him. This was particularly painful, since, as is often the case, they had a very close relationship when he was an infant. They had often felt fear and had hidden together from the violent abuser. As a child, George was too small to be able to defend himself or his mother. It was only as a full-grown man that he felt angry about how they had both been treated and, as a result, was perceived very differently as angry and dangerous. His desire to protect his mum was very significant in what happened next.

After he committed his offence, George knew he had done a bad thing, even though he was not intrinsically a bad man; he cared about the world and people's rights and felt very rejected by society. He did not know why he had lost control so suddenly; he just knew how unhappy and distressed he felt, and this is what we worked out together.

The impact of loss

Over the duration of our work, George began to understand and make links between the emotional impact of his losses and how he tried to numb those out and soldier on alone for years. His feelings of sorrow started to come through in his music. He reflected on how he had built up bitter resentment towards the abuser and we reflected on how he had restrained himself initially from acting aggressively back at that person. These issues were previously not understood, and family members had struggled to understand George when he isolated himself and ruminated, silently holding his anger inside him.

When his mum died, the most important relationship in George's life terminated – just when he felt he could have finally made her proud. He was unable to say goodbye to her. Feeling guilty and distressed, and having no one with whom to share his feelings, he became depressed, lost his job, was unable to pay the rent. He became disturbed in his behaviours; people complained and were afraid because he acted strangely, and he lost his home. Homeless, with no one to go to, no one with whom to grieve and mourn his loss, he became numbed-out, his feelings turned in on himself, and his depression deepened. He became increasingly isolated and anxious, and so unable to seek help. As he became more paranoid and distressed, the voices that he experienced as persecutory started talking about him as if he was bad, and he started to believe them and that they were real. His love of his mum had at that point turned to hatred of he knew not what. But he felt as if the whole world was against him and that people were like the abuser and out to get him. During our work, he was able to realise that what the voices were saying at the time of his mum's death was, in fact, rooted in a past reality of abuse.

> *Learning point 3*
> - What have you learnt from George's story?
> - What feelings do you consider to be okay to express through jointly creating music that match the mood in the here and now?
> - Think of the kinds of music that might match your mood in the here and now and help you overcome emotional pain and mourn instead of bottling up or ignoring sorrow.

Making sense of the offence through music therapy

In individual music therapy, George reflected on his hopeless and lost state and his shame before coming to the hospital. He described how he felt thoroughly misunderstood, and explained that the offence took place one day when he had, in fact, been contemplating taking his own life by jumping from a bridge. He saw some people who he thought were talking about him. He thought that he heard one of the men call out his name, and then he thought that he heard another man make an insulting sexual reference about his mother.

In fact, what had actually happened was that he had heard voices talking badly about his mum, which he attributed as coming from the person who he then attacked as if to defend his mother's honour and thus he killed him.

One of the people who was with the victim was, it later transpired, also called George. So, George really had heard one of the people use his own name. It then seemed that he had mistaken the derogatory rude comments about his mother as coming from the victim when they had actually come from the voices. This had triggered his rage, as it reactivated his anger both at his mother's death and his lack of access to help. The comment he heard made him believe and feel that the one person in his life whom he had loved more than anyone else had been profoundly insulted. He attacked thinking he was defending her honour and protecting himself from assault, as if he was still that abused child, and he fatally wounded the man.

It took years of work to put together the various aspects of this terribly tragic loss of life and the confusion between past experiences and the present in George's story with the incidents that led up to his offence. It was in music therapy that George had an epiphany in which, within the safety of a trusting therapeutic relationship, he was able to recognise that it was due to confusion over what his voices were saying (they had been telling him to attack the victim) and the reality of the situation that he had made such a horrendous mistake.

We both felt huge horror when George recognised in that therapy session, all those years after the offence, how he had felt controlled by the voices and how he had lost control. He realised that he had killed an innocent man because of how he had understood the voices, whereas he always thought he was doing the right things by doing what he was told. His voices seemed to have misled him.

Discussion

This work on the offence was a process over several years of individual therapy, because it needed to be done particularly sensitively. A powerful moment came about after I had connected with George's inner world by tuning in musically. In jointly creating the music, I had to be prepared to be emotionally strong enough in our music-making to enter George's inner world and lead him gently back to a safe and healthy place within himself, so that he could also relate to me.

The musical improvisations reflected his inner state, and his tortured forms of musical expression represented all that he had gone through and his shattered dreams. He had shared all those experiences with me. By our recording and playing back these improvisations in the sessions, George was better able to hear and to see himself.

It was only after we made sense of what had gone so wrong that George felt well enough and more at peace in his own mind to be able to join with others in G-CAMT. It was then that George discovered how to reconcile himself with other people: he was able to help others in this group as he had learned a lot of wisdom through his personal process of inner change. He felt valued again because others looked to him for advice without him being either too dominating or too withdrawn. Even if individuals felt differently about some things or disagreed, this could be reconciled in the sessions with help from the two music therapists. Everyone discovered how to understand each other better.

When George and I reviewed the overall therapy process, he reflected on how he had initially played music sadly, missing his mum. He recognised that the same feeling came up for him when he felt my musical support. This reminded him of how he used to feel 'supported' by her. In this way, George processed and shared his unresolved feelings of grief. Then he was able to release some of his pent-up resentment and to express his pain and angst. At one point I could hear how his music trilled indefinitely and precariously on two very high notes. I recall feeling as if this represented how George had teetered on a high-up ledge at that point, as if he was on that bridge and was about to jump. Yet, at the same time, he was also clearly in our music; we were there together, as though I had managed to invite him back to a safer place. It really felt as if I was saving his life.

The music directly represented what he had been talking and thinking about. I felt very emotional about this, and my supervisor could hear the same desperate qualities when I played back that musical improvisation in supervision. This helped me to feel less emotionally drained and alone in our difficult work.

George could play quite violently, but he played creatively and never damaged the musical instruments, and he could take our music to 'far-out' places. He came to a point of acceptance that, in the past, some of his hopes had, in fact, been unrealistic. He discovered how to differentiate his fantasies from his real life. His responses and emotions were initially jumbled up and chaotic; gradually they became more and more poignant, sorrowful and, finally, full of remorse and caring feelings.

In particular, improvising together helped George to reconnect first to me and then to others on the ward, rather than isolating himself. The positive nature of the therapeutic relationship enabled George to re-experience a different sort of trust, care and nurture, and eventually accept the things that could never be changed and to move on.

George had suffered a great deal in his life, as a result of which he had disconnected from all his feelings of pain. In music therapy, he was able to accept some feelings back within himself and thereby feel more whole and complete. George was now able to tolerate the sadness of his losses. My role was to contain, empathise with and sometimes challenge his experiences. Only then did George become able to speak up for himself and talk about how and why he had killed. This work was emotionally demanding for us both. While no one can condone or make excuses for an unlawful killing, George could be caring of his peers, of human rights and of me; he would try to better himself and he bared his soul in unravelling what had really happened, sharing his shattered dreams.

George developed feelings of remorse that he expressed eloquently within his music in his attempt to say sorry. Yet he remained aware of his impotence to ever put right what he had done. As our work progressed, he began to feel that he wanted to say sorry to the victim's family and to make amends, even though he knew that he could never undo what he had done wrong. This process is called restorative justice. It is a complex and prolonged process that has to be handled with great sensitivity to the feelings of the victim's family. George said that music therapy had literally 'resurrected' the good part of him. Finally, he was able to move on to conditions of lesser security near his home area.

> *Learning point 4*
> - In what ways does making music together in a clinical therapeutic setting reveal aspects of what happened long ago?
> - How is this remembered behaviour then ameliorated in the therapy?

Conclusion

George taught me more than anyone about the impact of deprivation, discrimination, rage, abuse, humility and the loss of love. When our work drew to a close, George was assessed as ready to move to conditions of lesser security. When saying goodbye, he was able to grieve naturally, not so much for the loss of me, but for the meaning and curative effect of our working relationship, which had facilitated his ability to mourn all the other losses. He no longer had to hold it all in and 'shut up and put up', as the abuser had said to that lovely little boy George, prior to robbing him of the innocence of childhood.

To mourn is often avoided because initially it feels so inconsolable. But even though we may fear that we might actually die if we were to allow ourselves to feel certain emotions, this is not actually the case. George was courageous in being able to share with me his initial feelings of shame and his whole life story, and, because he found he could do this safely and with understanding, he was able to overcome old feelings of humiliation. He felt supported through this to discover how to tolerate and work through pain and suffering to a more philosophical place, where his self-esteem developed, as others would even turn to him for advice.

It is important to remember that it is rare for people who experience distress with their voice-hearing experience to commit offences, as pointed out at the start of this chapter. In this case, George recognised how he had lost control when powerful negative emotions were accidentally triggered following the bereavement and other compounding issues.

We now know that group G-CAMT can help the individual to self-reflect (Sleight & Compton Dickinson, 2013) and discover how to manage better the instinctual impulses of fight, flight or freeze.

In fact, research shows that there may be more risk of potentially violent incidents from people who have not had G-CAMT while resident in secure hospitals (Kellet et al., 2019). A larger study is needed to explore how this, and other models of music therapy, could be helpful both in hospitals and in the community – for example, through social prescribing.

The goal for the future is that cognitive analytic music therapy can be included as a standard part of multidisciplinary hospital and community treatment, as the research shows that those receiving it become less withdrawn and more able to manage being with others, so that they can recover and move on more quickly.

With thanks to George for his informed consent for me to share his story, and to the many professional colleagues who helped along George's journey

Further reading

Campbell, N.C., Murray, E. & Darbyshire, J. (2007). Designing and evaluating complex interventions to improve healthcare. *British Medical Journal, 334,* 455–459.

Compton Dickinson, S.J. (2015). *A feasibility trial of group cognitive analytic music therapy in secure hospital settings.* Doctoral thesis. Anglia Ruskin University. https://arro.anglia.ac.uk/id/eprint/581523/

Compton Dickinson, S.J., Odell-Miller, H. & Adlam, J. (Eds.) (2013). *Forensic music therapy: A treatment for men and women in secure hospital settings.* Jessica Kingsley Publishers.

References

Blood, A.J. & Zatorre, R.J. (2001). Intensely pleasurable responses to music correlate with activity in brain regions implicated in reward and emotion. *Proceedings of the National Academy of Sciences, 98*(1), 11818–11823.

Compton Dickinson, S.J. & Hakvoort, L. (2017). *The clinicians guide to forensic music therapy: Two treatment manuals.* Jessica Kingsley Publishers.

Compton Dickinson, S.J. & Jolliffe, D. (2021). Enhancing empathy amongst mentally disordered offenders with music therapy. In D. Jolliffe & R. Farrington. (2021). *Empathy versus offending, aggression and bullying* (pp.142–154). Routledge.

Fachner, J. (2009). Music and altered states of consciousness: An overview. In: D. Aldridge & J. Fachner (Eds.). *Music and altered states: Consciousness, transcendence, therapy and addictions* (pp.15–37). Jessica Kingsley Publishers.

Hickling, F. & Rodgers-Johnson, P. (1995). The incidence of first contact schizophrenia in Jamaica. *British Journal of Psychiatry, 167*(2), 193–196.

Kellett, S., Hall, J. & Compton Dickinson, S.J. (2019). Group cognitive analytic music therapy: A quasi-experimental feasibility study conducted in a high secure hospital. Nordic Journal of Music Therapy, 28(3), 224–255.

Pettitt, B., Greenhead, S., Khalifeh, H., Drennan, V., Hart, T., Hogg, J., Borschmann, R., Mamo, E. & Moran, P. (2013). At risk, yet dismissed: The criminal victimisation of people with mental health problems. Victim Support/Mind. www.mind.org.uk/media-a/4121/at-risk-yet-dismissed-report.pdf

Sleight, V. & Compton Dickinson, S.J. (2013). Risks, ruptures and the role of the co-therapist. In S.J. Compton Dickinson, H. Odell-Miller & J. Adlam (Eds.), *Forensic music therapy: a treatment for men and women in secure hospital settings* (pp.169–183). Jessica Kingsley Publishers.

Tinnin, L. (1990). Mental unity altered states of consciousness and dissociation. *Dissociation, 3*(3), 154–159.

Conclusion
Isla Parker, Joachim Schnackenberg and Mark Hopfenbeck

This practical handbook offers fresh perspectives as to how creatively, courageously and earnestly voice hearers, activists, professionals and researchers have been seeking and finding new ways and insights into how to understand, deal or live with, and sometimes even learn from and be encouraged by, voices. Most of the contributing authors have spent a great deal of their lives working out new approaches, values and ideas, driven by the belief that more must be possible for people who are hearing voices and are distressed by them. It has become clear that for none of these authors has it been a question of how best to ignore voices. Many of the contributors have developed these practices in the face of, at times, strong opposition, as some of the views and approaches introduced in this book have questioned much of current mainstream practice.

For some contributors, the main aim of their interventions seems to be to help the voice hearer to be more assertive with the voices. For others, it has been about walking alongside the voice hearer as they learn to engage more constructively with the voices, and possibly even learn to relate to them as helpful sources of knowledge. For all, the aim is to show how the lives of voice hearers can improve so that they can live their lives to the full while accepting that they may need to learn to live with the voices, even if the voices do seem to disappear for a while, or completely for some, once they have been worked with constructively. Recovery is a loose term – it means different things to different people and can mean different things at different times. However, at its core, it represents the value and idea that people can move on to live the lives they want to without having to accept that they will always be impeded by a particular experience, such as hearing voices. This handbook offers a fresh person-centred approach to recovery, in that the individual can choose which strategies or therapies help them to live better with their voices. The individual may wish to meet a partner or have a child, or engage with a new hobby such as running or playing an instrument. They may wish to have a job or start their own business. Any one of these goals could help the person thrive and enjoy life.

Living with voices that can be noisy and experienced as negative and frightening is not easy. It takes courage, kindness and patience with oneself, as well as determination to try out a different approach to relating to voices. This handbook offers a lot of options – attending a hearing voices group, the Maastricht Approach, experience focused counselling, cognitive therapy approaches, compassion-focused therapy, psychodynamic therapy, dramatherapy and dance movement therapy, to name a few. The book also highlights the need to focus on language and values. Given the broad range of choices, there is something for everyone.

We have found in the course of collecting these chapters that not everyone agrees on the right way ahead or on the kind of language that it is appropriate to use. Some approaches may not agree that an openness to the links between trauma and the voices is the right way forward, let alone speaking curiously and openly with voices that may initially seem similar to an abusive person from the person's past. Others may not agree with the use of language that remains suggestive of disorder, pathology or even problems. This is okay. Not every approach is right for every person all of the time. It may also be that a person is initially cautious and then becomes more open to working in a more trauma-informed way as they go along. And vice versa. It is therefore a good idea for the voice hearer to keep checking out and clarifying with potentially accompanying persons, such as family, friends or mental health professionals, what every person finds helpful for themselves. It may be that they find a different approach that they prefer, but without first of all trying out a different approach, they would not know this to be the case.

Given that this is 'a practical handbook', the emphasis has been on providing practical strategies to try out. Voice hearers are increasingly empowering themselves to make changes, and today a number of voice hearers work as peers, trainers, coaches, supervisors, researchers, social activists, and so on. They are offering support to other voice hearers and anyone who might be accompanying or supporting other voice hearers who would like to improve how they relate to (their) voices, and make positive changes in their lives. Recovery and healing can occur in the context of everyday relationships, when the voice hearer builds a network of people who offer them support and company. If a voice hearer is feeling low and unmotivated, they may wish to suggest to a peer that they read one of the chapters in this handbook together, as this may offer them ideas to try out that will kick-start a new way of making a positive change in their lives – although they may of course find their own creative and helpful ways.

We believe that every voice hearer should have the opportunity to be loved, to love and to be able to work, if that is their choice. We also remember that hearing voices, having difficult relationships and difficult and traumatic experiences are a normal part of basic human existence. They do not belong to psychiatry or to therapists, and determining how to view and approach these experiences is not the privilege of certain professionals only. It is for voice hearers to decide how they want to relate to these experiences and if and whether they want a particular kind of support with them.

We look at this book as an invitation for a further exchange of ideas and dialogue and a statement to the wider world of mental health services and society that fundamental changes are both needed and possible. The future belongs to trauma-sensitive, recovery-orientated mental health and social action initiatives with a genuine belief in the inherent ability of every person to live their life to their full potential. It is likely to require a complete paradigmatic overhaul of today's hierarchical structures and systems, both towards the people using services and between professions. Support should be client led in a genuine collaborative system, not one in which the profession or title a person holds counts more than the lived experience of clients or, indeed, of other professionals; more than genuine, positive, client-led collaboration, real teamwork and more even than the latest research knowledge. Given how much has to change, it is not surprising that the kind of recovery-promoting relationships that are needed are still not the norm.

And yet, we are allowed to have hope because we are surrounded by modern heroes – voice hearers. In our experience, voice hearers are often survivors of untold horrors and traumas. They deserve to be treated like really strong people because they have survived often horrific and traumatic experiences in which they have been victims in their personal histories. They have often also had very traumatic mental health service experiences. The many stories of their great courage and suffering in their own recovery can but fill us with hope. If we want to look for strength and resilience and inspiration, we need look no further than to the people who have come so far. We do not mean just those who have come far in their recovery journey, but all voice hearers.

A final reason why we are allowed to have hope – as indicated in the introduction – is, of course, the voices themselves. When we did not want to hear the stories of trauma, hurt, assault and degradation, they have continued to insist that the truth must be heard. When we did not want to treat either voice hearers or voices with respect and sought to dismiss or eradicate them, they taught us to relate to them respectfully and sometimes even lovingly, so that we can understand that they can be used for good and can spur us all on to truly become the best we can all be.

The famous 14th century mystic and voice hearer Julian of Norwich, when she was close to despair at the sight of all the suffering around her, heard a comforting voice that helped her understand that there was a way through it all: 'And all shall be well and all shall be well and all manner of thing shall be well' (quoted in Spearing & Spearing, 1998, p.80). So we, too, do not want to give up the confidence that, despite all of the suffering, there can be a way forward.

We would like to thank all our authors for taking time to share their knowledge, experience and hope for recovery. To the voice hearers and their supporters who are dipping into this handbook, we would like to say: 'Carpe diem! Seize the day!' We hope that you have enjoyed reading this book, and good luck!

Reference

Spearing, E. & Spearing, A.C. (1998). *Julian of Norwich: Revelations of divine love*. Penguin Books.

Some resources

Intervoice (the umbrella organisation for the international Hearing Voices Movement) – www.intervoiceonline.org

Understanding Voices (a resource website hosted by Durham university) – https://understandingvoices.com/

Contact details

To contact the editors, email Joachim Schnackenberg via the efc Institute (www.efc-institut.de) at info@efc-institut.de

Afterword
Gail A. Hornstein

For more than a century, the phenomenon in which the 'senses are activated without there being an obvious external cause' (Chapter 26), often pejoratively labelled 'hallucinations' or 'false perceptions', has been seen as a defining symptom of mental illness. People who report such experiences are typically assigned a diagnosis of schizophrenia or other psychoses and they are prescribed neuroleptic medication to try to block out or stop their voices, visions or unshared experiences. Such interventions often fail or are rejected because of their toxic side effects. Even when these standard treatments are effective, they shed little light on the underlying mechanisms of voice hearing.

The development of the Hearing Voices Approach, beginning in the late 1980s, has been the prime catalyst for significant advances in the understanding of voice hearing, and this growth in knowledge over the past few decades now enables a book like this one to be written. By creating a compendium of approaches to understanding and coping with voices, and by addressing the specific needs of many different kinds of individuals, this book makes accessible for the first time – to professionals, to families, and, of course, to voice hearers themselves – a rich and creative range of alternatives.

These chapters describe many forms of psychotherapy, some familiar, like psychoanalytic and cognitive behavioural therapy (CBT), and others less well known, like values-based practice, experience focused counselling, and sound, music, drama and avatar therapy. Techniques that allow voice hearers to learn more about their experiences and better articulate their specific features, like the Maastricht Interview, voice dialoguing and the narrative genogram are also explored. Discussions of alternatives like hearing voices peer-support groups, Open Dialogue, meditation, and mindfulness complement chapters focused on the needs of specific subgroups of voice hearers, such as those from diverse ethnicities, children and young people and people with dementia. Regardless of their own particular backgrounds and interests, readers have the opportunity to widen their understandings.

Like the Hearing Voices Approach itself, the perspectives included in this book all start from the assumption that voice hearing, or any other kind of perplexing or unshared experience, has meaning, that it is not just a symptom of an illness, or possibly not even a sign of an illness at all, and trying simply to stop or block it out is not necessarily an appropriate or useful goal. Mental life is complex, and voice hearing is an experience that has existed throughout human history. The phenomenon means different things in different contexts and to different people. Sometimes it causes distress and sometimes it does not. Many people in the general population hear voices at least occasionally (estimates range from 4% to 10%); they just may not talk about it.

Voices that are demanding or threatening are understandably the source of greatest distress, both for voice hearers and for their families and carers. But this is where interpreting the meaning of the voices – especially their symbolic or metaphoric communications – can be most helpful. For example, threatening commands (for example, not to go out or not to trust someone) often have a protective function. Once the actual risk is understood, the threatening voice often modulates.

It is now clear that voice hearing in and of itself need not be distressing, and voices *per se* are often not the problem – it is the *relationship* between the person and their voices (e.g. bullying, inspiring, threatening, guiding and so forth), and how the voices are *interpreted* (e.g. as mental illness, a gift, a meaningful response to trauma and so forth) that determines how distressing the experience will be for a given person. Accordingly, many of the therapies described in this book focus on restructuring the relationship with and among the voices as a means of reducing the distress that negative voices can cause, rather than trying to stop them. As Dirk Corstens notes (Chapter 1), 'Voices need to be heard, but shouldn't be obeyed' – a distinction often not appreciated by voice hearers or by those seeking to help them. Techniques like talking with voices or voice dialoguing that enable the person to understand what the voices are trying to communicate can allow a detachment from the compulsion to enact in literal terms what they are saying.

The diversity described within the chapters of this book shows how crucial it is to suspend preconceived notions about voice hearing in general or the specific form it happens to take for an individual. The curiosity and openness to learning and deeper understanding highlighted by these authors can come from many sources – a psychotherapist, a soundscape, a hearing voices peer-support group. Each is helpful for some people in reducing distress from voices; no one method works for everyone. What especially does *not* work is a 'one-size-fits-all' attitude. As Mark Hopfenbeck notes (Chapter 27): 'Some will prefer to take medication; others will choose not to. Some will want to develop a relationship with their voices; others hate their voices and may not feel comfortable engaging with them.' In other words, for an intervention to be helpful, it must be consistent with the needs and choices of the individual. People who can describe their voices in vivid detail, for example, may particularly benefit from an approach like AVATAR or drama therapy; those with 'unusual sonic experiences' (Chapter 36) may relate more to sound therapy; people who feel isolated by their experiences may benefit most from peer support; those who want to explore the meaning of their voices may find psychotherapy or a hearing voices group most useful, and so on. It's often difficult to tell in advance what will help to reduce distress for a given person; that's why familiarity with a range of approaches and an open-minded attitude are so crucial.

Bill Fulford and David Crepaz-Keay (Chapter 13) make the key point that, although 'science' is often mistrusted, 'scientific advances open up choices in healthcare and with choices go values'. The transformative power of peer support, for example, has frequently been underestimated, with many clinicians seeing it primarily as social (rather than therapeutic) and as an adjunct – even if helpful – to 'real' interventions like medication or psychotherapy. But the findings of our US national study (Hornstein et al., 2020, 2021), based on the largest and most diverse sample of hearing voices group participants to date, demonstrate that these groups can, in and of themselves, foster significant and lasting change, even for people with diagnoses like 'chronic schizophrenia'. Voice hearers in some countries now have ready access to these groups, offering greater choice for people who have typically had few alternatives beyond medication or hospitalisation.

'Evidence-based treatments' are routinely hailed as key to scientific progress, but who decides, using what criteria, how 'evidence' will be defined? The many voice hearers who have ceased consulting mental health professionals or tapered themselves off medications that seemed more toxic than useful are not included in studies intended to assess the effectiveness of psychiatric treatment. The many voice hearers who attend hearing voices groups and are then able to return to work, school, or family responsibilities and are thus no longer in contact with mental health services are not included in studies evaluating standard interventions for voice hearers. As a consequence, the 'evidence base' for the approaches routinely used to ameliorate distressing voices is quite narrow, typically limited to samples of 'chronic' patients prescribed medication and/or CBT. Voice hearers and their families and allies may not even have heard of many of the alternatives described in this book, and mental health professionals may have little familiarity with the significant body of research that now supports these approaches.

This book joins a growing body of literature that starts from the assumption that people's actions and feelings always make sense (at least to them), even if others find those meanings hard to decipher. Human beings have a fundamental need to understand their own experiences – especially when confusing or frightening – and providing a framework for them to explore the significance of their own perceptions and feelings can lay the foundation for profound change.

The lack of attention – sometimes bordering on disrespect – to the *specificities* of their experiences that voice hearers have often received from mental health professionals or family members has until recently prevented the emergence of more varied and individualised approaches to understanding and coping with voices. This volume shows what's possible if you start from the assumption that even highly distressed people can articulate what is likely to be most helpful for them, what has not worked and, most importantly, what runs the risk of making things worse. Professionals often assume that they know which intervention will be most effective, but as activist Pat Deegan has noted (2005): 'Help isn't help if it's not helpful. Help that is not helpful can actually do harm.' The contributors in this book exemplify the flexible, creative and curious attitude that is key to discovering what is actually helpful for a given person, in welcome contrast to the all-too-common attitude that if one approach doesn't work, the problem should be declared 'chronic' and the person 'treatment resistant'. By emphasising the resilient and imaginative ways that voice hearers can cope with distress, these contributors remind us, as Dirk Corstens (Chapter 1) puts it, that 'Voice hearing is a natural and personal human experience. It does not belong to psychiatry.'

References

Deegan, P. (2005, September 6). *When help is not helpful.* [Blog]. www.commongroundprogram.com/blog/when-help-is-not-helpful

Hornstein, G.A., Branitsky, A. & Robinson Putnam, E. (2021). The diverse functions of hearing voices peer-support groups: Findings and case examples from a US national study. *Psychosis: Psychological, social and integrative approaches*, DOI: 10.1080/17522439.2021.1897653

Hornstein, G.A., Robinson Putnam, E. & Branitsky, A. (2020). How do hearing voices peer-support groups work? A three-phase model of transformation. *Psychosis: Psychological, social and integrative approaches, 12*(3), 201–211. doi: 10.1080/17522439.2020.1749876

Contributors

Rob Allison
Rob Allison is a mental health nurse and lecturer and has been interested in voice hearing throughout his nursing career. Over time, Rob came to conceptualise voices from a 'professional framework', but he found that this could marginalise an individual's account of voice hearing. Subsequently, he became aware of Voice Dialogue as a method of helping people to explore and develop more purposeful relationships with their voices. As part of Rob's PhD, he explored experiences of voice hearing from the perspectives of people who hear voices and mental health practitioners. He developed a novel theory of a tripartite relationship involving voice hearers, voices and practitioners, and guidance regarding how treatment experiences can influence voice hearing and be improved.

Deborah Altman
Deborah Altman has worked as a disability adviser in universities for almost 20 years. She is committed to offering all students the opportunity to discover the joy of studying and enabling them to fulfil their potential. She has a Master's degree in special and inclusive education, and further qualifications in supporting dyslexic students and those with autism spectrum conditions. Informed by the social model of disability, Deborah aims to address the socially constructed barriers that affect disadvantaged students. More recently, her explorations of the debates around conceptualisations of mental ill health and neurodiversity as disability or difference has helped to consolidate her approach to supporting students with hidden disabilities, including those who hear voices and students with chronic health conditions.

Daniel Baines
Daniel Baines is a fan of metalcore music who helped to create the peer support project Heavy Metal Therapy after finding metal music to be helpful for managing mental wellbeing and voices. He continues to support the project as Chief Metalcore

Advisor and shares his experiences with others in the hope of supporting them with their own struggles.

Dr Nicola Barclay
Nicola Barclay is a clinical psychologist in an NHS Early Intervention in Psychosis (EIP) service. She is interested in developing our understanding of how unusual sensory perceptions develop and, for those who find these experiences problematic, interventions to reduce distress and improve quality of life.

Assistant Professor Aaron P. Brinen
Aaron Brinen is an assistant professor in the Department of Psychiatry at Drexel University College of Medicine, Philadelphia. He trains residents in the cognitive behavioural therapy for psychosis (CBTp) section of their training. He teaches CBTp through the lens of recovery-oriented cognitive therapy. Additionally, Dr Brinen supervises residents in CBTp cases and an elective in dissemination. Dr Brinen is interested in researching the impact of recovery-oriented cognitive therapy on inpatient and outpatient individuals. Additionally, he is interested in the cross-over of different evidence-based treatments, particularly prolonged exposure for PTSD applied to individuals with both PTSD and a diagnosis of schizophrenia.

Peter Bullimore
Peter Bullimore is a voice hearer, but not just a voice hearer. He is proud to say that he is a voice hearer. Peter spent 10 years in the psychiatric system and was told that he would never work again. He has reclaimed his life from the mental health system and now works as a mental health consultant and trainer. He works 70–80 hours a week delivering training around the world on hearing voices, paranoia and childhood trauma.

Dr Mary Coaten
Mary Coaten recently completed her doctorate at the Institute for Medical Humanities, Durham University. She is a dance movement psychotherapist in the NHS. Her area of research is dance movement psychotherapy in acute psychosis. For the past decade, Mary has worked in the acute adult mental health inpatient setting, delivering dance movement psychotherapy groups. This work sparked her particular interest in the use of embodied and creative arts approaches for severe mental distress. She also works in a psychological therapies community team in an NHS trust, with a focus on trauma.

Ron Coleman
Ron Coleman's own route to recovery from the psychiatric system came from being a founder member, then national coordinator of the then UK Hearing Voices Movement. His own journey has given him many insights into the many difficult issues facing today's mental health services. Ron has published several books, including *Politics of the Madhouse* and *Recovery: An alien concept?* Currently Ron has reached an early retirement due to memory loss and other health problems.

This has not stopped him from writing, blogging, occasional appearances and a new passion for the politics of the dementia world, especially the voice of the protagonist. He is living as full a life as possible and is investigating artificial intelligence and neuroplasticity as a way of keeping independent for as long as possible.

Louise Combes
Louise Combes has worked as a dramatherapist at Aspire, Leeds Early Intervention in Psychosis since 2011. She specialises in working with clients who are not yet ready for talking therapies. With a multi-sensory approach, Louise gives people a choice of activities working with body movement, projecting ideas onto objects, or using roles as a way to express themselves and make positive changes. She is a registered dramatherapist, systemic practitioner, supervisor and trainer. Before her career in mental health, Louise worked in theatre, film and television and was head of communications at Comic Relief.

Dr Stella Compton Dickinson
Dr Stella Compton Dickinson is a London-based Health and Care Profession Council-registered music therapist, accredited supervisor, professional oboist and lecturer, and UKCP-registered cognitive analytic therapist and supervisor. She is co-author of *The Clinician's Guide to Forensic Music Therapy* (2017), and has her own private practice and 20 years' experience in the National Health Service as a clinician, head of arts therapies and clinical research lead. Her research was awarded the 2016 Ruskin Medal for the most impactful doctoral research.

Professor Chris Cook
Christopher C.H. Cook is Professor of Spirituality, Theology & Health and Director of the Centre for Spirituality, Theology & Health at Durham University. He is a Fellow of the Royal College of Psychiatrists, with research doctorates in medicine and theology. Ordained a priest in 2001, he is an Honorary Minor Canon of Durham Cathedral and Honorary Chaplain for Tees, Esk & Wear Valleys NHS Foundation Trust. His books include *Hearing Voices, Demonic and Divine* (2018), and *Spirituality, Theology and Mental Health* (2013), and he is co-editor of *Spirituality and Narrative in Psychiatric Practice: Stories of mind and soul* (2016).

Dr Dirk Corstens
Dirk Corstens has been a key collaborator in the Hearing Voices Project of Marius Romme and Sandra Escher at the University of Maastricht, Netherlands since qualifying as a social psychiatrist and psychotherapist in 1992. He is educated in cognitive, psychodynamic and systems therapy, transactional analysis, Voice Dialogue work, and Peer-supported Open Dialogue. He works now as a social psychiatrist and psychotherapist in Den Helder and Texel (Netherlands) in a community mental health team, and with Open Dialogue and individually with voice hearers. Dirk was the chair of the Intervoice Board 2009–2016 and recently temporarily again. Dirk developed the recovery programme 'Talking with Voices',

and is participating in research on this subject. He delivers courses on working and talking with voices.

Christine Cox
Christine Cox is a psychodynamic psychotherapist and counsellor, now retired from clinical practice. She has worked in mental health all her life, beginning as an occupational therapist working in psychiatric hospitals and later training to be a counsellor and psychotherapist. She worked for many years at the Isis Centre, an NHS counselling centre in Oxford, and concurrently developed a private practice in counselling and psychotherapy. She taught on the psychodynamic counselling training programme in the Continuing Education Department of the University of Oxford.

Professor Tom K.J. Craig
Tom Craig is Emeritus Professor of Social Psychiatry at the Institute of Psychiatry, Psychology and Neuroscience, King's College London, and Past-President of the World Association of Social Psychiatry. His clinical research focuses on developing and evaluating community-based psychiatric services and the promotion of these solutions at a national and international level. These programmes have included residential alternatives to the hospital asylum, specialised services for homeless mentally ill people, supported employment programmes, services for first episode psychosis and studies of the computer-based AVATAR programme for the treatment of auditory hallucinations.

Dr David Crepaz-Keay
Dr David Crepaz-Keay is Head of Empowerment and Social Inclusion for the Mental Health Foundation. He has been a technical advisor to the World Health Organization on empowerment issues. He worked with Public Health England on the 'Every Mind Matters' national campaign. David has received multiple psychiatric diagnoses and spent much time as a detained patient. He has a particular interest in hearing and seeing things, has been living with visions and voices for more than 40 years and has written and spoken widely on this and many other mental health concerns. He co-founded the National Survivor User Network.

Angie Culham
Angie Culham is a service user. Things were tough for her years ago. However, she is turning things around and she gives as much time as she can to helping others. Angie enjoys reading and writing poetry and meeting friends. She has met so many lovely people along the way and learned so much. Her own mental health has improved. It took a long time for Angie to admit that she heard voices, as there was a stigma about mental health. Now she is happy to talk about it, as she doesn't want anyone to hide how they feel.

Senait Debesay
Senait Debesay is a German-trained learning disabilities nurse (Heilerzieh-

ungspflegerin) and a state-recognised therapeutic educator (Diplom-Heilpädagogin). She first came across the experience focused counselling (EFC) approach in 2006 and has been applying EFC in a variety of settings with adults, children and young people who hear voices ever since. In 2007 she co-founded the efc Institute (www.efc-institut.de) to promote the development of training, education, research and supervision in EFC in German speaking countries and internationally. For several years now she has been pioneering the successful application of the EFC approach with children, young people and their families, as part of a child and young person's community based psychiatric service in Hanover, Germany. In the process, Senait has developed a particular interest in the potentially positive and supporting role of voices in a variety of attachment scenarios, as well as in the overcoming of adverse and traumatic life events. She has been a member of the Hearing Voices Movement since the year 2006 and has initiated various initiatives and support groups.

Dr Guy Dodgson

Guy Dodgson is a clinical psychologist in early intervention in psychosis (EIP) services. Guy has worked in EIP services for many years, and has researched why these services are effective. Working with people who have recently started to experience voices has led to Guy's interest in how voices develop and how voice hearers can make sense of, and manage, the experience.

Sheila Evenden

Having suffered from depression/severe OCD for most of her life, Sheila Evenden became involved in research about 12 years ago, purely by chance. She can honestly say that it is the best thing that has happened to her. As well as giving Sheila a sense of purpose, it means that, by participating in studies, she is able to use her illness in a constructive way, and therefore hopefully make a positive contribution to society. If Sheila going through all this means that someone else won't have to go through it in the future, Sheila thinks that it won't be a wasted life!

Jane Ford

Jane Ford, MA (Durham), BVA, AOTOS, BAST, ABRSM is a singing teacher, choral director and professional sound therapist. She is also secretary of the Therapeutic Sound Association and a sound therapy training provider. Her research interests include singing as an aid for dementia and Parkinson's disease as well as for general health and wellbeing, tuning fork therapy for treating depression and sound therapy in mental health. Jane works in hospices, care homes and secure hospitals, alongside her additional roles as singing teacher at Durham University and director of several choirs in the north east.

Professor Bill Fulford

Bill (KWM) Fulford is Fellow of St Catherine's College and Member of the Philosophy Faculty, University of Oxford; Emeritus Professor of Philosophy and Mental Health, University of Warwick, and Director of the Collaborating Centre for VBP, St Catherine's College, Oxford (valuesbasedpractice.org). His previous posts include Honorary Consultant Psychiatrist, University of Oxford, and Special Adviser for Values-Based Practice in the Department of Health. His publications include *Moral Theory and Medical Practice*, *The Oxford Textbook of Philosophy and Psychiatry*, *The Oxford Handbook of Philosophy and Psychiatry*, and *Essential Values-based Practice* (launch volume for the Cambridge University Press book series on values-based medicine).

Akiko Hart
Akiko Hart (she/her) is the CEO of the National Survivor User Network. She is a trustee of ISPS UK, the English Hearing Voices Network and National Voices, and sits on the Advisory Board of the Institute for Medical Humanities at the University of Durham. She has previously worked as the Hearing Voices Project Manager at Mind in Camden and Director of Mental Health Europe.

Dr Jacqueline Hayes
Jacqueline Hayes is a researcher and psychotherapist with lived experience of voice hearing. Currently teaching and researching at the University of Roehampton, London, she has previously held academic positions at the University of Manchester and University College London. Her work has been featured on BBC Radio 4's *Shortcuts* and in the media. Fascinated by social interaction, she is interested in how the social realities we live in become a part of us – the intersection between social, cultural and psychological. She runs a private practice in East Sussex where she lives with her family: partner Ben, daughter Carys, and baby bump who is due soon.

Dr Mark Hayward
Mark Hayward is a husband, father, Christian and supporter of West Ham United Football Club. He has worked as a clinical psychologist within NHS mental health services for the past 20 years. His roles combine clinical (Lead for the Sussex Voices Clinic – https://www.sussexpartnership.nhs.uk/sussex-voices-clinic); research (Director of Research for Sussex Partnership NHS Foundation Trust), and academic (Honorary Senior Research Fellow at the University of Sussex) activity. Mark is committed to increasing access to effective psychological therapies for people distressed by hearing voices.

Dr Charlie Heriot-Maitland
Dr Charlie Heriot-Maitland is a clinical psychologist, researcher and trainer. He currently holds an academic post at the University of Glasgow (MRC Clinical Research Training Fellow) and a clinical post at Balanced Minds (clinical psychologist and Director). In his academic work, Charlie is researching the application of compassion-focused therapy (CFT) approaches for people with distressing experiences in NHS psychosis services, as well as for children and families who have been referred to social services. He provides psychological therapies and supervision in a specialist CFT practice (Balanced Minds), and also runs compassion training workshops for practitioners and the general public.

Mark Steven Hopfenbeck

Mark Hopfenbeck has been an assistant professor at the Norwegian University of Science and Technology since 1996, and is Programme Director for the PGCert in dialogical practices, network meetings and relational competence, and the Programme Director for a PGCert in mindfulness. Mark is Norwegian coordinator of the Nordic Master's programme in dialogical and collaborative approaches to mental health and recovery. A Visiting Fellow at London South Bank University since 2017, he is lead trainer for PGCert in Peer-supported Open Dialogue, social network and relationship skills.

Professor Gail A. Hornstein

Gail Hornstein is Professor Emerita of Psychology at Mount Holyoke College (Massachusetts, US). Her research centres on the contemporary history and practices of psychology, psychiatry and psychoanalysis, and her articles and opinion pieces have appeared in many scholarly and popular publications. She is author of two books: *To Redeem One Person is to Redeem the World: The life of Frieda Fromm-Reichmann*, which questions standard assumptions about treatment through the story of a pioneering psychiatrist, and *Agnes's Jacket: A psychologist's search for the meanings of madness*, which shows how the insights of people diagnosed with psychosis can challenge fundamental assumptions about mental health, community and human experience. Her *Bibliography of First-Person Narratives of Madness in English*, now in its fifth edition with more than 1,000 titles, is used internationally by educators, clinicians, and peer organisations. She directs the Hearing Voices Research Project (a national research and training effort in the US, supported by the Foundation for Excellence in Mental Health Care), and speaks widely about mental health issues across the US, UK and Europe. www.gailhornstein.com

Charlotte Howard

Charlotte is an individual with personal mental health experiences that have required inpatient treatment in psychiatric services. She was introduced to the hearing voices group while an inpatient in a rehabilitation unit. Charlotte has aspirations to work in the adult mental health field and is currently studying through the Open University to gain qualifications for this.

Oana-Mihaela Iusco

Oana-Mihaela Iusco has been a voice hearer and experiencer of other unusual experiences and struggles since she was very young. She survived many traumatic events, suicide attempts and psychiatric service experiences. In 2015 she participated in an experience focused counselling (EFC) workshop, where she learned how to better make sense of her voices. This helped her to not just accept them but integrate them in her life, too. She thus found a way to overcome some of her experienced traumatic events with the aid of her voices. Since 2016 she has been a regular part of the efc Institute and (co-)delivered workshops for voice hearers and mental health professionals. She also works full time, is finishing her university studies and uses the experience of her own recovery process to help other voice hearers, psychiatry survivors and consumers.

Dr Lykourgos Karatzaferis
Lykourgos Karatzaferis is a social psychiatrist, a member of the social cooperative Psyhi, Logos, Epi-koinonia, and a member of the Hearing Voices Movement. He continues a never-ending education at Athenian Institute of Anthropos (AIA), which uses a systemic-dialectic psychosocial approach, according to which 'Anthropos' is conceptualised as a biopsychosocial, open, information-processing, decision-making anotropic system.

Dr Colin King
Colin King was diagnosed as a schizophrenic at 17 years of age. After enduring brutalised forms of institutionalised racism in the school and psychiatric systems that perpetuated racialised forms of misdiagnosis, Colin became a practitioner, commissioner and teacher. He resisted white voices and noises as he transited to becoming an activist through being a writer and the coordinator of the Whiteness and Race Equality network. Colin has 40 years' experience of being a misunderstood, demonised survivor, and he is currently writing within the oppressed zones of whiteness to produce two books on race and mental health. Currently Colin is a survivor of modern day drapetomania in his academic struggles with white institutions, and he is seeking liberation for his authentic voices to be recognised and heard as sane.

Ruth Lafferty
Voice hearing became a part of Ruth Lafferty's life in her late 40s. She was a practising psychotherapist and, while her voice hearing brought an end to that career, Ruth now uses the knowledge and understanding to help her with her voices and her voice dialogue training practice. Ruth's voices, along with her wonderful life partner, John, now support and encourage her in her new adventure. Ruth has just completed an MA in creative practice. Part of her area of research is the metaphors of trauma in land and seascapes. Her relationships, art and voice-training practices feed each other and provide a model of interdependency that Ruth fully endorses as a way of life.

Dr Anna Luce
Anna Luce is a clinical psychologist in an early intervention in psychosis team. Anna is keen to improve and expand the interventions and approaches she can offer to clients with psychosis and distressing voices, particularly around improving relationships with voices through understanding of their origin and possible functions (e.g. cognitive analytic therapy, Voice Dialogue and Open Dialogue).

Rufus May
Rufus May manages Bolton's acute services psychology team. Rufus has worked as a psychologist in the NHS since 1998. He has been a hearing-voices group facilitator since 2001. Rufus's interests include communication skills, voice

dialogue approaches, body work and creative approaches to using mindfulness. His passion for holistic psychological and social approaches to mental health is rooted in his own experiences at 18 of altered mind states and being treated for psychosis. With his partner Elisabeth Svanholmer, Rufus tries to create resources and training around holistic approaches to voice hearing and other experiences that can be challenging and misunderstood (see www.openmindedonline.com).

Caroline Moughton

Caroline Moughton read English at Cambridge. She worked as a librarian and then moved into an equality role. As Staff Disability Advisor at the University of Oxford from 2012–2018, Caroline was responsible for developing policy and for supporting individual members of staff with long-term health issues, many of whom had mental health conditions. Caroline recognised the importance of developing the university's support of staff experiencing mental ill health, and started work to raise awareness, develop the skills of managers and provide information and support for individuals. A key element of this was empowering individuals to share their stories, which proved very powerful.

Clifford O'Connor

Since college, Clifford has had a variety of jobs. He worked as a ski instructor, joined a high street bank, then trained (and qualified) as a helicopter pilot, before working for the police. He received a Distinction grade from the Open University for completing a design module, and has successfully registered designs with the UK Patent Office. Clifford then lived abroad until it became necessary to return and learn about mental health. Clifford has shared his own experiences with others, helped develop knowledge and skills, and worked part-time for the NHS and a university. He published a non-fiction book and currently works in a library.

Isla Parker

Isla Parker is a pen name. Isla is a freelance editor and writer who promotes the understanding of health issues and wellbeing. She undertook a degree in English, and found it interesting to study how literature explores illness. This led to Isla writing a novel for teenagers about anorexia, called *Size Zero?*, which is loosely based on her own experience. Isla has also co-edited *The Practical Handbook of Dementia* and *The Practical Handbook of Eating Difficulties* (both forthcoming). In her free time Isla enjoys playing the piano. She also takes part in an online writing group that has introduced her to writers from different countries.

Sasha Priddy

Sasha Priddy is a trainee clinical psychologist at the University of Sheffield. Prior to training, Sasha spent three years in the Psychosis and Complex Mental Health Faculty as a representative for the Pre-Qualification Group within the British Psychological Society. She has primarily worked in adult mental health services, across a range of settings, where she developed her interest in hearing voices groups.

Dr Kate Quinn

Kate Quinn is a clinical psychologist from the UK, working in NHS services in early intervention in psychosis. She is also a fan of heavy metal music. Kate's background is in working with young people who have extreme or unusual experiences that may be conceptualised as psychosis, such as hearing voices. She is interested in Voice Dialogue and community psychology approaches, and how we can engage young people in mental health support beyond the therapy room, such as via social media.

Olga Runciman

Olga Runciman is a psychologist and Open Dialogue family therapist. She is the owner of Psycovery, specialising in extreme states. She is a co-founder of the Danish Hearing Voices Network and the new International Institute for Psychiatric Drug Withdrawal. She is also a board member for Intervoice, Mad in America and the Danish Psychosocial Rehabilitation organisation. Olga works closely with WHO's global QualityRights initiative and the UN, particularly within the realms of human rights and psychiatry. Olga knows psychiatry from both the inside and the outside, having been on both sides, and today is in the unique position of being able to create a bridge between patient and professional.

Dr Mar Rus-Calafell

Dr Mar Rus-Calafell is a clinical psychologist. She is the independent research group leader of the Young Voices Research and Interventions (YVORI) research group, which is based at the Mental Health Research and Treatment Center, Ruhr-Universität Bochum. Prior to this, Mar was a post-doctoral researcher at the Oxford Cognitive Approaches to Psychosis group, Department of Psychiatry, University of Oxford, and a visiting Research Fellow at the Institute of Psychiatry, Psychology and Neuroscience, Kings College London. She was a key member of the AVATAR therapy team. Her research focus through her clinical and research career is the understanding and treatment of psychosis and the application of digital interventions, specifically virtual reality.

Dr Joachim Schnackenberg

Joachim Schnackenberg is a UK-trained mental health nurse and a German-trained social pedagogue/worker. He also conducted the first pilot mixed-methods randomised effectiveness study on experience focused counselling (EFC) as part of a PhD. In 2007, in consultation with Professor Marius Romme and Dr Sandra Escher and the German Hearing Voices Network, he co-founded a training institute (efc Institute – www.efc-institut.de) with his colleague Senait Debesay to provide education and training, consultation, supervision and research support to further develop EFC in the German-speaking countries and internationally. As a result, the EFC approach is now applied and further developed in a variety of mainstream acute, long-term rehabilitation and community services. He has been a member of the Hearing Voices Movement since 2000 and has been learning from voice hearers, such as Ron Coleman, and voices ever since. He has been applying the EFC approach in acute, community-based and long-term settings in different countries, particularly in Germany, Switzerland and England since 2000. In 2016, he also became the (part-time) director of hearing and voices and recovery in a psychiatric service in Kropp, Northern Germany.

David Storm
David Storm has worked in the NHS for 36 years, moving to Cumbria in 2004 and spending 25 years championing working with older people and people living with dementia who experience hearing voices or seeing visions. This has led to significant improvements in care offered across Cumbria, including delivering bespoke training to staff in the NHS and care homes, as well as supporting the development of non-traditional interventions. David was appointed Senior Associate of the Dementia Services Development Centre, University of Stirling in 2016, and Associate Director at Cumbria, Northumberland, Tyne & Wear NHS Foundation Trust in 2019.

Elisabeth Svanholmer
Elizabeth Svanholmer is interested in holistic approaches to challenging states of mind, and since 2005 has been involved with organising and facilitating hearing-voices training. This interest has come from Elisabeth's own experiences of hearing voices for as long as she can remember. Elisabeth is passionate about creating resources and supporting community development, such as organising meetings, setting up self-help groups, and providing peer supervision. Elisabeth believes that we can change the world one conversation at a time and this feels like a meaningful way for her to approach life and the messy world we live in. She regularly writes and shares blogs on various subjects, such as living with voices, sensitivity, bodywork, general wellbeing and reflections on life.

Dr Iseult Twamley
Iseult Twamley is a clinical psychologist. Since 2012, she has been Clinical Lead of the Cork Open Dialogue Implementation, Ireland, implementing Open Dialogue as part of the adult mental health service. She has trained and supervised Open Dialogue in the UK, Australia, Israel, Italy and the Netherlands. As a family member and trauma survivor herself, Iseult is passionate about collaborative and co-productive approaches to mental health. She credits her involvement with the Hearing Voices Network as challenging her previous 'education' and ethics and continues to seek opportunities to hear and learn from nonprofessional sources of wisdom.

Reshma Valliappan
Reshma Valliappan, aka Val Resh, is founder-director of The Red Door, which has been using creativity to redefine mental ill health and other disorders. She was awarded the Ashoka and Ink Fellow in 2014 in recognition of her work. A multi-disciplinary artist, Reshma is the protagonist of an award-winning documentary, *A Drop of Sunshine,* and author of a memoir, *Fallen, Standing: My life as a*

schizophrenist. Val's artwork and articles are published in many journals, textbooks and covers. She recently launched her art business, Val Resh, and commissions works, performs as SKii the mime, and speaks at TEDx.

Aimee Wilson

Aimee Wilson is a mental health blogger. Her blog, 'I'm not disordered' (www.imnotdisordered.co.uk), has half a million followers. Aimee began her blog when she was an inpatient in a psychiatric unit and undergoing trauma therapy. Aimee believes that blogging has been hugely instrumental in her recovery and helps her to maintain her mental health. She blogs on a variety of topics that relate to mental health, such as self-harming, stigma and recovery goals.

Name index

A

Aaltonen, J. 279
Abba, N. 316
Accepting Voices 13
Aderhold, V. 137
A Disorder for Everyone 25
Aeschylus 342
Afuape, T. 128
Alakare, B. 276
Alanen, Y.O. 275
Alderson-Day, B. 367
Aldridge, D. 374
Aleman, A. 2, 181
Alexander-Passe, N. 171
Alipor, A. 371
Allen, J.G. 273
Allen, P. 265
Allison, R. 343
All Party Parliamentary Group 211, 216
Andersen, T. 278
Anderson, A. 125, 256
Angermeyer, M.C. 5
Architects 361–362, 365
Arnkil, T.E. 130, 275, 276
Arseneault, L. 95
Asking Alexandria 361, 365
Association for Dance Movement Psychotherapy (ADMP) 352
A Straight Talking Introduction to Psychiatric Drugs 136

B

Bailey, T. 180–181
Baker, F. 307
Baker, P. 35, 220

Bakhtin, M. 307
Baldwin, C. 379
Ball, M. 337
Banerjee, S. 211
Barber, J. 90–91
Bardy-Linder, S. 316
Barker, M. 179
Barkus, E. 25
Barrett, F.S. 374
Bateman, A.W. 285
Bateson, G. 307, 309
Baumeister, D. 256
Beavan, V. 2, 35, 237
Beck, A.T. 229–230, 232
Becker, J. 374
Beethoven 266
Bell, V. 237
Bennett, D. 105
Bentall, R. 35, 141
Beresford, P. 46
Berrol, C. 352
Bikson, M. 121
Binns, C. 113
Bion, W. 290, 292
Biondo, J. 351
Birchwood, M. 236, 238, 247, 259, 298
Birtchnell, J. 240
Blood, A.J. 385
Boden, Z. 273
Bogen-Johnston, L. 249
Bogle, S. 273
Bollas, C. 291
Bowlby, J. 203
Boyce-Tillman, J. 368

Boydell, J. 259
Boyle, M. 1, 3, 4, 27, 124, 129, 136, 147, 180, 181, 274
Brabban, A. 257
Bracken, P. 131
Braehler, C. 302
Brauninger, I. 351
Breen, L.J. 83
Breggin, P.R. 361 70
Bring Me the Horizon, 365
British Comedy Guide 6
Brooker, D. 213
Bruner 307
Bryl, K. 351, 353
Bullimore, P. 4, 5, 313
Burr, J. 4, 180, 181, 182, 183, 185, 186, 187, 190
Burt, C.L. 106
Butler, J. 344, 345

C

Caddy, E. 88
Campbell, N.C. 393
Carter, S. 362–363, 364
Casson, J. 342, 343, 344, 348
Castelnovo, A. 76
Chadwick, P. 259, 316
Chaiklin, S. 353
Children Hearing Voices 208
Chin, J. 247
CIPD/Mind 166
Clark, D. 262
Clarke, D. 374
Clarke, D.M. 259
Clarke, E. 374
Clarke, L. 279
Coard, B. 106
Coaten, M. 353
Cohen, D. 70
Coleman, R. 4, 5, 184, 211, 212–213, 215, 220, 333, 376
Collaborating Centre for Values-based Practice in Health and Social Care 122
Colombo, A. 120
Compassion for Voices 302, 303
Compernolle, T. 343
Compton Dickinson, S.J. 385, 387, 393
Concise Medical Dictionary 287

Cook, C.C.H. 85, 86, 88, 90, 92
Cooke, A. 24, 25, 27, 353
Cooper, M. 359
Copeland, M.E. 166
Copolov, D. 264
Corrigan, P.W. 5
Corstens, D. 2, 3, 4, 21, 22, 25, 40, 81, 143, 149, 184, 195, 240, 247, 258, 306, 307, 334, 364, 367
Coyle, A. 76, 80
Craig, L. 161
Craig, T.K. 238, 239, 242, 243, 247, 331
Crawford, K. 37
Crepaz-Keay, D. 113, 122
Critical Mental Health Nurses Network (CMHNN) 124
Cultural Institute at King's 302, 303
Cunningham, T. 195

D

Dalai Lama 72
David, A.S. 237, 258
Davidson, L. 376, 378
Debesay, S. 191, 203
Deegan, P. 402
de Leede Smith, S. 25
Dent-Brown, K. 344
Deschrijver, M. 22
Deutsche Gesellschaft für Psychiatrie und Psychotherapie, Psychosomatik und Nervenheilkunde e.V. (DGPPN) 138, 139
Deutsche Gesellschaft für Soziale Psychiatrie (DGSP) 137, 139, 149
Dickens, C. 6, 259
Dillon, J. 4, 25, 26, 203
Dingle, G.A. 359
Division of Clinical Psychology 24
Dodgson, G. 264
Dornes, M. 203
Douglas, S. 220
Drama, Psychotherapy and Psychosis 342
Dudley, J. 316
Durham University 92,
du Sert, O.P. 242

E

Eacott, M.J. 266
Easton, S. 35

Eliade, M. 374
Ellerby, M. 302
Elliott, R. 81
Embracing Our Selves 335
Emily's Voices: A memoir 175, 379–380
Emunah, R. 344, 346
Engaging with Voices 302
England, A. 95
Escher, A.D.M.A.C. 2, 43
Escher, S. 3, 13, 15, 35, 36, 40, 45, 147, 181, 182, 184, 186, 187, 195, 203, 208, 213, 214, 240, 266, 315, 316, 329, 344, 377
Eysenck, H.J. 106
Eysenck, S.B.G. 106

F

Fachner, J. 385
Fairbairn, W.R.D. 286, 292
Farhall, J. 374
Faulkner, A. 129
Fernyhough, C. 4, 86, 181, 258, 265
Finkel, S.I. 212
Fletcher, P.C. 266
Fonagy, P. 285
Fossey, J. 221
Foucault, M. 104, 105
Fraser, A. 35
Freeman, A. 279
Freud, A. 289
Freud, S. 107, 288, 289
Fuchs, T. 351
Fulford, K.W.M. 120, 121
Furman, R. 381

G

Galasinski, D. 25, 27
Galton. F. 106
Gandhi, M. 6, 330
Garety, P.A. 259
General Medical Council (GMC) 121
Geretsegger, M. 359
Gerlach, J. 123
Gilbert, P. 295–296, 302, 303, 362, 364
Gillard, S. 276
Gioia, T. 374
Glicksohn, J. 374
God 5, 48, 85, 88, 89, 90, 91, 92, 182
Goffman, E. 5

Gómez, J.M. 273
Gordon, S. 264
Gotsis, I. 309, 314
Green, B. 97
Gregg, L. 97
Griffin, H. 179
Griffin, J.D. 266
Griffiths, R. 374
Grimby, A. 80

H

Hague, P. 40
Hall, W. 138, 139
Hakvoort, L. 387
Hamlet 342
Hammersley, P. 35
Handa, I.A. 119
Hanh, T.N. 319, 322
Harris, T.L. 376–378
Harrison, P. 180
Harrow, M. 138, 149
Hartigan, N. 247
Hayes, J. 76, 77, 78, 80, 81, 82
Hayward, M. 4, 81, 195, 228, 229, 240, 247, 252, 279
Hazell, C. 228
Healey, K. 26
Hearing the Voice 169
Hearing Voices Cymru 181
Hearing Voices Movement (HVM) 3, 4, 5, 6, 7, 8, 13, 21, 25, 40, 45–46, 63, 123, 130, 169–170, 180, 181, 182, 183, 195, 196, 211, 212–213, 305–307, 309, 315, 317, 325, 333, 376
Hearing Voices Network (HVN) 123–134, 145, 166, 174, 195, 269, 329
    Athenian Hearing Voices Network 306, 309, 313
    Danish Hearing Voices Network 320
Hearing Voices Network Aotearoa 45
Heriot-Maitland, C. 298, 302, 330
Herman, J. 187, 203
Hermans, H. 305
Herring, J. 121
Herrnstein, R.J. 107
Hickling, F. 385
Higgins, A. 276
Higgs, R. 46
Hildegard of Bingen 330

HM Government 172–173
Hobbes, T. 108
Holley, J. 276
Honig, A. 17
Hopfenbeck, M. 124, 276
Hornstein, G. 376, 401
Howard, S. 284
Huckvale, M. 242
Huhtaniska, S. 137
Hunt, H. 374
Hunt, S. 37

I

Intervoice 4, 6, 124, 169–170, 181, 398
Isik, B.K. 371
Isobel, S. 273

J

Jackson, H.J. 344
Jackson, L. 247
Jackson-Roberts, D. 369, 372–373, 374
Jacobs, M. 285
Jaynes, J. 13
Jennings, S. 341
Jensen, A. 106
Jeong, Y. 351
Jesus (Christ) 88, 90
Joan of Arc 6, 330
Johns, L.C. 121, 230, 367
Johnson, S.L. 259
Johnstone, L. 1, 3, 4, 27, 124, 128, 129, 136, 147, 180, 181, 274
Jolliffe, D. 385
Jones, C. 228
Jones, N. 24
Jones, S.R. 265,266
Julian of Norwich 397
Jung, C.G. 298, 330

K

Kabat Zinn, J. 317
Kalsched, D. 354
Kamp, K. 76
Kant, I. 108
Kellet, S. 393
Kelly, T. 24
Kempe, M. 89
Kennedy, A. 302
Kerri, M. 374

Keys to Safe Trauma Recovery 324
Kinderman, P. 24, 25, 27
Kinnair, D. 344
Kitwood, T. 221
Klein, M. 287
Knoll, E. 175, 179, 376, 379–380
Knols, M. 143
Koch, S. 351
Kokorikou, D. 313
Kolomvrezou, A. 313
Krippner, S. 369, 374
Krishna 87

L

Lady Gaga 6
Lafferty, R. 343
Lahad, M. 344
Lakeman R. 276, 280
Lanarkshire Health Board 121
Landy, R. 342–343, 344, 345, 346
Lang, P. 308–309
Langer, A.I. 316
Large, M. 94–95
Laroi, F. 2, 181
Larsen, E.B. 123
Layzell, S. 129
Leader, D. 79
Lebert, L. 279
Leff, J. 237–238, 242
Leucht, S. 3, 137, 181
Leudar, I. 76, 77, 78, 82
Leweke, F.M. 95
Lim, A. 258
Lincoln, T.M. 228, 229
Linscott, R.J. 2, 180
Living with Voices: 50 stories of recovery 13, 16, 19, 71, 329
Longden, E. 4, 19, 21, 25, 40, 46, 145, 269, 376
Ludwig, A.M. 368
Luhrmann, T.M. 25, 86, 89, 258, 273–274
Lysaker, P.H. 307, 378

M

Macauley, S., 212
Maise, M. 355
Making Sense of Voices 13
Malone, G. 342
Mantel, H. 259

Marconi, A. 94–95
Marineau, R.F. 343
Markou, S. 308–309
Marriot, A. 221
Martin, C.R. 194
Martin, L.A.L. 353
Matschinger, H. 5
May, R. 25
Mayhew, S.L. 302
McAdam, E. 308, 311–312
McCarthy-Jones, S. 2, 3, 5, 22, 25, 35, 141, 180, 237, 241, 246, 258, 265, 368, 375, 379
McEnteggart, C. 274
McGorry, P.D. 344
McGrath, J.J. 195
McLaughlin, T. 37
McLeod J. 359
Mead, G.H. 75
Meekums, B. 351, 353
Melley, J. 25
Mercadante, L. 85
Millham, A. 35
Mind 24, 32, 139
Mirza, K.A.H. 311–312
Mitchell, D. 259
Mohammed 88
Mollon, P. 285
Moncrieff, J. 3, 35, 70, 136, 137, 138, 139, 140, 146, 148, 149, 181
Moreno, J.L. 343
Morrison, A.P. 146, 229, 259
Morrison, T. 21
Moses 88–89
Moskowitz, A. 25
Murphy, R. 276
Murray, C. 107
Murray, R.M. 180, 181

N

National Collaborating Centre for Mental Health 115
National Institute for Mental Health in England (NIMHE)/Care Services Improvement Partnership (CSIP) 121
Nayani, T.H. 237, 258
Neale, A. 344
Neck Deep 360–361, 365
Nelson, B. 342

Nelson, H. 221
Nève-Hanquet, C. 310
NHS England 344
National Institute for Health and Care Excellence (NICE) 121, 344
Nietzsche 307
Nieuwenhuis, M. 380
Nonviolent Communication: A language of life 338

O

Ogden T.H. 292
Olson, M. 276, 278
Orestes 342
Our School by the Tower 342
Overcoming Distressed Voices 228

P

People Managers' Guide to Mental Health 166
Perry, A. 258
Peters, E. 228, 375
Pettitt, B. 384
Peyton, S. 338
Pilton, M. 266
Pluymaekers, J. 310, 313
Pohl, G. 203
Potter, D.J. 95
Priebe, S. 353
Purdon, C. 262

R

Rao, D. 5
Ratcliffe, M. 353
Razzaque, R. 147, 276
Read, J. 35, 184, 195, 259, 353
Read Johnson, D. 344
Recovery Movement 3
Rees, W.D. 80
Resnick, P.J. 237
Reynolds, V. 45–46
Richards, V. 24
Riggs, S. 105
Robbins, M. 13
Roe, D. 376, 378
Rogers, C.R. 75
Rogers-Johnson, P. 385
Röhricht, F. 344
Romme, M.A.J. 2, 3, 4, 13, 15, 16, 19, 25, 35,

36, 40, 43, 45, 71, 141, 147, 169, 181, 182, 184, 185, 186, 187, 195, 203, 208, 213, 214, 240, 266, 315, 316, 329, 344, 368, 370, 377
Roof, W.C. 87
Rosenberg, M. 337, 338
Rothschild, B. 324
Rueveni, U. 277
Rumney, B. (Dir) 342
Runciman, O. 4, 5
Rus-Calafell, M. 241
Russell, G. 302
Russo, J. 26, 46
Ryan, M-L. 378

S

Sabucedo, P. 78, 80, 82
Sackett, D.L. 121
St. Paul (Saul) 88–89
Samaha, A-N. 139
Savill, M. 353
Scharff, D.E. 286
Scharff, J.S. 286
Schlimme, J.E. 138, 139, 351
Schmais, C. 353
Schnackenberg, J. 1, 4, 180, 181, 182, 183, 185, 186, 187, 190, 194
Schubart, C.D. 95
Seikkula, J. 124, 130 , 275, 276, 278, 279, 307
Servonnet, A. 138, 139
Sevy, S. 95
Shafi, N. 381
Shakespeare 342
Sharma, H. 259
Sharman, L. 359
Shaw, C. 26
Shevlin, M.D. 258
Short Thought #2: Get to know your voices 332
Shulkes, D. 26
Silva, M. 273
Simmonds, J.G. 375
Slade, P.D. 221
Sleight, V. 393
Smith, D.B. 1
Smith, M. 184, 211, 220
Snell, T.L. 375
Socrates 6, 14
Sohler, N. 138

Spearing, A.C. 397
Spearing, E. 397
Speck, R. 277
Spencer, C. 97
Spring, B. 257
St. Anthony 89
Stanton-Jones, K. 352
Steel, C. 21, 190
Steffen, E.M. 76, 77, 78, 80, 81, 82
Steiner, J. 291
Stephanie, L. 316
Stern, D.N. 278
St. Francis 89
St. Katherine 89
Stockmann, T. 276
Stone, H. 20, 195, 196, 334
Stone, S. 20, 195, 196, 334
Strauss, C. 316
Subbiah, S. 203
Substance Abuse & Mental Health Services Administration (SAMHSA) 274
Swedenborg 330
Sweeney, A. 274

T

Taylor, K. 211, 212, 333
Telles-Correia, D. 26
The Body Keeps the Score 342
The Music of Madness 377
Therapeutic Sound Association 372
Thirioux, B. 342
Thomas, N. 375
Thomas, P. 131
Thomas, S. 82, 87–88
Tien, A.Y. 2
Timimi, S. 70, 139
Tinnin, L. 385
Torregrossa, L.J. 342
Treleaven, D. 323
Trimble, D. 278, 307
Troyer, J.M. 76
Turkington, D. 257, 279
Twamley, I. 5, 132

U

Understanding Voices 169, 398
United Nations Office of the High Commissioner 124

V

Valliant, G.E. 85
Valliappan, R. 52
van der Gaag, M. 228, 359
van der Kolk, B. 203, 342
van der Valk, R. 316
Van Dongen, E. 377, 378–379
van Os, J. 2, 121, 180, 181, 258, 259
Varese, F. 35, 127, 185, 266, 298
Vilhauer, R.P. 259
Virgin Mary 87
Voice Collective 170
von Peter, S. 277, 280
Vo Shakow, A 320, 325
Vygotsky, L.S. 75, 307

W

Waddingham, R. 26, 130
Wade, D. 95
Ward, C.A. 375
Ward, T. 241, 243
Waters, F. 4, 181
Watkins, J. 35
Weinmann, S. 137
Welch, P. 374
Wellcome Trust 92, 244
Wharne, S. 278
Whitaker, R. 145
Wilfer, A. 4
Wilkinson, S. 237, 367
Williams, H.L. 266
Wilson, B. 6
Windeatt, B.A. 89
Winkelman, M. 368
Winnicott, D.W. 75, 288, 293
Woods, A . 4, 5, 21, 26, 27, 237, 306, 376
Woolf, V. 259
Working to Recovery 212
Working with Voices 184

Y

Your Resonant Self 338

Z

Zatore, R.J. 385
Zubin, J. 257

Subject index

A

acceptance 15, 49, 52, 126, 184, 185, 211, 216, 217–20, 243, 283, 308, 316, 317, 325, 367, 370, 388
   of emotions 188
adversity 222, 223, 258
alcohol 60, 70, 97, 101, 156, 163, 257, 259
altered states of mind 290
angels 87, 91, 92, 114, 115
anger 19, 49, 60, 67, 80, 188, 204, 206, 216, 232, 243, 267, 268, 288, 289, 290, 291, 292, 307, 389–90
antipsychotics
   brain changes/volume reductions 3, 137, 181
   in dementia care 216
   and dopamine 138, 139
   efficacy 3, 137, 141, 148–49, 181
   mortality rates 3, 70
   national guidelines on prescribing 3, 6, 7, 115, 120, 139, 145, 149
   neurotoxicity of, 138
   stopping, 139, 140, 1412, 149
   symptomatic relief 136, 142–43
   tapering off, 19, 142, 401
   withdrawal symptoms 139
anxiety
   avatar therapy and, 241, 243
   cognitive model of, 259
   with dementia 214, 220,
   as defence (Freud) 289
   effects of trauma 273
   social, 53, 261
   treatment for, 146, 148
      poetry as, 381
   in voice hearing 17, 78, 97, 99, 157, 171, 173, 195, 230, 268, 285, 291, 321
art as therapy 52–54, 81, 154, 341, 354
   painting 48ff
assertiveness as response to voices 226, 239, 246–48, 279, 338, 395
   in relating therapy 249–52
attachment theory 191, 203, 209, 288, 299, 317
attitudes
   biomedical, 123, 159
   to cannabis use 96
   of caregivers/carers 187, 216, 278
   mindful, 317–18
   to hearing voices 14, 185, 330
AVATAR therapy 237–239
   evidence for, 242–43
avoidance 16, 184, 268, 273, 306, 307, 316
awareness
   as clinical skill 116–117
   conscious, 285
   practices 315, 323
   raising 174
   of self 387

B

beliefs
   about self 223
   about voices 46, 215, 222, 223–24, 230–32, 238
   challenging unhelpful,
      through CT-R 229–30, 232–35
      through AVATAR therapy 241–42
   distressing, 2, 222
   negative, about self 267, 321

unusual/non-shared, 36, 37, 44, 184, 353
questioning (CBT), 224–26
religious, 61, 85, 87, 91, 382
belonging 276, 309, 338, 364
binaural beat 371
biological
approach 2, 7, 35, 127
illness, voice hearing as, 136, 147, 180, 181, 214, 217, 220, 229–30
markers 3
biomedical model 35, 39, 123
bipolar disorder 136
black
despair 107
discrimination 107
empowerment 108
magic 48
men 108
stereotypes 106
voices 104, 107, 108, 113ff
black, Asian, minority ethnic 103
body/embodied (*see also* dissociation/ive) 31, 50, 66–67, 89, 98
in CFT 300, 308
in dance movement therapy 351–52, 353, 355, 356
in drama therapy 342, 346
effects of drugs on, 110, 140, 143, 148
language 250, 252
mindful scans 316
in psychodynamic theory 286–88
as sources of harm 324
tapping 322
trauma/threat effects on, 261–62, 297, 299, 385
use in mindfulness 318–19, 321, 324
brain
disorder(ed), 378
evolution of human, 297–298
voice-hearing processes in, 265–66
-wave activity 368, 373, 381
workings of, 259, 261–63
breath/breathing
exercises 164, 268, 300, 318–19, 320–21, 324, 347
rates 261, 299,
bullying/harassment 16, 120, 152, 163, 167, 171, 191, 238, 247, 268, 273, 291, 298, 400

C

cannabis
benefits of, 96
cutting down 100–101
experience of using, 96–98
harm-minimisation and, 99–100
ingredients 95
and psychosis 94–95
unhelpful effects 98–99
caregiver(s)/carers
attitudes of, 215, 216
dementia, experiences of 216–217
chair work 333, 343
chakra system 370
chants/ing 370
child/children/childhood
black, 106
and choice in therapy 208
and critical parent 21, 339
emotional development of (Klein), 287–88
Freudian theories of, 289–290
hearing voices 203–04
and abuse 209
attachments 209
coping with, 206
expression of, 204–05
and identity 207
and play 207–08
parental attitudes 208
object-relations and, 286–87
childhood abuse
emotional, 37, 204
and hearing voices 258, 385, 389–90
impact of, 393
physical, 16, 35, 37, 152
sexual, 16, 30–32, 35, 37, 57, 60, 62, 66, 67, 142, 190, 204, 239
and guilt 62
choice
and disclosure 170–72
in dramatherapy 344
and empowerment 373, 387
freedom of, 119, 401
of medication 136, 138, 143, 146
and mindfulness 321, 324
in trauma-sensitive approaches 274
civil rights movement(s) 3, 169, 181
cognitive behaviour therapy (CBT) 222ff

and beliefs about self 223–24
and conformation bias 225
and dissociation 266–67
evidence for, 401
integration with other models 364
in Open Dialogue 276
for psychosis (CBT-p) 232–36
in relating therapy 247
and relating to voices 226–27
collaborative/ation 41, 124, 397
   in emotion-focused counselling 184, 186
   in the HVM 307
   in Open Dialogue 124–25
   in trauma-informed approach 274
   with voices 201
communication
   challenging behaviour as, 213
   effects of cannabis on, 96
   through drama 342–43
   impact of voices on, 161
   metaphoric, 400
   through movement 352
   non-verbal, 226, 347, 353
   non-violent, 336–38
   online, 164
   in values-based practice 116–17, 118
   in Voice Dialogue 195–96
   voice hearing as, 72, 87, 278
   with voices 336–339
community
   hearing voices groups/networks as, 33, 39, 124, 125, 129, 278, 279, 329
   internal, of voices 200
   living in, 120, 196, 268, 337
   therapeutic sense of, 354
compassion/compassionate
   as courage 303
   definition of, 295–96
   in emotion-focused counselling 184
   -focused therapy 295ff, 299–301
   self-, 257, 316
   as social mentality 298–99
   'for voices' work (Gilbert) 267
   towards voices 72, 130
confidentiality
   in Freudian theory 289
   in university services 170
   in the workplace 160
conflict

   resolution 116
   of values 120
   voices and spirituality 91
connection
   in compassion-focused therapy 300
   in dance movement psychotherapy 352, 354–55
   in hearing voices groups 14, 15, 34, 39
   importance of, 52, 80, 147
      in bereavement 82
   with the 'other' 124
   between voices and life experiences 17, 211, 213, 264, 266
construct
   personal (Maastricht), 17–19, 21, 68, 184, 185, 190, 195, 204
coping strategies
   cannabis use as, 97
   helpful, 186–87
   in recovery 68–74, 360, 364
   unhelpful, 257, 260, 273
   with voices 36, 380
Covid-19 5, 79, 175, 249
   and online learning 177
   and work 164–65
creative/ity
   collage(s) 332, 339, 360
   drawing 332
   mapping 333
   painting 50–53, 72
   projection 341
   puppets 332
   sculpting 334
   ways to represent voices 331–34
   ways to work with voices 329ff
crisis
   point of (in Open Dialogue) 129, 130, 132, 275–278
   services 276
critical mental health 24
cultural
   bereavement 107, 108
   context, relevance to hearing voices 14, 41, 87, 90, 204, 238, 306–07, 382
   meanings of whiteness 103
   oppression 107
   wisdom and hearing voices 13
curious/curiosity
   'detective' 225–26

stance towards voices 125, 130, 132, 133, 183, 201, 222, 284, 330, 334

D

dance movement psychotherapy 351ff
daydreaming 283, 368
death
 of significant others, linked to voice hearing 35, 75, 104–05, 291-92, 390
 'post-death encounters' 76
 sudden, due to medication 70, 181
decision-making
 difficulties 163
 'mindfulness gauge' for, 324
 shared, 117–121
  in trauma-informed therapy 274
 values-based, 116
defence mechanisms 289
delirium 259
delusions 27, 36, 37, 48, 182, 291, 302
dementia
 discovery-based approach to, 213
 and identity 214–15
 labelling 212–13
 Lewy body, 63, 212
 lived examples of, 217–20
 structured interviewing 217
 use of antipsychotics 216
demons 13, 91, 92
depression 31, 49, 104, 214, 238, 259, 294, 298, 302, 347, 390
developmental model
 in dramatherapy 341
 in voice hearing 290
Devil, the 5, 90, 182, 373, 381
diagnosis (*see also* dementia)
 alternatives to, 274
 of borderline personality disorder 66
 as label 32, 130
 links with hearing voices 4, 103, 181, 214, 258
 psychiatric, 17, 82, 90, 144, 231
 racism and, 107
 'safety' of, 128, 130
 of schizophrenia/psychosis 5, 6, 18, 19, 22, 35, 49, 57, 67, 94, 104, 143, 147, 166, 171, 180, 320, 367, 369, 376, 378, 388, 399
 and stigma 5

dialogism 278
dialogical
 approach(es) 239
 engagement with voices 306
 human life as, 307
 work with voices 133
dialogical self theory (DST) 305
diary writing/journaling 15, 161
 'with voices' 336
disability
 adviser 175, 177, 178
 disclosure 155, 178
 discrimination 165
 hearing voices as, 169, 171
 legislation 152, 153
 rights 165
 reasonable adjustments 5, 155, 157, 165, 173, 175, 176, 178
 support notification (DSN) 175
 support services (university) 172–176, 179
disempowerment 273,
dissociation 187, 258, 262, 266, 268, 298
distraction
 from voices 234, 263, 264, 268, 269, 369
distress, sitting with, 24
dopamine 138, 139
dramatherapy for voices 341ff
dreaming state 368
drug(s)
 addiction/abuse 49, 60, 70, 96, 97
 -centred model 148
 law 99
 non-prescribed, 6, 33, 156, 220, 258, 259, 368
  cutting down, 100
 psychiatric (*see* antipsychotics)
drum(s) 372
 djembe 387

E

early intervention services 342, 359
 dramatherapy in, 344–345
ego 106, 289, 364
 'operating' 20
emancipation 13, 21, 39, 46
embodiment (of the voice/experience) 240, 241, 243, 349 (*see also* body)
 exercise 346–47

of feelings 342
emotional differentiation 79, 83
empathy 17, 284, 295, 302
employer 153, 154, 155, 156, 159, 160,
    confidentiality 171
    disclosing to, 165–66
employee
    rights 153
    support for, 159
employment
    and disability legislation 165
    experience 154
    history 154
    interviews, preparation for 155–56
    sickness absence 166–67
    supported, 276
emotional work 149
empowerment 19, 39, 241, 274, 276, 309, 316, 370, 372
    black, 108
    self- 34
engagement
    dialogical, with voices 306
    with medical services/professionals 70, 231, 232
    'psychology of', 196
    with suffering/distress 296
    voluntary, 7
environmental factors (in voice hearing) 180, 259
equality with professionals 103, 144, 145
Equality Act 2010 (UK) 172, 174
ethics/ethical values 27, 46, 71, 114, 115, 125, 131, 138, 243, 308
evidence-based practice 115, 117, 120, 121, 316, 344, 401
exclusion 46, 273, 385
external world 286
    of child 290

F

facilitator(s)/ing
    hearing voices groups 39ff, 41, 43, 45, 46, 334
    interviewing exercise 335–36
    Making Sense of Voices 240
    narrative genograms 310
    Talking with Voices 334, 337
    Voice Dialogue 21, 335

faith
    -healing 49
    in medical science 48
    religious, 48, 87, 88, 90, 91, 92
family
    black, 105
    conflict 77
    European norms of, 106
    inclusive practice with, 124
    inclusion, in Open Dialogue 132–33, 277
    meetings, in Open Dialogue 129
    and narrative genograms 305, 309
    relationships with/in, 129, 240, 330
    role in recovery 267, 268
    as support 92
    voices as, 5, 305
    voices of, 105
    white, 105
fantasy
    in children's lives 206
    of perfect self 292
    world 283
fear
    adults', of children's voices 205, 208
    of breakdown (Winnicott) 293
    cannabis as antidote to, 96
    cycle of, 260
    of disclosure 171
    of discrimination at work 153
    of failure 292, 293
    and fight, flee, freeze response 385–86
    -free interactions with voices 188
    internalisation and, 289–90
    of judgement 341
    managing, 268, 329
    of other people's reactions 17, 80
    as patient 129
    professionals', 132, 133, 191, 209
    protective function of, 183
    due to racism 105
    reduced, due to medication, 142
    responses to threat situations 261
    of voices 15, 17, 36, 63, 126, 184, 222, 256, 267
    of voice hearers 7, 17, 158
Findhorn community 88
fragmentation 291, 381
framework
    medical, 25

normalising, 190
peer-focused, of hearing voices groups 40
relational, 195
Open Dialogue, 276
'Three Phases of Voice Hearing' 43
of understanding 33, 142, 401

G

gods 85, 182,
grief 75ff
group processes 43–45
group cognitive analytic music therapy 387–88
groupwork/groups 5, 346, 388, 401
    compassion-focused therapy, 302
    mindfulness, 322
    peer support, for voice hearers 157, 164,
    placebo, 137
    self-help, 15, 56, 124, 147, 181
    for students 174, 179
    (see also hearing voices groups)
guilt
    and bereavement 77, 288
    and childhood sexual abuse 60
    in children 208
    layers of, 61–62
    trigger in hearing voices 18, 195
    vicious cycle of, 273

H

hallucinatory experiences 258, 259
hallucinations(s)
    auditory, 55, 76, 85, 229, 230
    command, 236
    'false perceptions' 399
    'hypervigilance', 264
    as messengers 213
    religious, 87
    'source-monitoring problem' 266
    terminology 25–27, 182, 184, 209
    visual, 48
harm-minimisation approach
    cannabis use 94, 96
harm-reduction
    cannabis use 100
harassment 120, 167, 171
healing
    communities as sites of, 129, 396
    conditions for holistic, 369

in dialogue 313
faith-, 49
function of voices 8
honouring stories 130
post-crisis, 129
potential 80–81
role-taking and, 345
'safe space' and, 371
self-, painting as 52
shamanic, 368
from trauma 277
hearing voices
    (see also hallucinations/coping/voices)
    and bereavement 5, 82
    as natural human experience 13, 15, 22,
        35, 73, 169, 203, 224, 248, 249, 251,
        402
    groups 30ff, 33, 40–41, 129, 401
        facilitating, 39ff
        mindfulness in, 315
        normalising effects of, 316
        resources for, 43
    interview 16–17, 148 (see also Maastricht Interview)
    as meaningful reaction 40, 41, 46, 237, 306, 400
    Movement 13, 123, 180, 306, 317, 376
        acceptance as principle in, 325, 329
        origins of, 40, 181, 195
        Ron Coleman and, 212–13
    network(s) 40, 145, 153, 170, 174
        principles of, 33–34
        and Open Dialogue 124–25
        Athenian, 306, 309
        Danish, 320
    as religious experiences 87
    sense making 40
    symbolic meaning of, 70, 82, 185, 400
heavy metal music 354, 356
hope
    and hearing voices groups 34, 44
    from projection (dramatherapy) 348
    safe spaces for, 279
    stress bucket model and, 257
    from survivors' stories 14, 16, 397
    in trauma-informed approach 274
hopelessness
    experience of voice hearers 129
    professionals as 'champions of', 70

voices as stories of, 195
human rights
   approach to mental health 124
   and Open Dialogue 279–80
   and 'supervision of solidarity' 46
hypervigilance
   -based voice hearing 264–65
   distraction technique 268
   as unhelpful coping strategy 257, 260, 273, 353

I
id 289
identity
   'ability spotting' 312
   black, 105
   formative influence of voices on, 207, 211
   group, shaping 41–42
   play and formation of, 208
   self-, in compassion-focused therapy 301
   and selves in Voice Dialogue 196, 307
   sexual, 62
   signifier, language as 24
   of voices 215, 218, 380
   voices as part of self-, 212, 214–15, 376
illusions (visual) 264
improvisation
   in dance movement therapy 356
   musical, 386, 389, 392
inclusive/inclusion 13, 17, 124,
   learning 179
   practice, in universities 176–77
inequality/ies
   in power 48, 184
   social, 180, 259
injustice
   race discrimination 108
   social, 273
inner critic 20–21
inner speech/internal voices 62, 68, 72, 75, 107, 264, 265–66
inner world 283, 287, 291, 292, 341, 391
   of child 286, 288, 290
innocence
   of childhood 393
   emotional, 55, 59, 60–62
integration
   of assertiveness skills 253
   of Open Dialogue with values-based practice 276
   repair and, 293–94
   of thoughts and feelings after trauma 385
   of voices into hearer's life 367, 368
interpersonal
   model in relating therapy 240
   skills 154
   trauma and voice hearing 258
   voice-hearing relationship 237, 283
intrusive
   thoughts 232, 262
   voices 91, 156, 158, 162, 175, 265, 269, 369
invalidation 273
involuntary treatment 115
isolation 129, 218, 230, 231, 256, 260, 268, 273, 276, 337, 388

J
job
   application 154–55
   interview 155–56

K
kindness 44, 295, 299, 317, 396

L
label
   black, 107
   illness 19
   psychiatric, 4, 32, 63, 109, 130, 376
labelling 65, 72, 172, 229, 399
   dangers of, 212–13
language 24ff
   beyond, 341, 345, 347
   body, 250, 252, 303
   children's, 204, 208
   of the client 370
   of disorder 25
   'from the gut' 188
   of illness 26, 173
   medical/pathologising, 71, 130, 144, 183, 184
   metaphorical, 72, 185, 187, 353
   musical, 378
   politics of, 26, 27, 396
   rules of, 24, 347
   shared, 129, 130, 132
   terminology 25, 26

unspoken, 369
use of, 83, 158–59, 200, 278, 379
of voices 76, 82, 199, 201, 338
life context 4, 17, 40, 57, 69, 75, 76, 79, 82, 115, 123, 142, 172, 181–85, 190, 191, 214, 238, 277, 294, 306
life history x, 7, 58, 86, 191, 211, 213, 216, 220, 239, 323, 360
lived experience 24, 40, 131, 154, 276, 352, 397
   of psychiatric services 41, 274
   race as, 105
living with voices 19–21, 22, 147, 161, 213, 396
   accounts of, 376, 382
   film about, 332
loneliness 256, 257, 273
loss 75, 82, 108, 213, 258, 288–89, 338, 389–90
   of appetite 101
   of autonomy 208
   of love 393
   of relationships 273
love 88, 288, 295, 302, 362, 396
   loss of, 393

M

Maastricht Approach 5, 13ff, 14, 182, 204
Maastricht Construct 184, 185, 190
Maastricht Interview 16, 36, 45, 68, 148, 184, 185, 186, 188, 189, 190, 203–04, 399
Maastricht Report 184, 185
mainstream
   healthcare 368
   mental health services 1, 4–5, 6, 126, 127, 171, 190, 351
   psychiatry 36, 39, 191
making sense of voices 5, 17–19, 22, 143, 180, 182, 213, 240
mantra 61, 72, 370–73
mapping
   mind-, 379
   in space (exercise) 333
   voices 301, 363
meaning-making 39, 239, 256ff, 278
medical model 27, 118, 119, 140, 143, 285, 294
medication (*see also* antipsychotics) 19, 136ff
   avoiding, 275, 279
   choice and, 146, 148–49, 170, 185, 276, 278, 367, 400, 401
   depot, 114
   effectiveness of, 136–140
   forced, 191
   prescribing practices 7–8, 35, 123, 140–44, 145, 146–48, 171, 229, 399, 401
   pros and cons of, 70, 144, 146, 164, 180
   reducing, 70, 185
   refusal 114–15, 117
   side/unwanted effects 35, 73, 123
   weight gain 142, 143
meditation 52, 69, 91, 321, 372
   breathing, 318, 321
memoirs 376
memories 67, 198
   dissociation and, 262
   early, 266
   painful/trauma, 239, 263, 266, 280, 323, 382, 385
      processing, 267, 386
   as triggers 386
   voices as/of, 211, 213, 372
Mental Health Act (UK) 64, 66,
mentalisation 284,
metalcore
   community 364, 365
   lyrics 364
   music 359, 360, 364
metaphor
   children's use of, 204
   in dance movement therapy 353–54, 357
   in dramatherapy 341, 348,
   in music therapy 388
mindfulness 72, 91, 101, 164, 233, 234, 262–64, 268, 315ff
   compassionate, 268
   evidence for, 315–16
   in groups 323
   and hearing voices 320–22
   musical, 387, 388
   practice 318–20
   principles of, 317–18
   problems with, 323
   trauma-sensitive approach to, 324
motivation 100, 209, 296, 322, 337
   and CT-R 233
   lack of, 232
mourning 288

the idealised self 292–93
as taboo 79–80
music
   choice of, in dance movement psychotherapy 354, 355, 356
   as distraction 269, 362
   as metaphor for experience 361, 363
   as non-shared experience 27
   therapeutic/helpful effects of, 53, 91, 101, 154, 162, 232, 233, 234, 268, 353, 357, 359, 364
   therapy 359, 368, 384ff
      with voice hearing 384–87, 388
      group cognitive analytic, 387–88
   voices' choices of, 365

N

narrative
   coherence of, in 'schizophrenia' 378
   genogram 305ff
      use with voice hearing 309–312, 313
   letter 360
   musical, 363
   personal, 55, 57, 206, 291, 377–80
      role in recovery 378–79
   'rescripting' 222
National Paranoia Network 37
neglect 16, 18, 209, 258, 273, 385
new age 87
non-judgemental
   approach 263, 334
      in groupwork 388
   attitude/stance 96, 315, 330
   spaces 40
non-shared realities x, 184, 305, 306, 309, 353
non-stigmatising approaches 257, 337–38, 386
non-violent communication 336
normalisation/normalising 171, 181, 186, 190, 257, 267, 316

O

object-relations theory 284, 286–87
Open Dialogue 123ff
   evidence for, 279–80
   peer-supported, 275–79
   principles of, 126
oppression 273

cultural, 107
ownership
   of experiences 41, 130
   of voices 68, 69, 71–74

P

pain 53, 59, 77, 78, 103, 178, 296, 312, 316–17, 324, 390, 391–93
panic 64, 259, 261, 321
   disorder 259
paradigmatic shift ix, 6, 123, 134, 181, 183, 190, 397
paradigm
   dominant, 7
   white, 109
paranoid/paranoia 31, 36, 37, 48, 52, 97, 98, 99, 291, 301, 316, 321
parts
   of body (mindfulness) 316, 318, 322
   emotional, 300, 301
   of self 284, 287, 289, 291, 332
   voices as, 66–67, 380
   in Voice Dialogue 20, 22, 196, 334–35, 364, 365
pathologising
   approach 1, 3, 7, 107
   language 26
   non-, 182, 209
peer support 6, 39, 40, 51, 69, 73, 274, 276, 307, 323, 388, 400, 401
   group 120, 157, 164, 174, 399
   movement 69
   worker 154
perception 2, 27, 76, 86, 212
person-centred
   approach 8, 118, 217, 220, 276, 277, 280
      to mindfulness 323, 325
      to recovery 378, 395
   Rogers 75
personality disorder 25, 40, 66, 136, 259
personality
   medicalisation of, 104
   psychoanalytic theory of, 240
   of voices 65, 67, 331
   in Voice Dialogue 334, 335, 364
play
   children's, 203, 322
   importance of, 207–08
   pedagogy of, 203

poems/poetry 97, 219, 360
  as therapy 381–82
police 66, 105, 120
polyphony 129–31, 132
postmodern/ist approach 125
post-traumatic stress disorder (PTSD) 266, 267, 353
poverty 273
power
  balance of, 227, 240, 298, 329, 377, 382
  beliefs about (relating therapy), 238, 240
  control over, 343
  dynamic 5, 238
    in Open Dialogue 125, 133
    in Voice Dialogue 334
  inequality with professionals 48, 79, 124, 126, 127, 128, 131, 132, 181, 184
  of 'no' 348
  of psychiatrists 144–45
  shared, 274
  structures 127, 132, 133
  of voices 15, 20, 44, 56, 105, 175, 198, 222, 223, 224, 231, 233, 235–36, 252, 268, 299, 321
  of words 26
Power Threat Meaning Framework 274
prayer
  as coping technique 91, 231
  voices heard in, 86, 87, 90
presence, sense of 76, 78, 80
prison (young black men) 104, 107, 108
projection 287–88, 289, 341, 349
  exercise 348
psychiatric system
  deaths in, 105
  survivors of, 278
psychiatrist/s
  advice to, 146–48
  how to deal with, 144–46
psychoanalytic
  approaches 240
  therapists 284
  therapy 399
psychodrama 81, 343
psychodynamic
  theories of voices 195, 283–84, 284–286, 291, 293
  therapy 275
  understanding of voices 283ff

psychoeducation 232, 256, 260, 267, 268
'psychosis'
  CBT for, 243
  compassion-focused therapy for, 301–02
  diagnosis of, 5, 6, 67, 94, 138, 185, 259, 267, 367
    impact of, 376
  dance movement therapy for, 353
  dramatherapy for, 343, 344
  early adversity and, 258
  early intervention in, 256, 341, 342
  as human reaction, 147, 148
  links with cannabis 94–95
  medication for, 141
  psychodynamic theories of, 291–92
  mindfulness and, 316
  psychosocial treatments for, 230
  sound therapy for, 369
  super-sensitivity, 139
  trauma and onset of, 274–75
  voices perceived as symptoms of, 35, 37, 115, 147, 256, 259
  of whiteness 108
puppets 332

R

racism 80, 106, 108, 273, 362
rage 292, 297, 386, 390, 393
reasonable adjustments (workplace) 5, 155, 157, 165, 173, 175, 178
recovery ix
  arts as tool for, 378–80
  contested definitions of, 48, 395
  embodiment of feelings and, 342
  hearing voices groups and, 34, 56, 69
  medication and, 138
  Movement x, 3
    and narrative genogram 313
  possibility of, 3, 147
  relationships and, 129, 396, 397
  sharing stories of, 19, 32, 69, 141, 143, 144, 147, 187, 190, 381
  social means to, 15, 17
  sound therapy and, 368, 373
  understanding voices and, 1, 13, 19, 20, 55, 182, 306, 307
  voices as contributors to, 6, 180, 184
recovery-oriented cognitive therapy (CT-R) 229ff

protocol for, 233–34
reflection (therapeutic) 239, 278, 313, 352, 372
refocusing 234, 235
relapse 54, 137, 139
relating therapy 81, 195, 240, 246ff
　basics of, 248
　evidence for, 252–53
religion/ious 13, 49
　coping 91–92
　and voices 85ff
repression 286, 287–88, 289
resilience 34, 37, 257, 397
rights-based
　mental health services 124
　practice 124
rhythm/rhythmic 353, 354, 355, 357, 372
role-play 226, 240, 247, 249, 301, 334
　in relating therapy 250–52
rumination 273

S

safe spaces 45, 197, 241, 280, 386
　in sound therapy 367ff
safety 7, 33, 42, 132, 183, 200–01, 278, 331, 337, 371, 385
　of diagnosis 128
　interpersonal, 274
　net, drumming as 372
saints 87, 89, 91
scientific
　advances 401
　discourse 1, 7, 136, 181, 183
　research 86–87, 149, 264, 297
　reliability 180
　validity 180, 376
schizophrenia (*see also* antipsychotics/psychosis) x, 1
　and cannabis use 95, 97
　contested validity of diagnosis 1, 48, 104, 141, 143, 147, 166, 180, 290, 376
　emotional disconnect in, 342
　and insight 378
　medication for, 136
　negative impact of diagnosis, 49, 53, 54, 181, 399
　non-medical management of, 138
　poetry as therapy for, 381
　voices as assumed symptom of, 2, 25, 35, 40, 67, 104, 171, 180, 182, 378
　as unhelpful label 4, 26, 144, 181, 376, 399
sculpting 333–34
security 48, 52, 59, 205,
　of care 392, 393
　social, benefits 160
self/selves 20, 21, 196, 201, 334, 335, 342, 364, 364
　alternative, 240
　compassionate, 299, 300, 301, 303
　idealised, 288, 292–93
　multiple, 300, 301
　sub-, 307
self-beliefs 222–27, 228
self-care 51, 196, 267, 268, 293
self-compassion 257, 316
self-expression 341, 372, 387,
self-help 55–56, 174
　book(s) 68, 228
　group(s) 15, 55, 56, 58, 69, 124, 147, 148, 181, 275, 306, 309, 329
　mutual, 274
　strategy 8
　talking with voices as, 336–37
self-injury/self-harm 57, 60, 61, 65, 107, 211, 320, 338, 367
sense-making 40
sensory experiences 2, 27, 40, 41, 258, 268
sexuality 61
shaman(s) 368
shame 17, 43, 60, 243, 249, 267, 268, 273, 288, 291, 298, 390, 393
silence 26, 43, 65, 91, 136, 162
sleep 52, 71, 97, 100, 101, 157, 163, 268, 321, 336
　deprivation 256, 258, 259
smoking
　cannabis 94ff
　tobacco 156, 315
social
　action 181, 397
　injustice 273
　network(s) 5, 16, 36, 123, 145, 146, 186, 207, 208, 275, 276–77, 279, 305, 317
　prescribing 393
　worker 32, 103, 105
social-rank-threat 299
sonic landscape 368, 372
sound/sound therapy 367ff

spirits 91, 182
spiritual/ity 85ff, 324
   coping 91–92
scientific research 86–87
splitting 286, 287–89
stigma 5, 17, 19, 67, 80, 158, 330
   around voices 70, 73, 80, 376, 382, 388
   in dementia 212
   self-, 158, 382
story/ies (see also narrative)
   co-creating, 129–30, 147
   in genograms 313
      'backlighting' 312
   -telling, 15, 16, 19, 144, 377–78
      importance of, 57–60, 61
      as means to ownership/agency 147, 376, 378
      through music 363–64, 378
      as recovery tool 378–79
   theatre as container for, 342
stress
   CT-R as means for reducing, 231–32
   CFT as treatment for, 302
   and dementia 214, 217
   managing, 268, 347
      at work 163, 167
      at university 175–76
   mindfulness and, 316, 324
   poetry and, 381
   sound therapy and, 367
   and trauma, 266, 273
   and voice hearing 71, 231, 290
stress-vulnerability model 257
student
   individual student support record (ISSR) 175
   peer support 174–75
   support recommendations (SSR) 175
   study support 175–78
   support/disability services 170, 175–76
suicide
   prevention 115, 119
   risk of, 115
   talking about, 132
   voices and, 65
superego 289, 290, 292
supervision
   in avatar therapy 239, 243
   in hearing voices groups 45–46
   in music therapy 386, 392
   in Open Dialogue 132
survivor(s)
   of childhood abuse 60
   -led research 307
   of mental health system 14, 60, 62, 71, 278
      black, 103, 108
   motto 278
   of trauma 27, 397
survival
   evolutionary, 297
   responses 264–65, 266
   role models 69
   strategies 273
symbol/ic 43, 70, 82, 185, 348, 353–57
   language 187, 400
symptom(s) (see also schizophrenia)
   as deficits 308
   of dementia 212, 216
   impact of emotion-focused counselling on, 184–85
   psychosocial models of managing, 138, 229–30, 232
   voices as, 19, 48–49, 50, 103, 104, 107, 119, 137, 178, 182, 191, 217, 220, 285
   withdrawal, 137, 139–40
systemic
   appreciative approach 308
   power 132
   therapy 268, 275, 343
   'way of thinking' 309

T

taboo
   and children's play 208
   mourning as, 79, 83
Talking with Voices 21, 196, 240, 247, 334ff, 400
   as self-help 336–37
   interview 334
technology 120, 243
   digital, 239, 240, 247
      use with voices 241–42
telepathy 182, 347
theatre 342, 345
therapeutic relationship 248–49, 284, 391, 392
   musical, 385

repair 293
threat
   mind state 300
   -response system 260–63, 264–65, 267, 299, 301, 303
   patterns 303
   voices as responses to, 200, 231, 258
time management 162, 163
trauma
   childhood, 203, 222, 259
   definition of, 273
   dialogical responses to, 275ff
   effects of, x, 261, 268
   -sensitive/informed approaches 3, 6, 7, 187, 188, 274–75, 276
   therapy 184, 267, 268
   voices, connection with, 3, 7, 17, 71, 105, 108, 127, 180, 184, 194–95, 214, 258, 266
triggers, for voices 16, 18, 36, 44, 154, 186, 216, 379
trust, in relationship 43, 45, 48, 56, 146, 191, 200–01, 203, 208, 215, 232, 246, 248, 274, 278, 279, 338, 345, 352, 353, 385, 392, 400
   violation of, 273
truth 126, 130, 256, 309
   voices speaking, 397
tuning fork 368, 371–73, 373

U

un/conscious 108, 283, 285, 287, 289, 290, 372, 380, 386
uncertainty 124, 130, 230
   tolerance of, 126, 128, 131–33, 183, 278
unexpressed emotion 187, 188, 206, 269–70, 351, 352, 385
United Nations 124 , 412
university
   disability support services 175–76
   inclusive practice 176–77
unshared realities/experiences 123, 124, 127, 128, 129, 174, 399, 400

V

values 24, 113ff, 217, 330, 395
   of the Hearing Voices Network 40, 41, 46, 305
   compared with HVN approach 126

   of metalcore 364
   of mindfulness 317
   in Open Dialogue 123ff
   statement 42, 43
   of Talking with Voices 337
   of Voice Dialogue 195
values-based practice 113ff, 276, 399
victim/victor 55ff
violence 8, 263, 273, 389
   domestic, 385
virtual 157, 177
   embodiment 241, 242
   reality 242
visualisation 241
Voice Dialogue 20, 21, 22, 55, 59, 81, 194ff, 247, 334–36, 359, 364
voice hearer(s)/ing
   media portrayal of, 13, 15, 66, 260, 261, 330
voices
   as animals 182, 204, 258
   attention seeking, 20, 65, 72, 73, 130, 161, 187, 188, 226, 233, 235, 268, 364
   challenging, 127, 131, 325
   command/ing, 18, 27, 50, 52, 57, 58, 65, 82, 236, 381
   content of, 32, 36, 72, 74, 91, 199, 230, 239, 265, 291, 353, 381
   credibility of, 231, 232, 233
   critical, 20, 86, 91, 155, 159, 161, 162, 163, 164, 199, 201, 223, 230, 246, 247, 290, 291, 301, 336, 337–39, 369
   decoding, 185, 201
   demonic, 85, 91, 92
   divine, 85, 87
   eradication of, 14, 149, 229
   external, 51, 62, 68, 71, 72, 86, 105, 108, 231, 286, 291, 302, 307
   fear of, (see fear)
   function of, 59, 184, 185
   inner, 21, 75, 85, 88, 265, 267, 278, 285
   intentions of, 6, 21, 155, 185, 192, 197, 199, 205, 222, 237, 336, 338
   interviewing, 130, 335–36
   mapping, 301, 333
   meaning of, 2, 4, 7, 8, 17, 19, 22, 35, 41, 45, 69–70, 74, 76, 82, 86, 87, 149, 181, 184, 205, 214, 220, 235, 256ff, 284, 306, 400, 401

misattribution 86
as monsters 204
negotiation with, 55, 119, 156, 199, 200, 334, 337
normalising, 171, 181, 184, 186, 190, 257, 267, 316
negative, 15, 27, 44, 53, 57, 58, 86, 163, 190, 238, 240, 243, 244, 312, 353, 379, 388, 396, 400
  impact of, 161, 170, 181, 207, 213, 215, 223, 230
profiling, 55, 198, 215–16, 219, 220
revelatory, 91–92
sabotaging, 227, 293
sculpting 333–34
significance of, 8, 34, 87
as social network 305
structured time with, 56–57
as symptoms (*see* symptoms)
white, 105, 107, 108
voice hearing
and abuse 298, 336
and agency 26, 27, 34, 118, 130, 277, 317, 378, 382
protective, 20, 21, 155, 185, 195, 200, 218, 339, 400
voice profiling 55, 57, 198, 215–16, 219, 220
voodoo 48

W

whiteness 103ff
work
  bullying at, 167
  disclosure at, 165–66
  emotional, 149
  managing, 160–63
  paid, 5, 31, 53, 143, 152ff
    applying for, 153–56
    managing voices in, 156–163, 164
  sickness absence from, 166–67
WRAP/WAP 154, 166
writing as therapy 15, 81, 142, 187, 219, 268, 301, 336, 357, 376ff, 385

Y

yoga 101, 188, 318, 319, 323, 324